Yearbook of Anesthesiology 12
2023

Indian College of Anaesthesiologists Board of Trustees

1. Dr VP Kumra, New Delhi, India
2. Dr Manorama Mittal, New Delhi, India
3. Dr B Radhakrishnan, Kerala, India
4. Dr Jayashree Sood, New Delhi, India
5. Dr LD Mishra, Lucknow, Uttar Pradesh, India
6. Dr Vijay Vohra, New Delhi, India
7. Dr Roshan Lal Garg, New Delhi, India
8. Dr Surinder Mohan Sharma, New Delhi, India
9. Dr Bimla Sharma, New Delhi, India
10. Dr Pradeep Jain, New Delhi, India
11. Dr SK Malhotra, Chandigarh, India
12. Dr Raminder Sehgal, New Delhi, India
13. Dr Muralidhar Kanchi, Bengaluru, Karnataka, India
14. Dr Sunila Sharma, New Delhi, India
15. Dr Kumar Belani, Minneapolis, Minnesota, USA
16. Dr Sunanda Gupta, Udaipur, Rajasthan, India

Yearbook of Anesthesiology 12
2023

Editors

Mukul Chandra Kapoor
Chief Consultant, Professor, and Head
Department of Anesthesiology and Critical Care
Amrita Institute of Medical Sciences and Amrita Hospitals
Faridabad, Haryana, India

Baljit Singh
Professor and Head
Anesthesiology and Intensive Care
SGT University
Gurugram, Haryana, India
CEO, Indian College of Anaesthesiologists
Former Professor Anesthesiology
GB Pant Hospital
New Delhi, India

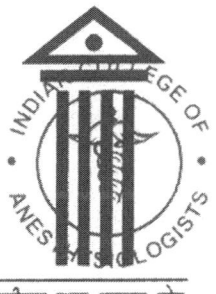

Indian College of Anaesthesiologists

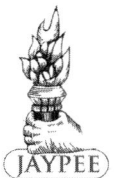

JAYPEE BROTHERS MEDICAL PUBLISHERS
The Health Sciences Publisher
New Delhi | London

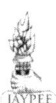 **Jaypee Brothers Medical Publishers (P) Ltd**

Headquarters
Jaypee Brothers Medical Publishers (P) Ltd
EMCA House, 23/23-B
Ansari Road, Daryaganj
New Delhi 110 002, India
Landline: +91-11-23272143, +91-11-23272703
+91-11-23282021, +91-11-23245672
Email: jaypee@jaypeebrothers.com

Corporate Office
Jaypee Brothers Medical Publishers (P) Ltd
4838/24, Ansari Road, Daryaganj
New Delhi 110 002, India
Phone: +91-11-43574357
Fax: +91-11-43574314
Email: jaypee@jaypeebrothers.com

Overseas Office
JP Medical Ltd
83 Victoria Street, London
SW1H 0HW (UK)
Phone: +44 20 3170 8910
Fax: +44 (0)20 3008 6180
Email: info@jpmedpub.com

Website: www.jaypeebrothers.com
Website: www.jaypeedigital.com

© 2023, Jaypee Brothers Medical Publishers

The views and opinions expressed in this book are solely those of the original contributor(s)/author(s) and do not necessarily represent those of editor(s) or publisher of the book.

All rights reserved. No part of this publication may be reproduced, stored or transmitted in any form or by any means, electronic, mechanical, photocopying, recording or otherwise, without the prior permission in writing of the publishers.

All brand names and product names used in this book are trade names, service marks, trademarks or registered trademarks of their respective owners. The publisher is not associated with any product or vendor mentioned in this book.

Medical knowledge and practice change constantly. This book is designed to provide accurate, authoritative information about the subject matter in question. However, readers are advised to check the most current information available on procedures included and check information from the manufacturer of each product to be administered, to verify the recommended dose, formula, method and duration of administration, adverse effects and contraindications. It is the responsibility of the practitioner to take all appropriate safety precautions. Neither the publisher nor the author(s)/editor(s) assume any liability for any injury and/or damage to persons or property arising from or related to use of material in this book.

This book is sold on the understanding that the publisher is not engaged in providing professional medical services. If such advice or services are required, the services of a competent medical professional should be sought.

Every effort has been made where necessary to contact holders of copyright to obtain permission to reproduce copyright material. If any have been inadvertently overlooked, the publisher will be pleased to make the necessary arrangements at the first opportunity.

Inquiries for bulk sales may be solicited at: jaypee@jaypeebrothers.com

Yearbook of Anesthesiology 12 2023

First Edition: 2022

Second Edition: **2023**

ISBN: 978-93-5465-959-1

Printed at Replika Press Pvt. Ltd.

Dedicated to

Anesthesiology and Critical Care Physicians who toil hard to sustain life. The Anesthesiologists remain behind the screen and seldom get the appreciation they deserve from their patients. Critical Care Physicians are constantly on their toes, see much mortality, and get appreciated often. However, they also face the ire of the patient's relatives and, at times, violence when their patients die!

Contributors

Adam C Adler
Associate Professor Anesthesiology
Texas Children's Hospital
Baylor College of Medicine
6621 Fannin Street, Suite #A3300
Houston TX, 77030
adam.adler@bcm.edu

Alok Kumar
Senior Adviser
Anesthesiology and Cardiothoracic
Anesthesiology
Army Hospital (R&R)
New Delhi, India
mipayal07@gmail.com

Amit Mathew
Associate Professor
Christian Medical College
Vellore, Tamil Nadu, India

Anil Parakh
Head
Department of Anesthesiology
Global Hospitals
Mumbai, Maharashtra, India
anilparakhglobal@gmail.com

Anoushka Afonso
Associate Professor
Department of Anesthesiology
and Critical Care
Director
Enhanced Recovery Programs Faculty
Director
Memorial Sloan Kettering Pipeline
Program Memorial Sloan Kettering
Cancer Center 1275 York Avenue
C-336 New York, NY 10065, USA
afonsoa@mskcc.org

Arvind Chandrakantan
Associate Professor
Anesthesiology and Pediatrics
Texas Children's Hospital
Baylor College of Medicine
6621 Fannin Street, Suite #A3300
Houston TX, 77030, USA
chandrak@bcm.edu

Balavenkata Subramanian Jagannathan
Senior Consultant Anesthesiology
Ganga Hospital
Coimbatore, Tamil Nadu, India
drbalavenkat@gmail.com

Baljit Singh
Professor and Head
Anesthesiology and Intensive Care
SGT University
Gurugram, Haryana, India
CEO
Indian College of Anaesthesiologists
Former Professor
Anesthesiology
GB Pant Hospital
New Delhi, India

Barry L Friedberg
President
Goldilocks Anesthesia Foundation
drbarry@goldilocksfoundation.org

Basavaraju Karan
Specialist (Anesthesiology)
Sultan Qaboos Comprehensive Cancer
Care and Research Centre
Muscat, Oman
karanbasavraj@gmail.com

Bindiya Salunke
Associate Professor
Department of Anesthesia, Critical Care
and Pain
Tata Memorial Hospital
Mumbai, Maharashtra, India
bindi02@gmail.com

C Adam Coridan
Resident Physician
Department of Anesthesiology
and Perioperative Medicine
Penn State Milton S Hershey Medical
Center
Hershey, PA 17033-0850, USA

Contributors

Cody Tidwell
Resident Physician
Department of Anesthesiology
University of Minnesota
Minneapolis, MN
tidwe027@umn.edu

Dheeraj Arora
Senior Consultant
Cardiac Anesthesiology and Critical Care
Amrita Institute of Medical Sciences and Amrita Hospitals
Faridabad, Haryana, India
dheerudoc@yahoo.com

Federico Semeraro
Consultant
Anesthesia and Intensive Care
Department of Anesthesia and Intensive Care and EMS
Maggiore Hospital Bologna
Bologna, Italy
federicofsemeraro@gmail.com

Gautam Gondal
Fellow DM Critical Care
Department of Anesthesiology, Critical Care and Pain
Tata Memorial Hospital
Homi Bhabha National Institute
Mumbai, Maharashtra, India

Gautam Khanna
Senior Consultant
Anesthesiology and Critical Care
Amrita Institute of Medical Sciences and Amrita Hospitals
Faridabad, Haryana, India
gautam.77k@gmail.com

Jayakrishnan S
Resident Anesthesiology
Army Hospital (R&R)
Delhi Cantt, New Delhi

Jigeeshu V Divatia
Director
Homi Bhabha Cancer Hospital and RC
Mullanpur and Sangrur, Punjab
Professor and Head
Department of Anesthesia, Critical Care and Pain
Tata Memorial Hospital
Mumbai, Maharashtra, India
divatiajv@tmc.gov.in
jdivatia@yahoo.com

Jitin Narula
Consultant
Cardiac Anesthesiology and Critical Care
Amrita Institute of Medical Sciences and Amrita Hospitals
Faridabad, Haryana, India
jatin.narula.13@gmail.com

Joanna S Rodriques
Consultant Anesthesiologist
Khar Hinduja Hospital
Mumbai, Maharashtra, India

KR Balakrishnan
Chairman—Cardiac Sciences
MGM Hospital
Chennai, Tamil Nadu, India

Kumar Belani
Professor of Anesthesiology
Division Head
Pediatric Anesthesiologist-in-Chief
(M Health Fairview Masonic Children's Hospital)
Adjunct Professor in Medicine and Pediatrics and Environmental Health Sciences
Schools of Medicine and Public Health
Distinguished International Professor, AHC
University of Minnesota
Mayo B-574, 420 Delaware Street SE, MMC 8294
Minneapolis, MN 55455
belan001@umn.edu

Madhanmohan Chandramohan
Junior Consultant Anesthesiology
Ganga Hospital
Coimbatore, Tamil Nadu, India
dr.madhanmohanc@gmail.com

Maria Bustillo
Professor of Neuroanesthesiology
Weill Cornell University
New York, USA
bustilo@med.cornell.edu

Mukul Chandra Kapoor
Chief Consultant, Professor, and Head
Department of Anesthesiology and
Critical Care
Amrita Institute of Medical Sciences
and Amrita Hospitals
Faridabad, Haryana, India
mukulanjali@gmail.com

Nishanth Baliga
Assistant Professor
Department of Anesthesiology, Critical
Care and Pain
Tata Memorial Hospital
Homi Bhabha National Institute
Mumbai, Maharashtra, India

Parli Raghavan Ravi
Senior Consultant (Anesthesiology)
Sultan Qaboos Comprehensive Cancer
Care and Research Centre
Muscat, Oman
parliravi@gmail.com

Pradeep Sharma
Assistant Professor and Classified
Specialist (Anesthesiology and
Neuro-Anesthesiology)
Department of Anesthesiology and
Critical Care
Command Hospital
Pune, Maharashtra, India

Praveen Neema
Professor of Cardiac Anesthesiology
Department of Cardiac Anesthesia
Amrita Institute of Medical Sciences
Kochi, Kerala, India
praveenneema@gmail.com

Rahul Pillai
Associate Professor
Christian Medical College
Vellore, Tamil Nadu, India

Rahul Yadav
Professor
Department of Anesthesiology
and Critical Care
Armed Forces Medical College
Pune, Maharashtra, India
docrahulyadav@gmail.com

Raj Sahajanandan
Professor
Christian Medical College
Vellore, Tamil Nadu, India
rajsahajanandan@gmail.com

Rajini Kausalya
Head and Senior Consultant
(Anesthesiology)
Sultan Qaboos Comprehensive Cancer
Care and Research Centre
Muscat, Oman

Rakesh Garg
Additional Professor
Department of Onco-Anesthesia and
Palliative Medicine
Dr BR Ambedkar Institute Rotary
Cancer Hospital
All India Institute of Medical Sciences
New Delhi, India
drrgarg@hotmail.com

Rashmi Datta
Professor and Head
Department of Emergency Medicine
Hamdard Institute of Medical Sciences
and Research
New Delhi, India
drrashmidatta@gmail.com

Contributors

Roelof MAW van Wijk
Head
Department of Anesthesia and Interim Head of Intensive Care
Critical Care and Perioperative Services
The Queen Elizabeth Hospital
Adelaide, Australia
Clinical Associate Professor
Discipline of Acute Care Medicine
University of Adelaide
Adelaide, Australia
roelof.VanWijk@sa.gov.au

Roopali Phulli
PDCC Fellow Onco-Anesthesia
Rajiv Gandhi Cancer Institute and Research Center
New Delhi, India

Ruparna Khurana
Senior Resident
Department of Onco-Anesthesia and Palliative Medicine
Dr BR Ambedkar Institute Rotary Cancer Hospital
All India Institute of Medical Sciences
New Delhi, India
ruparna@gmail.com

Sanjib Das Adhikary
Professor
Department of Anesthesiology, Orthopedics and Rehabilitation
The Pennsylvania State University
Vice Chair for Research and Innovation
Division Director for Orthopedic Anesthesia and
Regional Anesthesia and Acute Pain Medicine
Department of Anesthesiology and Perioperative Medicine
H-187 Penn State College of Medicine
Milton S Hershey Medical Center
500 University Drive
Hershey, PA 17033-0850, USA
sadhikary1@pennstatehealth.psu.edu

Santosh V
Consultant Anesthesia
MGM Hospital
Chennai, Tamil Nadu, India

Serjey Ghercuic
Clinical Research Coordinator
Department of Anesthesiology
University of Minnesota
Minneapolis, MN

Shaloo Garg
Professor and Senior Consultant
Department of Anesthesiology and Critical Care
Amrita Institute of Medical Sciences and Amrita Hospitals
Faridabad, Haryana, India
shaloopradeep@gmail.com

Sheila Nianan Myatra
Professor
Department of Anesthesiology and Critical Care
Tata Memorial Hospital
Mumbai, Maharashtra, India
sheila150@hotmail.com

Suresh Rao KG
Co-Director
MGM Hospital
Chennai, Tamil Nadu, India
sureshraokg@gmail.com

Tommaso Scquizzato
Cardiac Arrest Researcher
Department of Anesthesia and Intensive Care
IRCCS San Raffaele Scientific Institute
Milan, Italy
scquizzato.tommaso@hsr.it

Venkatesan Thiruvenkatarajan
Senior Consultant Anesthetist
Department of Anesthesia
The Queen Elizabeth Hospital
Adelaide, Australia

Clinical Associate Professor
Discipline of Acute Care Medicine
University of Adelaide
Adelaide, Australia
venkatesan.Thiruvenkatarajan@sa.gov.au

Vijaya Gottumukkala
Professor
Department of Anesthesiology
and Perioperative Medicine
Director, Program for Advancement
of Perioperative Cancer Care
Division of Anesthesiology, Critical Care
and Pain Medicine
Associate Head, Institute for Cancer
Care Innovation
Lead, Institutional Enhanced Recovery
Program
The University of Texas MD Anderson
Cancer Center
Unit-409, 1515 Holcombe Blvd
Houston, Texas 77030-4009, USA
vgottumukkala@mdanderson.org

Vinh Huu Nguyen
Assistant Professor
Pediatric Anesthesiologist
Section Chief Solid Organ Transplant
Co-Chief Clinical Director of East Bank
University of Minnesota Anesthesia
Department
420 Delaware St SE, Minneapolis,
MN 55455, USA

Vipin Kumar Goel
Junior Consultant Anesthesiology
Ganga Hospital
Coimbatore, Tamil Nadu, India
drvipingoel@gmail.com

Foreword

I am delighted to write a foreword for the 12th edition of the *Yearbook of Anesthesiology*. The vision of the Indian College of Anaesthesiologists is to impart high-quality anesthesia knowledge to all anesthesiologists. *Yearbook of Anesthesiology* 12th edition covers varied topics of great relevance to the students, practicing anesthesiologists, and those working in tertiary care hospitals.

The chapters include topics that only experienced anesthesiologists could have contributed. I am pleased to see that senior and experienced anesthesiologists, both national and international, have contributed and shaped this edition as extraordinary.

I take this opportunity to thank the contributors and the editor and co-editor, Dr Mukul Chandra Kapoor and Dr Baljit Singh, for this edition.

Jayashree Sood
MD FFARCS PGDHHM FICA
CEO
Indian College of Anaesthesiologists
Honorary Secretary, Board of Management
Member, Sir Ganga Ram Trust Society
Chairperson
Institute of Anesthesiology, Pain and Perioperative Medicine
Sir Ganga Ram Hospital
New Delhi, India

Preface

Unless you try to do something beyond what you have already mastered, you will never grow.

–Ronald E Osborn

The Indian College of Anaesthesiologists (ICA) proudly presents the 12th edition of the popular *Yearbook of Anesthesiology*. This book remains the most popular and sought-after update for anesthesiologists and students of anesthesiology and critical care. The reader base of the book has continued to rise steadily with each succeeding edition. This 12th edition is different from earlier editions and has a significant focus on emerging technologies and techniques.

This edition is focused on professionals who want to keep up-to-date with developments in the field of Anesthesiology and Critical Care. It is suitable as a textbook for postgraduate training in the clinical aspects of anesthesiology and recent advances in the field. The book attempts to cover topics from all subspecialty spectrums of anesthesiology. The book also forays into the future and discusses the challenges likely to be faced by the profession of anesthesiology and critical care.

A large segment of anesthesiology work has shifted outside the traditional domain of the operating room. Anesthesiologists are increasingly required to cover non-operating room anesthesia (NORA). Advanced therapeutic long-duration interventions are commonly performed today in patients with significant underlying comorbidities. NORA in such critically balanced patients offers unique challenges in a relatively unfamiliar environment. This book covers NORA for complex gastroenterological procedures. The opioid epidemic in the West has restricted the use of opioids in patients. This book also covers the role of opioid-free anesthesia in NORA.

Managing the airway is the primary responsibility of anesthesiologists, and proficiency in securing it can be challenging at times. We discuss the current recommendations to secure the difficult airway. We also foray into managing airway reconstruction surgeries where airway access is not just tricky but is also shared. We also present a relatively new field in airway surgery, managing children with obstructive sleep apnea.

Technology is making significant forays in healthcare. The increased use of ultrasound in the operating rooms and intensive care units has improved outcomes by aiding early diagnosis and intervention. Point of Care Ultrasound (POCUS) has changed patient management protocols. Anesthesiologists and Critical Care Physicians need to be more familiar with this advance. Similarly, artificial intelligence (AI) is slowly creeping into all spheres of medicine. Multiple monitors and automated intervention systems have already entered our domain. Many software programs, based on different algorithms, are available today to aid diagnosis and monitoring. Many robots are under development with the capability of performing anesthesia-related procedures. Anesthesiologists need to marry up with AI and help develop better algorithms for these machines.

Organ transplants are increasingly performed for end-stage organ disease. The profile of organs that can be transplanted is expanding. The COVID-19 disease made many victims lung cripples. There was a multifold rise in lung transplants across the country. We discuss the anesthetic management of patients for lung transplants. We also discuss the management of another less frequently done transplant, the pancreatic transplant.

The profile of neurosurgery is expanding. New challenges are emerging in Neuroanesthesia as a result. The therapeutic options in managing Functional Movement Disorder are expanding, and new surgical options are available. We discuss the anesthetic management of patients coming for functional movement disorder surgery. With better diagnostics and evaluation, more children with neural tube defects are getting identified early. These neonates and infants have immature systemic physiology elevating their risk of perioperative complications. We discuss the anesthetic management of these patients for spinal surgeries. With improved hardware and better expertise, work in vascular neuro-intervention has increased. We discuss the management of these interventions.

Acute respiratory failure is commonplace in intensive care units. The incidence of acute respiratory was relatively high during the COVID-19 epidemic. We discuss the different modalities involved in the physiology of acute respiratory failure. We also discuss non-invasive ventilation support in patients with acute respiratory failure. We also discuss intraoperative ventilation modes to prevent postoperative respiratory morbidity.

Many exciting developments are taking place to facilitate the care of patients for surgery. Enhanced recovery after surgery (ERAS) is now widely practiced worldwide. We discuss the role of ERAS in oncosurgery as it facilitates earlier return to planned adjuvant therapies and improved cancer outcomes. Anesthesiologists are being encouraged to don the role of perioperative physicians. Perioperative surgical homes (PSH) is an extension of this. It is expected that PSH will not only improve patient satisfaction but also outcomes. We discuss various aspects of PSH to increase awareness of this emerging patient management technique.

New themes have emerged, and new methods and technologies have been adopted. Old ideas have fallen by the wayside. The book is also available as a Kindle edition. The text is made accessible to anyone, independent of prior technical knowledge. Those with a background in anesthesiology should find the book a valuable introduction to the diverse applications of technology in health.

An investment in knowledge always pays the best interest.

–Benjamin Franklin

Mukul Chandra Kapoor
Baljit Singh

Contents

1. **Acute Respiratory Failure: Pathophysiology, Causes, and Diagnosis** 1
   Roopali Phulli, Praveen Neema
   - Pathophysiology of Acute Respiratory Failure in Coronavirus Disease 2019 (COVID-19) *13*
   - Diagnosis *15*

2. **Noninvasive Ventilation for Acute Respiratory Failure** 18
   Gautam Gondal, Nishanth Baliga, Sheila Nianan Myatra
   - Pathophysiology of AHRF *19*
   - Advantages of NIV over IMV *20*
   - Role of NIPPV in Acute Respiratory Failure *20*
   - Role of HFNO in Acute Respiratory Failure *25*
   - NIV in COVID-19 *28*

3. **Ventilation Strategies to Prevent Postoperative Pulmonary Infection** 34
   Mukul Chandra Kapoor
   - Postoperative Pulmonary Infections *35*
   - Risk Factors for Postoperative Pulmonary Complications *37*
   - Role of Mechanical Ventilation in Lung Injury *37*
   - Evidence-based Strategies for Intraoperative Lung Protective Ventilation *41*
   - Lung Protective Ventilation During Different Stages of General Anesthesia *44*

4. **Anesthetic and Intensive Care Management for Lung Transplant** 50
   Suresh Rao KG, Santosh V, KR Balakrishnan
   - Preoperative Assessment *51*
   - Intraoperative Management *52*
   - Maintenance of Anesthesia *53*
   - Mechanical Circulatory Support *54*
   - Surgical Consideration and Anastamosis *54*
   - Postoperative Analgesia *55*
   - ECMO Postlung Transplant *58*
   - Weaning of Mechanical Ventilation *58*
   - Hemodynamic Management *58*
   - Fluid Management *59*
   - Infection and Sepsis Management *59*

5. **Pediatric Obstructive Sleep Apnea: A Comprehensive Review** 62
   Arvind Chandrakantan, Adam C Adler
   - Pediatric OSA *63*

6. **Assessment of Functional Capacity** 78
   Gautam Khanna

7. **Role of Adjuncts for Regional and Neuraxial Anesthesia** 87
   Balavenkata Subramanian Jagannathan,
   Madhanmohan Chandramohan, Vipin Kumar Goel
   - Classification   89
   - Multimodal Perineural Adjuvant   96

8. **Myocardial Injury after Non-cardiac Surgery** 102
   Alok Kumar, Jayakrishnan S
   - Definitions   103
   - Etiopathogenesis   105
   - Risk Factors and Assessment   106
   - Management   108
   - Future Perspectives   111

9. **Anesthesia Management for Carotid Endarterectomy and Stenting** 114
   Dheeraj Arora, Jitin Narula
   - Anatomy   115
   - Carotid Endarterectomy: Surgery   115
   - Anesthesia Management   116
   - Anesthesia Techniques   116
   - Monitoring   119
   - Postoperative Management   120
   - Carotid Artery Stenting   121

10. **Anesthetic Implications in the Intravascular Treatment of Cerebral Aneurysms and Arteriovenous Malformations** 127
    Anil Parakh, Joanna S Rodriques
    - Anesthetic Considerations   128
    - Complications and their Management   131
    - Intracranial Aneurysms   132

11. **Anesthetic Considerations for Functional Neurosurgery** 140
    Maria Bustillo
    - Functional Neurosurgery   141
    - Deep Brain Stimulation   144
    - Magnetic Resonance Imaging-guided Focused Ultrasound   147
    - Additional Indications for Focused Ultrasound   149

12. **Anesthetic Implications in Pediatric Spinal Neurosurgery** 151
    Pradeep Sharma, Rahul Yadav
    - Common Neurosurgical Entities in the Spinal Region   153
    - Primary Spinal Cord Tumors   155
    - Spinal Cord Injury in Pediatric Age Group   156
    - Craniovertebral Junction Anomalies   156

- Spinal Deformity *156*
- Spinal Cord Vascular Malformations *157*
- Preoperative Evaluation *157*
- Preoperative Fasting *158*
- Premedication *159*
- Anesthesia Concerns *159*
- Preparation of Operating Room for Surgery *159*
- Induction of General Anesthesia *160*
- Airway Management *161*
- Maintenance of Anesthesia *162*
- Intraoperative Complications *166*
- Emergence and Tracheal Extubation *166*
- Postoperative Management *167*

13. Awake Tracheal Intubation 171
Bindiya Salunke, Jigeeshu V Divatia

- Indications *173*
- Contraindications *173*
- Fasting Guidelines *174*
- Components of Awake Tracheal Intubation *174*
- Failed Awake Intubation Rescue *180*
- Managing Complications *181*
- Tracheal Extubation *181*
- Documentation *181*

14. Anesthesia for Tracheal Reconstruction Surgeries 185
Raj Sahajanandan, Rahul Pillai, Amit Mathew

- Applied Anatomy *186*
- Preoperative Evaluation *186*
- Optimization *189*
- Multidisciplinary Discussion *190*
- Airway Management Strategy *191*
- Anesthetic Management *197*
- Special Considerations *198*
- Evolving Techniques *199*
- Case Scenarios *199*
- Role of ECMO *200*
- Emergence *201*
- Extubation *202*

15. Anesthesia for Pancreas and Islet Cell Transplantation 206
Cody Tidwell, Vinh Huu Nguyen, Serjey Ghercuic, Kumar Belani

- Diabetes Mellitus *207*
- Pancreas Anatomy and Physiology *209*
- Patient Selection *210*
- Immunosuppression and Prophylaxis *211*
- Overview of Surgical Technique *211*
- Preoperative Evaluation *213*
- Anesthetic Considerations *213*
- Postoperative Complications *215*

16. **Anesthetic Implications in Gastroenterological Interventions Outside the Operating Room** 218
    Venkatesan Thiruvenkatarajan, Roelof MAW Van Wijk
    - Preprocedural Risk Assessment and Optimization   *219*
    - Monitoring   *220*
    - Pharmacological Principles of Sedation   *221*
    - Organizational Logistics of Gastroenterological Procedures in Suites Outside Operating Room   *222*
    - Oxygen Supplementation and Airway Management Strategies to Mitigate Hypoxemia   *224*
    - Oxygen Delivery During Gastroenterological Interventions   *224*
    - Considerations of Capnography Monitoring   *232*
    - Assessment and Considerations of Aspiration Risk   *233*

17. **Opioid-free Anesthesia with Friedberg's Triad** 239
    Barry L Friedberg
    - Friedberg's Triad 1.0: Measure the Brain   *240*
    - Friedberg's Triad 2.0 Preempt the Pain   *249*
    - Friedberg's Triad 3.0 Emetic Drugs Abstain   *252*
    - Challenging Cases   *253*

18. **Environmental and Occupational Considerations of Anesthesia** 257
    Parli Raghavan Ravi, Rajini Kausalya, Basavaraju Karan
    - Earth Atmosphere   *258*
    - Earth's Energy Expenditure   *259*
    - Terminology and Definitions   *260*
    - Montreal Protocol for Ozone Layer   *260*
    - Kyoto Protocol   *260*
    - Climate Chemistry and Inhaled Anesthesia Agents   *261*
    - Global Warming and Inhalation Anesthetic Agents   *261*
    - Strategies to Reduce Environmental Hazards in Anesthesia   *264*
    - Waste Prevention: Avoid, Reduce, Reuse, Recycle, and Reprocess   *264*
    - Education and Advocacy   *266*
    - Global Consensus Statement from the World Federation of Anesthesiologists on Environmental Protection   *266*
    - Other Environmental Hazards Exposure to Anesthesiologist   *266*
    - Substance Use, Abuse, and Addiction   *268*
    - Radiation   *269*
    - Surgical Smoke   *269*

19. **Enhanced Surgical Recovery Programs and Cancer Outcomes** 274
    Anoushka Afonso, Vijaya Gottumukkala
    - Preoperative Preparation   *276*
    - Intraoperative Management   *281*
    - Postoperative Care   *285*

20. **Perioperative Surgical Homes** 292
    Rashmi Datta
    - Traditional Perioperative Management   *294*

- Evolution of the Concept *295*
- Elements of Perioperative Surgical Home *298*
- Perioperative Surgical Home Team *299*
- Benefits of Perioperative Surgical Home *302*
- Barriers to Implementation *303*

21. Overview of Point-of-Care Ultrasound for the Anesthesiologist 309
C Adam Coridan, Sanjib Das Adhikary

- Point-of-Care Ultrasound for Diagnostic Evaluation *311*
- Point-of-Care Ultrasound for Procedures *317*

22. Artificial Intelligence In Anesthesia 326
Shaloo Garg

- Artificial Intelligence *328*
- Applications of Artificial Intelligence *331*
- Limitations and Ethics *337*
- Future of Artificial Intelligence *337*
- Artificial Intelligence, 5g, and Anesthesia *338*

23. Technologies Likely to Impact Cardiopulmonary Resuscitation in the Near Future 343
Tommaso Scquizzato, Federico Semeraro

- Preventing Cardiac Arrest *344*
- Technologies for Recognizing Cardiac Arrest *345*
- Technologies for CPR and Defibrillation *346*
- Technologies in Advanced Life Support *348*

24. Comprehensive Care at the End-of-Life 354
Rakesh Garg, Ruparna Khurana

- Case Vignette *354*
- Definitions and Implications of Operational Terms *356*
- End-of-Life Care–Recognition and Management *357*
- Death Rattle *359*
- Pain *360*
- Nausea and Vomiting *361*
- Breathlessness *361*
- Delirium *361*
- Massive Hemorrhage *362*
- Psychological Issues *362*
- Spiritual Distress *363*
- Good Death *363*
- Advance Directives and Advance Care Planning *363*
- Do Not Intubate/Do Not Attempt Resuscitation (DNI/DNAR) *364*
- Euthanasia and Physician-assisted Suicide *365*
- Palliative Sedation *366*
- Artificial Hydration and Nutrition *366*
- Where Do We Stand Today? *367*

Index *371*

CHAPTER

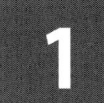

Acute Respiratory Failure: Pathophysiology, Causes, and Diagnosis

Roopali Phulli, Praveen Neema

■ ABSTRACT

Acute respiratory failure is a major cause of morbidity and mortality in critical care unit. Acute respiratory failure involves diverse mechanisms such as gaseous exchange abnormality of lung parenchyma, inability to move air in and out of the lung and increased respiratory muscles workload. A sound knowledge of underlying pathophysiology and mechanisms of respiratory failure and their assessment is necessary for the diagnosis and rationale management which can potentially improve the patient outcome.

Keywords: Acute respiratory failure; Physiology of respiration; Ventilation-perfusion mismatch; Atelectasis; COVID-19; Critically ill.

■ KEY POINTS

- Acute respiratory failure is a major cause of admission to critical care units.
- Acute respiratory failure is a major cause of morbidity and mortality in critical care units.
- Acute respiratory failure involves diverse pathology.
- A sound knowledge of physiology of respiration is necessary to understand basic mechanisms of respiratory failure.
- Arterial blood gas analysis identify basic mechanism of respiratory failure.
- Early detection of the underlying mechanism of acute respiratory failure allow rational management.

■ INTRODUCTION

Acute respiratory failure is a major cause of morbidity and mortality in patients admitted to critical care units (CCU). Acute respiratory failure involves diverse pathology, including gaseous exchange abnormality of lung parenchyma as occurs in pulmonary congestion, pulmonary edema, pneumonia, atelectasis, or it can be secondary to the inability to move air in and out of the lung as observed in cases of neurological disorders (Guillain-Barré syndrome), phrenic nerve injury, neuromuscular disorder (myasthenia gravis), muscle fatigue, status asthmaticus, chronic obstructive pulmonary disease, drug overdose (narcotic), or it can be because of increased respiratory muscles workload as occur in loss of integrity of chest wall or airway, in the presence of inability to clear the airway of secretions, or in the presence of a foreign body in the airway.[1]

Overview of the Respiratory System

The respiratory system performs the vital function of gaseous exchange.[2] Oxygen is transported through the upper airways to the alveoli, where it diffuses across the alveolocapillary membrane and enters the capillary blood.[1] In the alveoli, O_2 combines with hemoglobin and is transported as oxyhemoglobin by the arterial blood to the tissues. In the tissues, O_2 enters in Krebs' cycle and generates high energy adenosine triphosphate (ATP) from pyruvate, essential for all metabolic processes. The cellular metabolism yields mainly CO_2, which diffuses from the tissues into the capillary blood, where a major portion of it is hydrated as carbonic acid and transported to the lungs by the venous blood. In the lungs, CO_2 diffuses into the alveoli and finally exhaled into the atmosphere (Expiration).

Respiration is accomplished and regulated by an intricate set of structures.[3] These structures include: (1) the lungs; (2) the conducting airways; (3) the thoracic wall that acts as bellows and protects the lungs; (4) the respiratory muscles that moves air in and out of the lungs; and (5) the respiratory centers with their sensitive receptors and communicating nerves that control and regulate ventilation. These functional components can be affected by many pathologic processes. The interactions of musculoskeletal, cardiopulmonary, and nervous systems can be disrupted by anesthetic agents, disease, and surgery.[1]

Significant impairment in the gaseous exchange capacity of the respiratory system leads to its failure.[1] Traditionally, respiratory failure has been a clinical diagnosis. Nowadays, arterial blood gas analysis is easily available, therefore, respiratory failure is considered in terms of impairment of its actual gaseous exchange functions, i.e., oxygenation failure (arterial hypoxemia) or CO_2 removal failure (ventilatory failure, hypercapnia) or failure of both the functions.[1] The physiology of respiration and pathophysiological mechanisms that lead to respiratory failure is reviewed in this chapter. Disorders that cause different types of respiratory failure are also briefly mentioned. An overview of the assessment of respiratory failure and diagnosis is also presented.

Physiology of Respiration

The alveolus with its capillary network constitutes the functioning unit of the lung. The transport of air from the atmosphere to the alveoli (ventilation) and the supply of blood to the pulmonary capillaries (perfusion) is governed by many factors.[1] Exchange of gases between the alveolar air and the pulmonary capillary

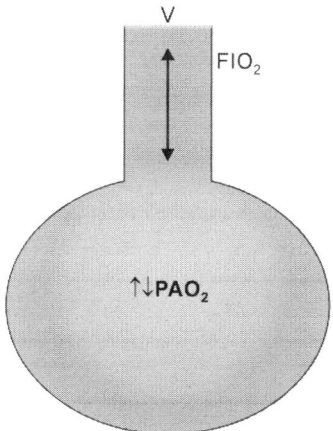

Fig. 1: Schematic diagram shows the effect of ventilation and inspiratory O_2 concentration on PAO_2.

blood constitutes external respiration. The gas exchange between a solution and its surrounding is governed by Henry's Law. The law states that when a solution (e.g., pulmonary capillary blood) is exposed to a gas (e.g., alveolar gas), the gas molecules dissolve, and equilibrate with the solution (capillary blood); similarly, gas molecules dissolved in the capillary blood equilibrates with the surrounding alveolar gas. Because of ventilation, the partial pressure of O_2 in the alveoli (PAO_2) is higher than its partial pressure at the venous end of the pulmonary capillary blood (PvO_2), and O_2 moves down the pressure gradient resulting in a lower PAO_2 and a higher partial pressure of O_2 in the blood leaving the pulmonary capillaries. Similarly, CO_2 moves out from the pulmonary capillary blood into the alveoli, causing a decrease in partial pressures of CO_2 in the pulmonary capillary blood and higher partial pressure of CO_2 in the alveoli ($PACO_2$).[1] After equilibration, the PAO_2 decreases and $PACO_2$ increases, whereas the partial pressure of O_2 increases and CO_2 decreases in the blood leaving the pulmonary capillaries,[4] and the PO_2 and PCO_2 in the blood leaving pulmonary capillaries and the PAO_2 and $PACO_2$ are equal.

The partial pressure of O_2 and CO_2 in the pulmonary capillary blood leaving the alveoli is decided by O_2 and CO_2 delivery to the alveolus and O_2 and CO_2 removal from the alveolus.[1] The partial pressure of O_2 in the inspiratory air (FIO_2) and the sweep rate of air (ventilation, V), are the determinants of O_2 delivery to the alveolus **(Fig. 1)**. An increase in FIO_2 and an increase in ventilation increases PAO_2.[1] The quality, quantity, and the saturation of the hemoglobin (SvO_2) of the blood perfusing the alveoli determines the extent of extraction of O_2 from the alveolus, a decrease in SvO_2 increases O_2 extraction, and an increase in SvO_2 decreases O_2 extraction. The SvO_2 is affected by the extraction of the O_2 in the tissues (metabolism), which is affected by the supply of O_2 to the tissues (cardiac output)[1] **(Fig. 2)**. The absolute quantity of hemoglobin in the circulating

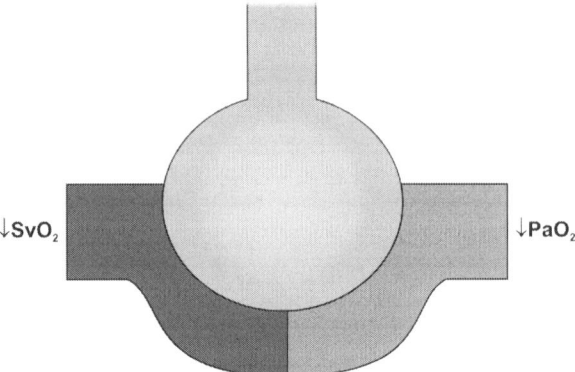

Fig. 2: Effect of decreased venous saturation on the arterial partial pressure of O_2.

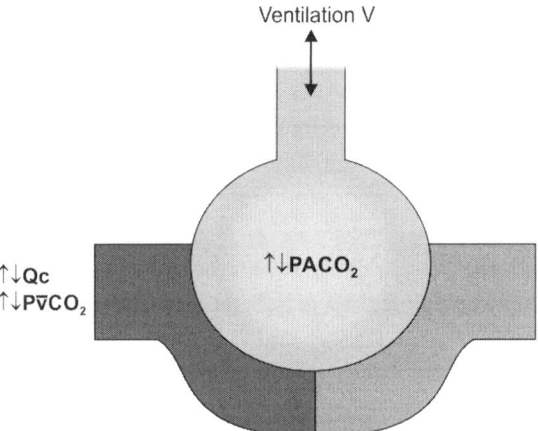

Fig. 3: Effect of cardiac output and partial pressure of venous CO_2 on the partial pressure of O_2 in alveoli.

pulmonary capillary blood also increases or decreases the extraction of O_2 in the alveoli, though this particular factor is less important.

The PAO_2 is further affected by the partial pressure of CO_2 in the pulmonary capillary blood.[1] A decrease in tissue metabolism or a decrease in cardiac output results in a decreased amount of CO_2 transported to the pulmonary capillary blood, and an increase in tissue metabolism or an increase in cardiac output results in an increased amount of CO_2 transported to pulmonary capillary blood. A decreased or an increased amount of CO_2 in the pulmonary capillary blood results in a decreased or an increased diffusion of CO_2 to alveoli and a parallel change in $PACO_2$. Similarly, a decrease in ventilation decreases CO_2 removal from the alveoli and an increase in ventilation increases CO_2 removal from the alveoli. A decreased removal cause an increase in $PACO_2$ and an increased removal cause a decrease in $PACO_2$ **(Fig. 3)**. A decrease in $PACO_2$ results in an increase in PAO_2 and an

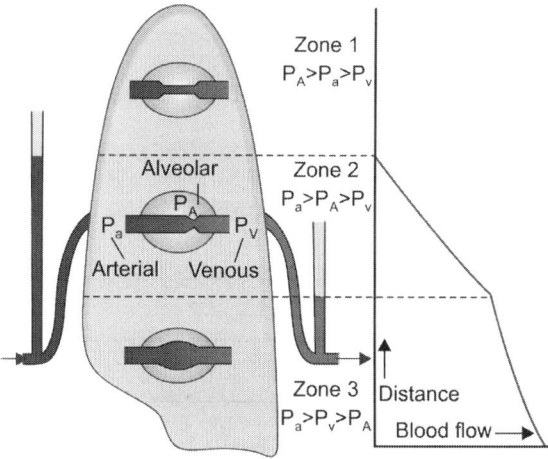

Fig. 4: Schematic diagram shows the relation between pulmonary arterial pressure, pulmonary venous pressure, and alveolar pressure and their effect on pulmonary capillary flow.

increase in $PACO_2$ results in a decrease in PAO_2 affecting O_2 diffusion into pulmonary capillary blood (Refer: Alveolar gas equation).

The distribution of ventilation and perfusion further influences the PAO_2 and $PACO_2$ and PO_2 and PCO_2 in the pulmonary capillary blood leaving the alveoli. The major determinants of the distribution of pulmonary blood flow include cardiac output, pulmonary artery pressure, gravity, posture, and interaction of pulmonary artery pressure with alveolar pressure and pulmonary venous pressure **(Fig. 4)**. In general, perfusion is more at the lung bases than the apex.[1] This difference increases with a decrease in cardiac output and hypotension and with positive pressure ventilation and positive end-expiratory pressure (PEEP).

The distribution of ventilation is maximum at the bases and designed to match the perfusion. The lungs are suspended in the thoracic cage by the trachea, and its surface adheres to the inner surface of the thoracic wall, and its bases rest on the diaphragm. The intrapleural space separates the lungs from the chest wall. The suspended lung is pulled down from the pleural surface by its own weight resulting in maximum pulling pressure at the apex of the lung, which keeps decreasing toward its base resulting in a maximal (negative) intrapleural pressure at the apex and least at the base. Because of maximum negative intrapleural pressure at the apex, the alveoli have higher volume than the alveoli at the base **(Fig. 5)**. As the alveoli at the base are small, they have a greater capacity to expand, whereas the larger alveoli at the apex have a lesser capacity to expand; in other words, the alveoli at the apex of the lung sit on the flatter part of the compliance curve whereas the alveoli in the middle and at the base sit on the steeper part of the compliance curve **(Fig. 6A)**. During inspiration, the thoracic cage volume increases due

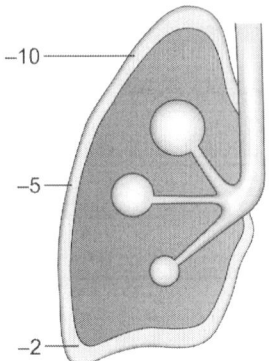

Fig. 5: Bigger alveolar size at apex as compared to base, an effect of higher negative intrapleural pressure at apex.

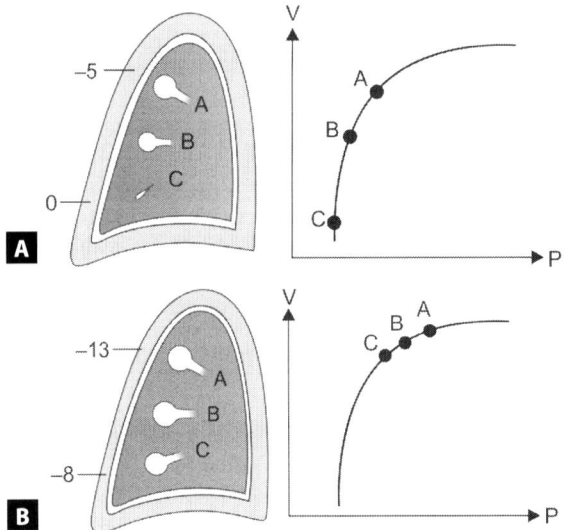

Figs. 6A and B: (A) Alveolar (lung) compliance at base and at apex of the lung; (B) Greater expansion of alveoli at base as compared to apex, an effect of higher compliance of alveoli at bases.

to descent of diaphragm and outward expansion of the chest wall, which further increases negative intrapleural pressure resulting in the downward and outward expansion of the lungs causing passive inward movement of the air in the lungs and expanding alveoli maximally at the base as compared to the apex **(Fig. 6B)**. The distribution of ventilation is further affected by the regional forces, the health of lung parenchyma, and the resistance offered by the airways. External pressure on the lung parenchyma due to the pleural collection, chest wall tumor, bulla, etc., cause compression atelectasis of lung parenchyma.

In contrast, pulmonary congestion, consolidation, etc., decreases the compliance of the affected lung. Both the conditions divert ventilation to

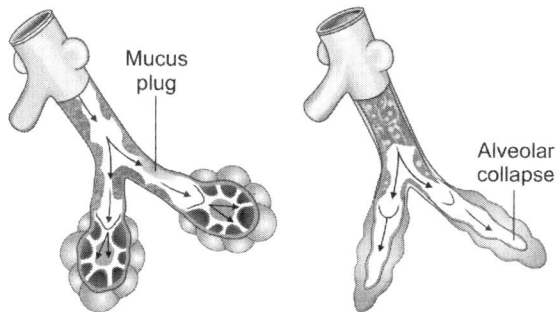

Fig. 7: Mucus plug causing absorption atelectasis.

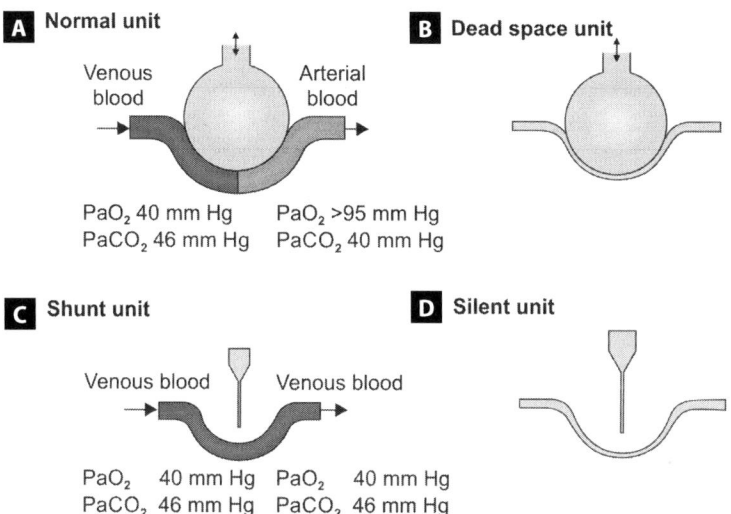

Figs. 8A to D: Various relationships of ventilation and perfusion.

compliant regions of the lung. The presence of secretions or mucus plugs or foreign bodies in the airways increases the workload of the respiratory muscles. It results in preferential ventilation of the alveoli having open airways, whereas the underventilated alveoli collapse over a period due to absorption of the remaining gases in the alveoli (absorption atelectasis; **Fig. 7**).

An efficient gaseous exchange will take place, if a perfect matching exist between ventilation and perfusion in each of the functioning unit of the lung.[1] The partial pressure of O_2 and CO_2 of the capillary blood leaving an alveolus is primarily determined by the ventilation-perfusion (V/Q) ratio of that alveolus.[5] The V/Q matching in an alveolus can exist in one of the four relationships **(Figs. 8A to D)**: (1) the normal unit in which ventilation and perfusion are matched; (2) the dead-space unit in which the alveolus is normally ventilated, but there is no capillary blood flow; (3) the shunt unit in which the alveolus is not ventilated, but there is normal capillary blood flow;

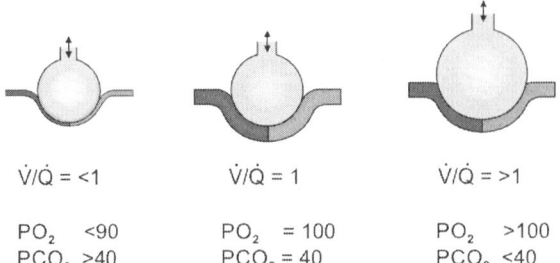

Fig. 9: Effect of ventilation perfusion mismatch on PaO_2 and PCO_2.

and (4) the silent unit in which the alveolus is unventilated, and the capillary has no perfusion.[1] The complexities of the V/Q relationship are caused primarily by the spectrum between the two extremes of dead space and shunt units. The lung consists of millions of alveoli with its network of capillaries. The V/Q relationship can exist in various combinations in health and disease. The partial pressure of O_2 and CO_2 in the blood leaving the pulmonary capillaries and joining the pulmonary veins reflects the heterogeneity of ventilation and perfusion in the alveoli, the functional units of the lung.[1]

Effect of Ventilation-Perfusion Imbalance

The PAO_2 and $PACO_2$ in each alveolus and therefore of the capillary blood leaving an alveolus is primarily determined by the V/Q ratio of the alveolus. As the V/Q ratio decreases to <1, the partial pressure of the O_2 falls, and that of CO_2 increases in the blood exiting the alveolus. The opposite occurs as the V/Q ratio increases **(Fig. 9)**. Any pathological process that affects the airways, lung parenchyma, and vasculature of the lungs will cause an imbalance between V/Q and will produce areas of abnormal V/Q ratio. The extent to which gas exchange is impaired depends on the V/Q mismatch. The partial pressure of O_2 and CO_2 in the pulmonary venous blood reflects the total heterogeneity of V/Q in the alveoli. Areas of low V/Q ratio suffer from low ventilation as compared to perfusion resulting in complete mop up of oxygen by the hemoglobin but hypoxemia as the available O_2 is not enough to fully oxygenate the flowing blood. Because of the poor ventilation, CO_2 diffused in the alveoli is not washed out as much as in well-ventilated regions, causing an increase in $PACO_2$ in the areas of low ventilation resulting in decreased diffusion gradient of CO_2 between capillary blood and alveoli. Therefore, the capillary blood leaving areas with a low V/Q ratio will have arterial hypoxemia and hypercapnia. Areas with a high V/Q ratio do not adversely affect the arterial blood gas tensions; they oxygenate the flowing capillary blood to the level equal to PAO_2 in the area; similarly, CO_2 is removed to the extent equal to $PACO_2$ in the area. The lung areas with low V/Q contribute blood with a low partial pressure of O_2 to the pulmonary venous blood, whereas the areas with a high V/Q ratio contribute blood with a high partial pressure of O_2. The areas of high and low V/Q ratios do not counterbalance each other for two reasons—first, the areas of low V/Q generally receive more blood flow than the areas of high V/Q; second, because of the nonlinear shape of the O_2-hemoglobin dissociation curve,[6] the higher partial pressure of O_2 in the blood leaving areas of high V/Q ratio does not translate into a proportionate increase in hemoglobin saturation and O_2 content and therefore provides little extra O_2 to the blood leaving the areas of high V/Q. As mentioned earlier, in the shunt units, the perfused alveoli with no ventilation, the venous blood passes unchanged through these units. This is an intrapulmonary right to left shunt and causes hypoxemia by adding the venous blood to the arterial blood. Ventilation-perfusion mismatch usually does not lead to an increase in the partial pressure of CO_2 because stimulation of the chemoreceptor increases minute ventilation to maintain partial pressure of CO_2 within the normal range. Moreover, CO_2 diffuses much faster as compared to O_2. However, an increase in partial pressure of CO_2 will occur if an increase in the ventilation is limited by respiratory depression, neuromuscular disability, or excessive work of breathing.

Effect of Low-hemoglobin Saturation in the Pulmonary Capillary (Venous) Blood

Hemoglobin saturation in the mixed venous blood that perfuses through pulmonary capillaries is about 75%. Low cardiac output, increased tissue metabolism/extraction and anemia are the reasons for low-hemoglobin saturation. Low-hemoglobin saturation per se does not affect oxygenation in the alveoli, provided ventilation is adequate. However, V/Q mismatch exists in the presence of low cardiac output. Low-hemoglobin saturation produces arterial hypoxemia by three mechanisms. First, the blood leaving the areas of low V/Q will have a lower partial pressure of O_2 because of the lower equilibration partial pressure (hemoglobin with low saturation will extract more O_2 before becoming saturated, thereby reducing PAO_2). Second, the effect of the shunt units will be exaggerated due to low saturation of venous blood. Third, decreased arterial O_2 content will lead to a further decrease in O_2 supply to the tissues. If tissue O_2 consumption remains unchanged, venous O_2 saturation will further decrease. A low-cardiac output state compounds the effects of low V/Q and shunt areas.

Evaluation of Ventilation-Perfusion Imbalance

Diffusion of gases reaches equilibrium one-third of the way through the capillary/alveolar interface. In normal circumstances, deoxygenated blood from the pulmonary arteries has a PVO_2 of 40 mm Hg, and alveolar air has a PAO_2 of 100 mm Hg, resulting in a movement of oxygen into capillaries until arterial blood equilibrates at 100 mm Hg (PaO_2) provided O_2 availability in the alveoli is not limiting. Similarly, the partial pressure of CO_2 decreases from a $PVCO_2$ of 46 mm Hg to a $PaCO_2$ of 40 mm Hg in alveolar capillaries due to a $PACO_2$ of 40 mm Hg provided capillary perfusion and ventilation is not limiting.

The severity of V/Q imbalance can be assessed by several measurements based on ideal alveolar gas equation, which represents mixed alveolar gas in the absence of V/Q imbalance. The PAO_2 is calculated from a modified alveolar gas equation. $PAO_2 = (PB - PH_2O) FiO_2 - PaCO_2/R$ (Where PB is the barometric pressure, PH_2O is the water vapor pressure in the alveoli, R is the respiratory quotient, and $PaCO_2$ is the partial pressure of CO_2 in the arterial blood). The different measurements used in the clinical practice to evaluate V/Q imbalance are:

1. Alveolar-arterial O_2 partial pressure difference ($PAO_2 - PaO_2$)
2. Venous admixture effect or shunt effect – $Qva/Qt = (Cc'O_2 - CaO_2)/(Cc'O_2 - CvO_2)$ (Where Qva is the venous admixture, Qt is cardiac output; $Cc'O_2$, CaO_2, and CvO_2 are O_2 content in ideal pulmonary capillary blood (blood leaving the alveoli with a perfect match between ventilation and perfusion), O_2 content of arterial and mixed venous blood). Calculating venous admixture at 100% inspiratory O_2 tension ($FiO_2 = 1$) eliminates the contribution of low V/Q units and measures the true shunt fraction (Qs/Qt).
3. Dead space effect, the volume of inspired air that does not participate in gaseous exchange $V_D/V_T = PaCO_2 - PECO_2/PaCO_2$ (Where V_D is wasted ventilation; dead space, V_T is tidal volume, $PaCO_2$ and $PECO_2$ are partial pressure of CO_2 in arterial blood and mixed exhaled gas).

Unfortunately, the clinical usefulness of all three measurements is limited because they are influenced by the changes in minute ventilation, cardiac output, and V/Q imbalance.

Classification of Respiratory Failure

On the basis of arterial blood gas analysis, respiratory failure is divided into three types: Type I or oxygenation failure, Type II or ventilatory failure, and Type III or combined oxygenation and ventilatory failure.

Type I Respiratory Failure (Oxygenation Failure; Arterial Hypoxemia)

Type I failure is characterized by an abnormally low partial pressure of O_2 in the arterial blood (PaO_2 <60 mm Hg while breathing room air). The partial pressure of O_2 in the arterial blood reflects: (1) Partial pressure of O_2 in inspiratory gas; (2) minute ventilation; (3) quantity of blood flowing through pulmonary capillaries; (4) O_2 saturation of the hemoglobin in the blood flowing through pulmonary capillaries (an effect of tissue metabolism, anemia and cardiac output); (5) diffusion across the alveolar membrane; and (6) V/Q matching. Arterial hypoxemia can be caused by any disorder that produces areas of low V/Q or a right to left intrapulmonary shunt and is characterized by increases in PAO_2–PaO_2 difference, venous admixture, and V_D/V_T.

Pathophysiologic mechanisms of arterial hypoxemia:
- Decreased PAO_2:
  - Hypoventilation
  - Decreased FiO_2
  - Under ventilated alveoli (areas of low V/Q)
- Intrapulmonary shunt (areas of zero V/Q):
  - Small airway obstruction causing a segmental collapse
  - Pulmonary collapse or consolidation (pneumonia)
  - Endobronchial intubation
  - Excessive positive end-expiratory pressure in the presence of segmental atelectasis
- Decreased mixed venous O_2 content (low-hemoglobin saturation):
  - Decreased cardiac output
  - Increased metabolic rate
  - Decreased arterial O_2 content

Causes of type I (oxygenation) respiratory failure:
- Adult respiratory distress syndrome (ARDS)
- Asthma
- Pulmonary edema
- Excessive intravenous fluid administration
- Chronic obstructive pulmonary disease (COPD)
- Interstitial fibrosis
- Pneumonia
- Pneumothorax
- Pulmonary embolism
- Pulmonary hypertension.

Type II Respiratory Failure (Ventilatory Failure: Arterial Hypercapnia)

The partial pressure of CO_2 in the arterial blood reflects the efficiency of the ventilatory mechanism that clears (washes out) CO_2 produced during tissue metabolism. Type II failure can be caused by any disorder that decreases central respiratory drive, interferes with the transmission of signals from the central nervous system to muscles of respiration (diaphragm and intercostals), or impedes the ability of respiratory muscles to expand the lungs and chest wall. Type II failure is characterized by an abnormal increase in the partial pressure of CO_2 in the arterial blood ($PaCO_2$ >46 mm Hg), and is accompanied by simultaneous falls in PAO_2 and PaO_2. Therefore, PAO_2 – PaO_2 difference remains unchanged.

Common causes of type II respiratory failure:
- *Disorders affecting central ventilatory drive:*
  - Brainstem infarction or hemorrhage
  - Brainstem compression from supratentorial mass
  - Drug overdose, narcotics, benzodiazepines, anesthetic agents, etc.
- *Disorders affecting signal transmission to the respiratory muscles:*
  - Myasthenia gravis
  - Amyotrophic lateral sclerosis
  - Guillain-Barré syndrome
  - Spinal-cord injury
  - Multiple sclerosis
  - Residual paralysis (Muscle relaxants)
- *Disorders of respiratory muscles or chest wall:*
  - Muscular dystrophy
  - Polymyositis
  - Flail Chest
- *Increased work of breathing:*
  - Airway obstruction (Foreign body airway, intratracheal tumor, obstructive sleep apnea, inability to clear airway secretions, and external airway compression)
  - Pulmonary congestion/edema.

Type III Respiratory Failure (Combined Oxygenation and Ventilatory Failure)

Combined respiratory failure shows features of both arterial hypoxemia and hypercapnia (decrease in PaO_2 and increase in $PaCO_2$). Assessment based on the alveolar gas equation shows increases in PAO_2–PaO_2 difference, venous admixture, and V_D/V_T. In theory, any disorder causing Type I or Type II respiratory failure can cause Type III respiratory failure.

Common causes of type III respiratory failure:
- Adult respiratory distress syndrome
- Asthma
- Chronic obstructive pulmonary disease.

Cardiovascular and Respiratory Responses to Arterial Hypoxemia

The peripheral chemoreceptors located in the arch of the aorta and at the bifurcation of the carotid artery recognize low PaO_2 (hypoxemia) and send afferent signals to the brain. Recognition of hypoxemic state results in cardiovascular system adjustments to deliver more blood to tissues to compensate for reduced O_2 delivery. The acute central cardiovascular response to hypoxic stress triggers an increased heart rate at an unchanged stroke volume mediated primarily by increased sympathetic neural discharge as a function of increasing hypoxic severity. Lower levels of hypoxic exposure may result in some degree of systemic vasodilation. With the increasing severity of hypoxia, the peripheral vasculature constricts to redistribute oxygen delivery to critical organs, the heart,[7] and the brain.[8] Hypoxemia increases minute ventilation and consequently the work of breathing, potentially leading to greater muscle fatigue.

PATHOPHYSIOLOGY OF ACUTE RESPIRATORY FAILURE IN CORONAVIRUS DISEASE 2019 (COVID-19)

The acute respiratory distress syndrome (ARDS), originally described in 1967 by Petty and coworkers,[9] is a syndrome of acute respiratory failure that presents with progressive hypoxemia and increased work of breathing. The characteristic pathological changes that occur in the lungs of an ARDS patient are described in three phases, namely (1) acute (inflammatory, first 1-6 days); (2) subacute (proliferative, next 7-14 days); and (3) chronic phases (resolution, after 14 days).[10] The acute phase presents with alveolar and interstitial edema along with the accumulation of neutrophils, macrophages, and red blood cells in the alveoli. There is evidence of endothelial and epithelial injury, mostly seen with denuding of the alveolar epithelium. There are prominent hyaline membranes noted in the alveoli; therefore, ARDS is also known as hyaline membrane disease. In the subacute phase, there is a proliferation of alveolar epithelial type II cells, with a resolution of some of the edema. There may also be infiltration of fibroblasts and collagen deposition. In the chronic phase, there is a resolution of the acute neutrophilic infiltrate with more mononuclear cells and alveolar macrophages in the alveoli, and often more fibrosis with ongoing evidence of alveolar epithelial repair. In many patients, resolution progresses without fibrosis, with gradual resolution of the edema and acute inflammation.

First case of COVID-19 caused by coronavirus 2 (SARS-CoV-2) appeared in Wuhan, China. Although most patients have a favorable prognosis, pneumonia and severe hypoxemia associated with SARS-CoV-2 infection can lead to ARDS, which is associated with a high mortality rate.[11] There have been many studies comparing the respiratory mechanics in COVID-associated ARDS versus classical ARDS. Some authors described COVID-19-related ARDS patients with intriguingly high compliance as compared to non-COVID ARDS,[12-14] others reported cases with very low compliance.[15] Gattinoni and colleagues proposed an integrative concept[14] hypothesizing a progressive transition from a phenotype characterized by low elastance, low lung weight, low recruitability, and low ventilation-to-perfusion ratio (phenotype L) to a phenotype characterized by high elastance, high lung weight, high right-to-left shunt, and high recruitability (Phenotype H), the transition being mainly driven by the extent of the patient's ventilatory response and its ability to promote self-inflicted lung injury.[16] There is a subgroup of patients with COVID-19-related ARDS who have disease characterized by low static compliance of the respiratory system and high D-dimer concentration and have a markedly increased mortality compared with other patients.[17] Although Grasselli and colleagues could not demonstrate a direct link between D-dimer concentrations and thrombotic burden, they found that the ventilatory ratio, a marker of dead space, was higher in patients with COVID-19-related ARDS who had very high D-dimer concentrations irrespective of the patients' static compliance.[17] This was supported by CT angiogram studies showing filling defects or occlusions of the pulmonary vasculature that were more prominent in patients with high D-dimer concentrations. It suggested that intravascular pathology plays a major role in increasing dead space and causing hypoxemia (decreased PaO_2/FiO_2) in COVID-19-related ARDS. Additionally, this could explain that static compliance and PaO_2/FiO_2 were not correlated in COVID-19-related ARDS but in classical ARDS.

Assessment of Pulmonary Function in Critically Ill Patients

The primary aim of the respiratory system is the gaseous exchange (cardiopulmonary interaction). Airways provide a conduit for air passage from the environment to the lungs, the neuromuscular system ensures ventilation, and the lung parenchyma provides the surface for interaction between ventilation and perfusion. The health of the lung parenchyma and the airways determines the load (work of breathing) placed on the neuromuscular system; increased load due to lung disease or airway disease can stress and precipitate the failure of the neuromuscular system. Deterioration in pulmonary function in critically ill patients can be because of the inadequacy of airways, lung parenchyma, cardiopulmonary interaction, and neuromuscular system. The assessment of pulmonary function is of particular importance in: (1) deciding the necessity of ventilatory support, (2) assessing response to therapy, (3) optimizing ventilator management, and (4) deciding on weaning from the ventilator.

Clinical assessment of the respiratory system is often focused on auscultatory findings; however, considerable information can be obtained from careful inspection and examination of the breathing pattern. Presence of wheeze, crepitations, increased respiratory rate, suprasternal and intercostal indrawing/recession, accessory muscle activity (sternomastoid), and rib cage–abdominal paradox indicates increased work of breathing. Various tests are described to assess different components. Measurement of airway resistance and lung compliance allow evaluation of load put on the neuromuscular component while assessment of the function of the respiratory center and the strength of respiratory muscle allow evaluation of the efficiency of the neuromuscular component. Measurement of airway occlusion pressure (AOP) at 0.1 seconds in a mechanically ventilated patient is closely related to the intensity of respiratory neural drive.[18] The occlusion pressure is measured by transiently and surreptitiously occluding the airway during early inspiration and measuring the change in airway pressure after 0.1 seconds before the patient reacts to the occlusion. Although AOP 0.1 values represent negative pressure, it is customary to report it in positive units, which in the normal subject during relaxed breathing is 0.93 ± 0.48 (SD) cmH$_2$O.[19] A high AOP 0.1 value during acute respiratory failure indicates increased respiratory drive and neuromuscular activity and, if sustained, may result in inspiratory muscle fatigue. Modern ventilators provide a facility for the measurement of airway resistance and lung compliance, and AOP. Respiratory muscle strength is assessed by measuring the maximum inspiratory and expiratory pressure (P$_i$max and P$_e$max,) generated against an occluded airway. These measurements can be obtained readily with an aneroid manometer.[20] The maximum force generated by the inspiratory or expiratory muscle is related to their initial length.

Consequently, these measurements are made at residual volume (P$_i$max) or total lung capacity (P$_e$max). P$_i$max and P$_e$max in healthy adult men are approximately 111±34 and 151±68 cm of H$_2$O, respectively.[21]

The values tend to decrease with age and are lower in women.[22] In ambulatory patients with neuromuscular disease free of lung disease, hypercapnia is likely to develop when P$_i$max is reduced to one-third of the normal predicted value. The respiratory system performs continuously, and for sustained ventilation, the muscles of respiration must perform (endurance) without getting fatigued. A number of techniques, such as transdiaphragmatic pressure measurement, phrenic nerve stimulation, and determination of tension–time index, are used to detect the presence or development of muscle fatigue.[23] Diaphragmatic ultrasonography is found helpful in the assessment of diaphragmatic function. The method assesses changes in the thickness of the diaphragm during inspiration and easily recognizes diaphragm palsy.[24] Vital capacity (VC) is the only lung volume commonly measured in the CCU. In a study of patients with Guillain-Barré syndrome, VC measurement was found a reliable predictor of respiratory failure hours before actual intubation,[25] and a fall in VC to <15 mL/kg indicates the need for endotracheal intubation.

■ DIAGNOSIS

As discussed earlier, the diagnosis of respiratory failure is based on an analysis of arterial blood gas, but it is important to suspect it clinically. The patients with respiratory failure will have clinical features of underlying disease; additionally, they may have hypoxemia and hypercapnia. The compensatory responses to hypoxemia such as tachypnea, tachycardia, hypertension, intercostal muscle retraction, and use of accessory muscles during inspiration may also be present. Cerebral hypoxia produces changes in mentation that can range from mental confusion and restlessness to delirium. A decrease in peripheral oxygen saturation (SpO_2 <92%) indicates the presence of arterial hypoxemia. Hypercapnia exerts its major effects on the central nervous system. As the $PaCO_2$ increases, patients typically progress through the stages of lethargy, stupor, and finally, coma (CO_2 narcosis). Other symptoms are secondary to catecholamine release and concomitant hypoxemia. The patient is often described as "fatigued" or "tired out". However, the clinical manifestations described are nonspecific and may occur without respiratory failure. Therefore, the diagnosis of respiratory failure must be confirmed by arterial blood gas analysis.

CONCLUSION

Respiratory failure is a medical emergency and a real threat to the life of patient. Many diseases of diverse etiology are associated with respiratory failure. A sound knowledge of underlying pathophysiological mechanisms producing disturbances in gaseous exchange allows the selection of optimal management strategy.

Disclaimer: A major part of this chapter is taken from the review article "Respiratory failure" published by the corresponding author of this chapter in Indian Journal of Anaesthesia and cited as reference 1 in this chapter.

Conflict of interest: None.

REFERENCES

1. Neema PK. Respiratory failure. Indian J Anaesth. 2003;47:360-6.
2. Kreit JW, Rogers RM. Approach to the patient with respiratory failure. In: Ayres S, Holbrook G (Eds). Textbook of Critical Care. Philadelphia: WB Saunders; 1995. pp. 680-87.
3. Papadakos PJ. Perioperative evaluation of pulmonary disease and function. In: Murray MJ, Coursin DB, Pearl RG, Prough DS (Eds). Critical Care Medicine. Philadelphia: Lippincot-Williams and Wilkins; 2002. pp. 374-84.
4. Shapiro BA, Peruzzi WT. Physiology of respiration. In: Shapiro BA, Peruzzi WT (Eds). Clinical Application of Blood Gases. Baltimore: Mosby; 1994. pp.13-24.
5. West JB. Ventilation-perfusion relationships. Am Rev Respir Dis. 1977;116:919-25.
6. Stoelting RK. Pulmonary gas exchange and blood transport of gases. In: Stoelting RK (Ed). Pharmacology and Physiology in Anesthetic Practice. Philadelphia: JB Lippincott; 1987. pp. 721-33.
7. Kaijser L, Grubbstrom J, Berglund B. Coronary circulation in acute hypoxia. Clin Physiol. 1990;10:259-63.

8. Norcliffe LJ, Rivera-Ch M, Claydon VE, Moore JP, Leon-Velarde F, Appenzeller O, et al. Cerebrovascular responses to hypoxia and hypocapnia in high-altitude dwellers. J Physiol. 2005;566:287-94.
9. Ashbaugh DG, Bigelow DB, Petty TL, Levine BE. Acute respiratory distress in adults. Lancet. 1967;2:319-23.
10. Bachofen M, Weibel ER. Alterations of the gas exchange apparatus in adult respiratory insufficiency associated with septicemia. Am Rev Respir Dis. 1977;116:589-615.
11. Yang X, Yu Y, Xu J. Clinical course and outcomes of critically ill patients with SARS-CoV-2 pneumonia in Wuhan, China: a single-centered, retrospective, observational study. Lancet Respir Med. 2020;8:475-81.
12. Gattinoni L, Coppola S, Cressoni M, Busana M, Rossi S, Chiumello D, et al. COVID-19 does not lead to a "typical" acute respiratory distress syndrome. Am J Respir Crit Care Med. 2020;201:1299-300.
13. Tobin MJ. Basing respiratory management of COVID-19 on physiological principles [editorial]. Am J Respir Crit Care Med. 2020;201:1319-20.
14. Gattinoni L, Chiumello D, Caironi P, Busana M, Romitti F, Brazzi L, et al. COVID-19 pneumonia: different respiratory treatments for different phenotypes? Intensive Care Med. 2020;46(6):1099-102.
15. Pan C, Chen L, Lu C, Zhang W, Xia JA, Sklar MC, et al. Lung recruitability in COVID-19-associated acute respiratory distress syndrome: a single-center observational study. Am J Respir Crit Care Med. 2020;201:1294-97.
16. Brochard L, Slutsky A, Pesenti A. Mechanical ventilation to minimize progression of lung injury in acute respiratory failure. Am J Respir Crit Care Med. 2017;195:438-42.
17. Grasselli G, Tonetti T, Protti A, Langer T, Girardis M, Bellani G, et al. Pathophysiology of COVID-19-associated acute respiratory distress syndrome: a multicentre prospective observational study. Lancet Respir Med. 2020;8:1201-8.
18. Whitelaw WA, Derenne JP. Airway occlusion pressure. J Appl Physiol. 1993;74:1475.
19. Tobin MJ, Gardener WN. Monitoring of the control of breathing. In: Tobin MJ (Ed). Principles and Practice of Intensive Care Monitoring. New York: McGraw-Hill; 1998. pp. 415-64.
20. Tobin MJ. State of the art: respiratory monitoring. Am Rev Respir Dis. 1988;138:1625.
21. Koulouris N, Mulvey DA, Laroche CM, Green M, Moxham J. Comparison of two different mouth-pieces for the measurement of $P_i$max and $P_e$max in normal and weak subjects. Eur Respir J. 1988;1:863.
22. Chen HI, Kuo CS. Relationship between respiratory muscle function and age, sex and other factors. J Appl Physiol. 1989;66:943.
23. Tobin MJ, Laghi F. Monitoring of respiratory muscle function. In: Tobin MJ (Ed). Principles and Practice of Intensive Care Monitoring. New York: McGraw-Hill; 1998. pp. 945-88.
24. Gottesman E, McCool FD. Ultrasound evaluation of the paralyzed diaphragm. Am J Respir Crit Care Med. 1997;155:1570.
25. Chevrolet JC, Deleamont P. Repeated vital capacity measurement as predictive parameter for mechanical ventilation need and weaning success in the Guillain-Barré syndrome. Am Rev Respir Dis. 1991;144:814.

CHAPTER 2

Noninvasive Ventilation for Acute Respiratory Failure

Gautam Gondal, Nishanth Baliga, Sheila Nianan Myatra

ABSTRACT

Noninvasive ventilation is mechanical ventilation (MV) without the use of an invasive artificial airway (endotracheal tube or tracheostomy tube]. Noninvasive ventilation is able to offer the same physiological effects of invasive MV delivered via endotracheal intubation (ET) but avoids the life-threatening risks associated with the use of an artificial airway. Noninvasive positive-pressure ventilation (NIPPV) and high-flow nasal oxygen (HFNO) are the two most commonly used noninvasive techniques to support patients with acute respiratory failure. The conditions associated with acute respiratory failure that are known to benefit the most with NIPPV are acute cardiogenic pulmonary edema and acute exacerbations of chronic obstructive pulmonary disease (AECOPD) with hypercapnic acidosis (pH between 7.25 and 7.35). The major indication for the use of HFNO includes acute hypoxemic respiratory failure.

Keywords: Noninvasive ventilation; Respiratory failure; COVID-19; High-flow nasal oxygen (HFNO); Noninvasive positive pressure ventilation (NIPPV).

KEY POINTS

- Noninvasive ventilation (NIV) should be offered in a controlled environment with intense monitoring to reduce the risk of NIV failure and in facilities where prompt intubation is possible.
- The conditions associated with acute respiratory failure that are known to benefit the most with noninvasive positive-pressure ventilation (NIPPV) are acute cardiogenic pulmonary edema and acute exacerbation of chronic obstructive pulmonary disease (AECOPD) with hypercapnic acidosis (pH between 7.25 and 7.35).
- NIPPV is commonly used in patients with mild-to-moderate ARDS; however, in severe ARDS the risk of NIPPV failure is high.
- Randomized trials and observational studies in patients with hypoxemic respiratory failure consistently demonstrate improved oxygenation and decreased need for intubation with the use of HFNO when compared with low flow oxygen systems.

- The mode of NIV (NIPPV or HFNO) should be individualized based on the clinical presentation of the patient and the current evidence supporting the use of the modality.

INTRODUCTION

Acute hypoxemic respiratory failure (AHRF) is the most common form of respiratory failure accounting for a large proportion of intensive care unit (ICU) admissions worldwide.[1] Approximately 60% of patients with AHRF require invasive mechanical ventilation (IMV).[2] IMV is associated with adverse events including ventilator-induced lung injury (VILI) and ventilator-associated pneumonia (VAP).[3] Patients with acute respiratory failure on IMV have high-hospital mortality rates of up to 30%.[4] Noninvasive ventilation (NIV) is able to offer the same physiological effects of IMV delivered via endotracheal intubation (ET) but avoids the life-threatening risks associated with the use of an artificial airway. Noninvasive positive-pressure ventilation (NIPPV) and high-flow nasal oxygen (HFNO) are the two most commonly used noninvasive techniques to support patients with acute respiratory failure. Use of helmet continuous positive airway pressure (CPAP) has shown promising results; however, more robust data and universal availability are required before it can be recommended for routine use. In this chapter, we will discuss the current evidence for the use of NIV in various conditions.

PATHOPHYSIOLOGY OF AHRF

Acute hypoxemic respiratory failure usually refers to a patient with an increased breathing frequency and low-oxygen saturation or ratio of arterial partial pressure of oxygen (PaO_2) to inspired oxygen fraction (FiO_2): PaO_2/FiO_2 while receiving supplemental oxygen (e.g., breathing frequency of >25 breaths/min with a PaO_2/FiO_2 of <300 mm Hg). Direct or indirect lung injury accounts for essentially all causes of AHRF through different pathophysiological pathways. All AHRF causes, however, lead to pulmonary edema caused by lung inflammation that results in aeration loss with hypoxemia, altered respiratory mechanics, and increased respiratory drive.

Acute respiratory distress syndrome (ARDS) is a subset of AHRF. The ARDS definition requires the presence of bilateral pulmonary infiltrates on chest imaging, with hypoxemia not fully explained by fluid overload or cardiac dysfunction and assessed under positive pressure ventilation with at least 5 cmH_2O of positive end-expiratory pressure (PEEP). The severity of hypoxemia is classified by the PaO_2/FiO_2, as mild (PaO_2/FiO_2 of 201–300 mm Hg), moderate (PaO_2/FiO_2 of 101–200 mm Hg), and severe (PaO_2/FiO_2 ≤ 100 mm Hg).[5]

ADVANTAGES OF NIV OVER IMV

With NIV similar physiological effects can be achieved as with IMV delivered via a tracheal tube (i.e., unloading of respiratory muscles, improvement of gas exchange, and augmentation of alveolar ventilation), while avoiding the complications associated with the use of an invasive artificial airway. By avoiding tracheal intubation, NIV eliminates the risks associated with upper airway trauma, improves patient comfort, and minimizes the risk of complications of IMV such as ventilator-associated pneumonia (VAP) and the need for sedation. It preserves airway clearance, and allows intermittent ventilation so that normal activities such as eating, drinking, and communication are possible; additionally, breaks from ventilation can be used for administering nebulized medication, physiotherapy, and expectoration. In this chapter, we will discuss two NIV therapies: (1) NIPPV and (2) HFNO, the two most commonly used NIV in ICU.

ROLE OF NIPPV IN ACUTE RESPIRATORY FAILURE

The conditions associated with acute respiratory failure that are known to benefit the most with NIPPV are acute exacerbations of chronic obstructive pulmonary disease (AECOPD) with hypercapnic acidosis (pH between 7.25 and 7.35) and acute cardiogenic pulmonary edema (ACPE).[6] **Figure 1** shows a patient on NIPPV.

Acute Exacerbation of Chronic Obstructive Pulmonary Disease with Hypercapnic Respiratory Acidosis

An initial trial of bilevel NIPPV [also known as bilevel positive airway pressure (BiPAP)] should be given for patients with AECOPD complicated by hypercapnic acidosis ($PaCO_2$ >45 mm Hg or pH <7.35). Evidence from large randomized trials and meta-analyses has consistently indicated that BiPAP improves clinical outcomes in patients having an AECOPD complicated by

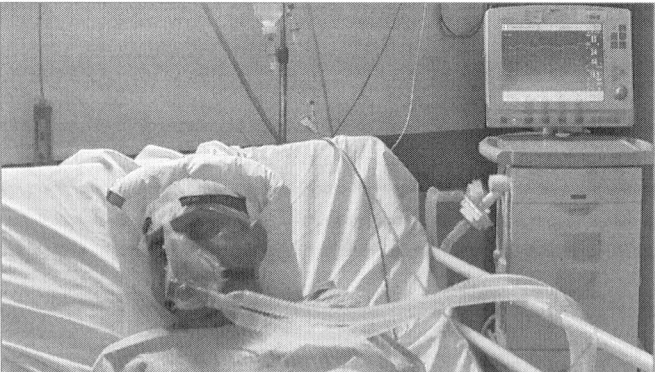

Fig. 1: Patient on noninvasive positive pressure ventilation (NIPPV).

hypercapnic acidosis. A meta-analysis of 17 randomized trials of patients with AECOPD and acute hypercapnia ($PaCO_2$ >45 mm Hg) reported almost 50% reduction in mortality in patients treated with NIPPV plus standard therapy compared with standard therapy alone.[7,8]

While data in the past suggested that patients with severe exacerbations were more likely to benefit from bilevel NIPPV, a Cochrane analysis done in 2017 consisting of 17 trials reported no differences between those with mild (defined as a pH between 7.3 and 7.35) or severe exacerbations (defined by those with a pH <7.3).[9] Guidelines on the use of NIPPV also recommend its use in patients of AECOPD with hypercapnic acidosis (pH between 7.25 and 7.35).[6]

Acute Nonhypercapnic Respiratory Failure due to AECOPD

For patients with acute nonhypercapnic respiratory failure due to AECOPD, the derived benefit from bilevel NIPPV is uncertain compared with patients who have acute hypercapnic respiratory failure due to AECOPD. The American Thoracic Society guideline group advises against using NIPPV in this population of patients, though backed by low quality of evidence.[10] Data that support not administering NIPPV in this population include several small randomized or prospective trials that reported poor tolerance of bilevel NIPPV as well as no impact of NIPPV on mortality.[7] However, it may be tried on an individualized basis in an effort to prevent the development of acute hypercapnia.

Acute Cardiogenic Pulmonary Edema

Noninvasive positive-pressure ventilation improves ACPE due to preload reduction, preventing alveolar collapse at end-expiration, and by decreasing left ventricular afterload while also reducing the work of breathing. In patients with ACPE, a trial of NIPPV with the mode of CPAP is beneficial. Meta-analyses of small randomized trials in patients with ACPE report that NIPPV decreases the need for intubation, improves clinical and laboratory indices of respiratory failure (such as heart rate, dyspnea, acidosis), and reduces mortality.[10] A meta-analysis of 13 trials that included 1,369 patients found that patients with ACPE who received CPAP plus standard care had a lower hospital mortality than those who received standard care alone.[11] Several studies have found that patients with ACPE who present with acute hypercapnic respiratory failure derive the greatest mortality benefit with the use of NIPPV.

Acute Hypoxemic Nonhypercapnic Respiratory Failure NOT due to ACPE

Due to the diverse causes of this scenario, an individualized approach is recommended. The choice of initial therapy may include HFNO, NIPPV, or low-flow oxygen. One should take into consideration the cause of the AHRF prior to initiating therapy. One should start therapy with NIPPV or HFNO as early as possible and have a low threshold to perform intubation. This cautious approach to NIPPV is because data are not as supportive in this population compared with patients who have acute hypercapnic respiratory failure due to AECOPD or acute respiratory failure due to ACPE. The benefit from NIPPV varies due to the wide range of underlying etiologies. A study done by Duan et al., reported a failure rate of 61% for those with acute respiratory failure due to septic shock compared with 23% in those with acute respiratory failure who did not have sepsis.[12] The evidence for use of HFNO in this scenario is more robust and is recommended for AHRF, which will be discussed later in this chapter.

Pneumonia

Benefit from NIPPV in patients with pneumonia is variable. Some data suggest that bilevel NIPPV is beneficial in patients with AHRF due to pneumonia provided they are able to manage their secretions. In a trial done by Ferrer et al., that demonstrated benefit from NIPPV in patients with AHRF of varying etiologies, the mortality benefit and reduced intubation rate associated with NIPPV use were most evident in the subgroup of patients with pneumonia.[13]

Several small randomized trials have also reported decreased ICU mortality, decreased intubation rate, and improved oxygenation in patients with community-acquired pneumonia who receive NIPPV compared with standard therapy. In a large database analysis, the benefit of NIPPV was less effective in patients older than 65 years who had acute respiratory failure due to pneumonia.[14]

Research has also demonstrated a high failure rate of NIPPV in patients with Middle-East respiratory syndrome (MERS) and influenza; because of these experiences in the past, NIPPV should be used cautiously in patients with AHRF from COVID-19.[15]

The Immunocompromised Patient

Although NIPPV is frequently used in immunocompromised patients for the treatment of AHRF, the evidence for its use is conflicting. This may be due to the wide array of etiologies of acute respiratory failure in patients who are immunosuppressed or the higher likelihood that acute respiratory failure will progress due to the immunosuppression itself. NIPPV should be administered cautiously, preferably in an ICU in this population ensuring that patients are aggressively monitored. Few studies demonstrated increased mortality in patients who got intubated in these immunocompromised patients. A randomized controlled trial which looked at the effect of NIV on mortality in patients with AHRF among immunocompromised patients compared to standard oxygen therapy found that there was no difference in mortality and intubation rates between the two groups.[16]

Acute Respiratory Distress Syndrome

In the LUNG SAFE study, it was shown that NIPPV is commonly used in patients with ARDS, but with an increase in the severity of ARDS there is an increased risk of NIPPV failure. Patients with PaO_2/FiO_2 ratio of less than 150 had higher ICU mortality when treated with NIPPV compared with subjects treated with invasive ventilation.[1] Hence, the current recommendation for the use of NIV is for patients with mild-to-moderate ARDS.

Acute Exacerbation of Asthma

Bilevel NIPPV is commonly used in patients with AHRF from severe asthma exacerbation, but the evidence for use of NIPPV in this population is scarce. In a trial of 30 patients who presented to the emergency department with a severe asthma exacerbation that was not responding to inhaled bronchodilator therapy, use of bilevel NIPPV was associated with a reduction in the rate of hospitalization and improved predicted forced expiratory volume in 1 second.[17] However, in a meta-analysis of five trials, that included this trial, NIPPV did not reduce the intubation rate; mortality could not be assessed since there were no deaths in any of the studies analyzed.[18] Thus, more evidence is needed to determine the value of NIPPV in patients with acute respiratory failure due to an acute asthma exacerbation.

Postextubation Respiratory Failure

Noninvasive positive-pressure ventilation has been used in patients who develop acute respiratory failure in the first 24–72 hours following extubation. NIPPV has also been used as a tool to prevent reintubation in patients at high risk of developing acute respiratory failure following extubation. Vaschetto et al., evaluated the effect of extubation without performing a spontaneous breathing trial followed by NIPPV application in 130 nonhypercapnic patients ventilated more than 48 hours and excluded patients of acute respiratory failure secondary to neurologic disorders, status asthmaticus, COPD, and cardiogenic pulmonary edema and obese patients. It was observed that early extubation reduced the duration of IMV but did not affect ICU length of stay. Further research is needed to validate these risk factors and determine if there are other populations who would benefit from postextubation support.[19]

Oxygenation Before and during Intubation

Prior to intubation, patients with hypoxemic respiratory failure are typically preoxygenated with 100% oxygen in order to prevent arterial oxygen desaturation during the procedure. NIPPV can also be used in this setting.

A randomized trial compared standard preoxygenation (with a bag mask valve) to preoxygenation with NIPPV. The NIPPV group had fewer oxyhemoglobin desaturations during intubation and higher oxyhemoglobin saturation at the end of preoxygenation, during intubation, and following intubation. Other studies have described NIPPV as a tool to prevent desaturation during intubation, including nasal intubation. The OPTINIV study showed that the use of HFNO for apneic oxygenation and NIPPV for preoxygenation was more effective in reducing the severity of desaturation as compared to NIPPV alone.[20] Subgroup analyses of the FLORALI-2 trial demonstrated a potential benefit for NIPPV among patients with a P/F ratio <200.[21,22]

Intubation Refusal or Palliation

Noninvasive positive-pressure ventilation has been used in patients who decline ET. Observational studies indicate that up to 43% of such patients survive to hospital discharge, but the mortality rate during the next 6 months is high.[23] NIPPV reduces the symptoms of dyspnea in patients receiving palliation for end-stage pulmonary diseases. Therefore, NIPPV should be applied to reduce the symptoms of breathlessness even in patients with a do-not-intubate (DNI) order. In an observational study of 36 patients with a DNI order, NIPPV delivered via an oronasal mask resulted in an improvement in eight patients while the remainder improved only after switching to a full-face mask.[24]

Postoperative Respiratory Failure

Noninvasive positive-pressure ventilation is not routinely applied as a primary prevention strategy, but is used as a secondary intervention for the treatment of hypoxemic respiratory failure. A trial of 293 patients, which compared the use of NIV in hypoxemic respiratory failure following abdominal surgery with low-flow oxygen, showed that the patients who received NIV delivered via a face mask had fewer reintubations (33 vs. 45%). NIV was also associated with more ventilator-free days (25 vs. 23 days), and fewer healthcare-associated infections (31 vs. 49%) but was not associated with a mortality benefit.[25] In certain high-risk patients like obesity, thoracic surgery, upper abdominal surgery, cardiovascular surgeries in whom incidence of postoperative atelectasis and subsequent respiratory failure is high, postextubation application of NIV/HFNO is reasonable though evidence is lacking.

Contraindications

Absolute contraindications for NIPPV include:
- Hypotension, postcardiac arrest, or unstable hemodynamic status.
- Inability to protect airway (impaired swallowing and cough)
- Trauma or burns involving the face

- Facial, esophageal, or gastric surgery
- Altered sensorium and decreasing level of consciousness (reduced ability to clear secretions, which may lead to aspiration).

Relative contraindications for NIPPV include uncooperative patients, copious secretions, and anxiety.[26]

Risks of NIPPV Failure

1. *PaO_2-FiO_2 Ratio (PFR):* The more severe (lower) a patient's PaO_2/FiO_2, the higher the risk he or she has of NIV failing. Most studies found through multivariate analyses that a PaO_2/FiO_2 less than 150 mm Hg at baseline and up to 1 hour after NIV initiation predicts NIV failure.[27]
2. *Tidal Volume:* A posthoc analysis of the FLORALI study found that a tidal volume of more than 9 mL/kg of predicted body weight at 1 hour was associated with the need for intubation. This may be due to the high underlying respiratory drive of patients in AHRF.[28]
3. *Severity Scores:* The most common scores used in studies of NIV include the Simplified Acute Physiology Score II, Sequential Organ Failure Assessment score, and Acute Physiology and Chronic Health Evaluation II score. The higher the severity score, the higher the risk of poor outcomes.[27]
4. *Etiology:* Patients with community acquired pneumonia, ARDS with PFR less than 150, and immunosuppression with de novo respiratory failure have a higher risk of failure of NIPPV therapy. Pneumonia as the etiology of respiratory failure is independently associated with the risk of NIV failing.[27] The LUNG-SAFE study found that patients with PaO_2 FiO_2 less than 150 mm Hg had higher ICU mortality when treated with NIV compared with subjects treated with invasive ventilation. Data have been published in subjects with immunosuppression and respiratory failure treated with high-flow nasal cannula (HFNC), which demonstrate that HFNC may be preferred instead of NIV for patients with immunosuppression.[1]
5. *Combined Factors:* The HACOR Score: Duan et al., have tested and validated this score that uses heart rate, acidosis, consciousness, oxygenation, and RR (HACOR). A HACOR score of greater than 5 after 1 hour of NIV treatment had a diagnostic accuracy to predict NIV failure of 81.8% in their testing cohort and 86% in their validation cohort. Subjects with a HACOR score greater than 5 at 1 hour also had higher hospital mortality than subjects with a HACOR score less than 5.[29]

ROLE OF HFNO IN ACUTE RESPIRATORY FAILURE

With the use of conventional devices oxygen flow is limited to no more than 15 L/min. However, the inspiratory flow of patients with respiratory failure varies widely in a range from 30 to more than 100 L/min. The difference between patient inspiratory flow and delivered flow is large, and as a result, the FiO_2 delivered is variable and often lower than expected. As an alternative to conventional oxygen delivery for hypoxemic patients HFNO oxygen therapy has been developed.

The components of the apparatus are listed here **(Fig. 2)**:
- An air/oxygen blender
- An active heated humidifier
- A single-heated circuit
- A nasal cannula.

Using the air/oxygen blender, FiO_2 is set from 0.21 to 1.0 in a flow of up to 60 L/min. Active humidifier heats and humidifies the gas, which is delivered through the heated circuit. The physiological effects of high flow, heated and humidified gas include reduction of anatomical dead space, PEEP effect, a constant FiO_2, and good humidification. Itagaki et al., found that thoracoabdominal synchrony is better with HFNC than with face mask delivery. The PEEP effect of HFNC at 35 L/min flow is approximately 2.7 ± 1.04 cmH_2O with the mouth closed and 1.2 ± 0.76 cmH_2O with the mouth open. Corley et al., evaluated end-expiratory lung volume using electrical lung impedance tomography and found that end-expiratory lung volume was greater with HFNC than with low-flow oxygen therapy.[30] Humidification of the gas improves mucociliary function, facilitates clearance of secretions, is associated with less atelectasis and reduces the work of breathing.

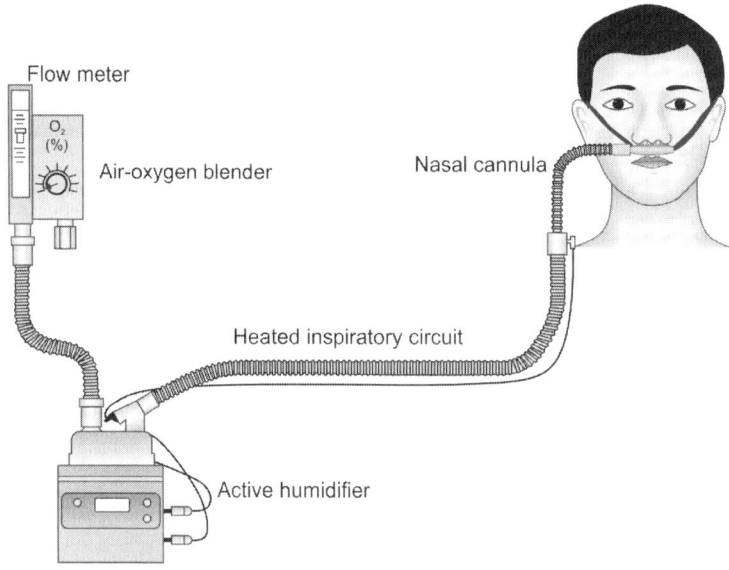

Fig. 2: Parts of HFNO equipment.

The flow rate should be initially set at 20–35 L/minute and then escalated as per patient tolerance. The flow rate can then be increased in 5 to 10 L/min increments, if on clinical examination there is no improvement of respiratory distress. The FiO_2 (range 21–100%) should then be set to target a desired oxygen saturation. Increasing the flow rate and FiO_2 will both result in improved peripheral oxygen saturation, but to reduce oxygen toxicity the flow can be increased first up to the maximum value and then the FiO_2 can be increased.

The major indications for the use of HFNO include:

Nonhypercapnic Hypoxemic Respiratory Failure

Randomized trials and observational studies in patients with hypoxemic respiratory failure consistently demonstrate improved oxygenation and decreased need for intubation when compared with low flow oxygen systems. But studies have failed to show consistent and convincing benefit on mortality, ICU, and hospital length of stay, dyspnea and comfort. A meta-analysis of 14 trials that compared HFNC with conventional oxygen therapy (i.e., low-flow systems) in patients with AHRF due to several etiologies showed little or no impact on intubation rates (26% each) but reported improved dyspnea and comfort.[31] A recent meta-analysis with 21 studies demonstrated fewer treatment failures when compared with standard oxygen therapy (RR 0.62, 95% CI 0.45–0.86; 15 studies, 3,044 participants; low certainty) with no significant effect on mortality, development of pneumonia, or ICU length of stay.[32]

Immunocompromised Patients

Patients who are immunosuppressed who have hypoxemic respiratory failure, administration of HFNO should not be routine and the threshold to intubate should be low. A multicenter randomized trial of 778 immunocompromised patients with hypoxemic respiratory failure reported that despite improved PaO_2:FiO_2 ratios and respiratory rates, HFNO did not alter mortality, intubation rates, length of stay, ICU-acquired infections, patient comfort, or dyspnea scores.[33] This is in contrast with the results of a prior prospective study of 1,611 immunocompromised patients with AHRF, which reported that HFNC reduced intubation rates.[34]

Patients with a Do Not Resuscitate or Intubate Order

Evidence of symptomatic relief of dyspnea using HFNC in this population is lacking. A systematic review, which included six studies and 293 patients, showed that use of HFNC was associated with improved oxygenation and reduced respiratory rate, but there was no difference in the reduction of dyspnea or the dose of morphine administered.[35]

Optimizing Oxygenation and Ventilation During Tracheal Intubation

The PEOXYFLOW trial failed to show improvement in oxygenation among hypoxemic patients undergoing endotracheal intubation. Guitton et al., conducted the PROTRACH study to evaluate the effect of HFNC in patients without pre-existing hypoxemia undergoing tracheal intubation in the ICU, but in this study also HFNC failed to increase the lowest oxygen saturation during intubation. The OPTINIV study showed that by adding HFNO for apneic oxygenation to NIV for preoxygenation was more effective in reducing the severity of desaturation compared to NIV alone. In a multicenter study of 124 patients undergoing intubation who had severe hypoxemia (PaO_2:FiO_2 ratio <300 mm Hg, respiratory rate >30 breaths/minute, and a FiO_2 >50% to achieve a saturation of >90%), HFNC did not reduce the lowest saturation during intubation when compared with preoxygenation using a conventional high-flow oxygen face mask. The results of the FLORALI 2 trial suggest that HFNC was inferior to NIV to improve oxygenation, and NIV may be the best method of preoxygenation to reduce oxygen desaturation during TI of critically ill patients.[22]

Postextubation Support

An individualized approach should be followed to administer the mode of postextubation support. Meta-analysis done recently comparing postextubation support with the use of NIPPV and HFNC has found no difference in outcomes between the two. Both HFNC and NIPPV reduced reintubation rates after extubation.[36]

Postoperative Respiratory Failure

High-flow nasal oxygen may be an alternative to NIV, particularly in those in whom NIV is not tolerated. HFNC has been shown to be superior to conventional oxygen therapy and may be an alternative to NIPPV in patients who are not able to tolerate NIPPV. The studies of HFNC in this population are very heterogeneous and imprecise.[37]

NIV IN COVID-19

The decision to initiate noninvasive modalities of ventilation in patients with COVID-19 should be made based on the clinical status and comorbidities (i.e., OSA, hypercapnia, and heart failure) of the patient, the risk of exposure to health care workers, best use of resources, and patient tolerance. Both HFNC and NIPPV have been used in critically ill patients with COVID-19. NIPPV should be used if the patient has a comorbidity for which there is proven efficacy of NIV [e.g., acute hypercapnic respiratory failure from an AECOPD, ACPE, underlying sleep-disordered breathing (e.g., obstructive sleep apnea or obesity hypoventilation), or respiratory muscle weakness].

In a randomized trial of 220 patients with COVID-19 and AHRF, intubation rates were lower with oxygen delivery through HFNC compared with standard low-flow delivery, with each adjusted to maintain peripheral oxygen saturation greater than 92% (43 vs. 51%; hazard ratio 0.62, 95% CI 0.39–0.96; number needed to treat 7). HFNC also reduced the time to clinical recovery (11 vs. 14 days), but the mortality difference was not statistically significant (8 vs. 16%).[38]

In the RECOVERY-RS trial involving 1,273 patients with AHRF due to COVID-19 who required oxygen at FiO_2 of at least 0.4, patients were randomly assigned to NIV (administered as CPAP), HFNC, or conventional oxygen therapy (via facemask or low-flow nasal cannula).[37] NIV reduced tracheal intubation compared with conventional oxygen (33 vs. 41%, 95% CI 0.53–0.96). By contrast, intubation rates were similar with HFNC and conventional oxygen (41% each). Mortality rates were similar in all three groups (17, 19, and 20%, respectively). In a posthoc analysis comparing NIV and HFNC, intubation rates were lower in the NIV group (32 vs. 41%; 95% CI 0.46–0.99). The limitations of this trial include lack of blinding, substantial crossover between groups (17%), low recruitment, and no standardized criteria for intubation.[39]

The HENIVOT trial enrolled a total of 110 patients with moderate or severe AHRF due to COVID-19 and reported that among patients receiving helmet NIV or HFNC, there was no difference in the number of days free of respiratory support at 28 days [20 days (helmet NIV) vs. 18 days (HFNC)]. However, patients receiving helmet NIV had lower rates of intubation (30 vs. 51%) and experienced more days free of IMV (28 vs. 25 days). Although encouraging, the trial was performed by experts in the delivery of helmet NIV and as such, may not be easily generalizable.[40]

The COVIDIVCUS trial which enrolled 546 patients reported no difference in the 28-days cumulative need for mechanical ventilation among patients who received HFNC, NIV, or low-flow oxygen.[41]

High-flow nasal cannula and NIV are considered aerosol-generating procedures. Thus, when HFNC or NIV are used standard precautions should be undertaken such as using full personal protective equipment, isolation rooms for patients, and use of helmet NIV. A surgical mask may be placed on the patient during HFNC when health care workers are in the room or when the patient is being transported. If NIPPV is being used, the mask should have a good seal and not have an antiasphyxiation valve or port. In NIPPV, use of a dual limb circuitry with a filter on the expiratory limb on a critical care ventilator may decrease dispersion compared with single limb circuitry on portable devices.[42]

CONCLUSION

Noninvasive ventilation offers a great advantage in avoiding complications related to IMV. Hence, this mode of ventilation should be offered in a controlled environment with intense monitoring to reduce the risk of NIV failure and in facilities where prompt tracheal intubation is possible. The mode of NIV (NIPPV or HFNC) should be individualized based on the clinical presentation of the patient and the current evidence supporting the use of the modality. Use of Helmet CPAP has shown promising results; however, more robust data and universal availability are required before it can be recommended for routine use.

REFERENCES

1. Bellani G, Laffey JG, Pham T, Fan E, Brochard L, Esteban A, et al. Epidemiology, patterns of care, and mortality for patients with acute respiratory distress syndrome in intensive care units in 50 countries. JAMA. 2016;315(8): 788-800.
2. Schettino G, Altobelli N, Kacmarek RM. Noninvasive positive-pressure ventilation in acute respiratory failure outside clinical trials: experience at the Massachusetts General Hospital. Critical Care Med. 2008;36(2):441-7.
3. Liang Y, Zhu C, Tian C, Research P, Lin Q, Li Z, et al. Early prediction of ventilator-associated pneumonia in critical care patients: a machine learning model. BMC Pulm Med. 2022;22(1):250.
4. Esteban A, Anzueto A, Frutos F, Alía I, Brochard L, Stewart TE, et al. Characteristics and outcomes in adult patients receiving mechanical ventilation: A 28-day International Study. JAMA. 2002;287(3):345-55.
5. Acute Respiratory Distress Syndrome Network; Brower RG, Matthay MA, Morris A, Schoenfeld D, Thompson BT, Wheeler A. Ventilation with lower tidal volumes as compared with traditional tidal volumes for acute lung injury and the acute respiratory distress syndrome. N Engl J Med. 2000;342(18): 1301-8.
6. Gupta S, Ramasubban S, Dixit S, Mishra R, Zirpe KG, Khilnani GC, et al. ISCCM guidelines for the use of non-invasive ventilation in acute respiratory failure in adult ICUs. Indian J Crit Care Med. 2020;24(S1):S61-81.
7. Rochwerg B, Brochard L, Elliott MW, Hess D, Hill NS, Nava S, et al. Official ERS/ATS clinical practice guidelines: noninvasive ventilation for acute respiratory failure. Eur Resp J. 2017;50(2):1602426.
8. Brochard L, Mancebo J, Wysocki M, Lofaso F, Conti G, Rauss A, et al. Noninvasive ventilation for acute exacerbations of chronic obstructive pulmonary disease. N Engl J Med. 1995;333(13):817-22.
9. Osadnik CR, Tee VS, Carson-Chahhoud KV, Picot J, Wedzicha JA, Smith BJ. Non-invasive ventilation for the management of acute hypercapnic respiratory failure due to exacerbation of chronic obstructive pulmonary disease. Cochrane Database Syst Rev. 2017;2017(7): CD004104.
10. Nava S, Hill N. Non-invasive ventilation in acute respiratory failure. Lancet. 2009;374(9685):250-9.

11. Weng CL. Meta-analysis: Noninvasive ventilation in acute cardiogenic pulmonary edema. Ann Intern Med. 2010;152(9):590.
12. Duan J, Chen L, Liang G, Shu W, Li L, Wang K, et al. Noninvasive ventilation failure in patients with hypoxemic respiratory failure: the role of sepsis and septic shock. Ther Adv Resp Dis. 2019;13:1753466619888812.
13. Ferrer M, Esquinas A, Leon M, Gonzalez G, Alarcon A, Torres A. Noninvasive ventilation in severe hypoxemic respiratory failure. Am J Resp Crit Care Med. 2003;168(12):1438-44.
14. Stefan MS, Priya A, Pekow PS, Lagu T, Steingrub JS, Hill NS, et al. The comparative effectiveness of noninvasive and invasive ventilation in patients with pneumonia. J Crit Care. 2018;43:190-6.
15. Lansbury L, Rodrigo C, Leonardi-Bee J, Nguyen-Van-Tam J, Lim WS. Corticosteroids as adjunctive therapy in the treatment of influenza. Cochrane Database Syst Rev. 2019;2(2):CD010406
16. Lemiale V, Mokart D, Resche-Rigon M, Pène F, Mayaux J, Faucher E, et al. Effect of noninvasive ventilation vs oxygen therapy on mortality among immunocompromised patients with acute respiratory failure: a randomized clinical trial. JAMA. 2015;314(16):1711-19.
17. Soroksky A, Stav D, Shpirer I. A pilot prospective, randomized, placebo-controlled trial of bilevel positive airway pressure in acute asthmatic attack. Chest. 2003;123(4):1018-25.
18. Lim WJ, Mohammed Akram R, Carson KV, Mysore S, Labiszewski NA, Wedzicha JA, et al. Non-invasive positive pressure ventilation for treatment of respiratory failure due to severe acute exacerbations of asthma. Cochrane Database Syst Rev. 2012;12:CD004360.
19. Vaschetto R, Longhini F, Persona P, Ori C, Stefani G, Liu S, et al. Early extubation followed by immediate noninvasive ventilation vs. standard extubation in hypoxemic patients: a randomized clinical trial. Intensive Care Med. 2019;45(1):62-71.
20. Bauchmuller KB, Glossop AJ, de Jong A, Jaber S. Combining high-flow nasal cannula oxygen and non-invasive ventilation for pre-oxygenation in the critically ill: Is a double-pronged approach warranted? Intensive Care Med. 2017;43(2):288-90.
21. Frat JP, Ricard JD, Quenot JP, Pichon N, Demoule A, Forel JM, et al. Non-invasive ventilation versus high-flow nasal cannula oxygen therapy with apneic oxygenation for preoxygenation before intubation of patients with acute hypoxemic respiratory failure: a randomized, multicenter, open-label trial. Lancet Resp Med. 2019;7(4):303-12.
22. de Jong A, Casey JD, Myatra SN. Focus on noninvasive respiratory support before and after mechanical ventilation in patients with acute respiratory failure. Intensive Care Med. 2020;46(7):1460-63.
23. Schortgen F, Follin A, Piccari L, Roche-Campo F, Carteaux G, Taillandier-Heriche E, et al. Results of noninvasive ventilation in very old patients. Ann Intensive Care. 2012;2(1):5.
24. Lemyze M, Mallat J, Nigeon O, Barrailler S, Pepy F, Gasan G, et al. Rescue therapy by switching to total face mask after failure of face mask-delivered noninvasive

ventilation in do-not-intubate patients in acute respiratory failure. Crit Care Med. 2013;41(2):481-8.
25. Jaber S, Lescot T, Futier E, Paugam-Burtz C, Seguin P, Ferrandiere M, et al. Effect of noninvasive ventilation on tracheal reintubation among patients with hypoxemic respiratory failure following abdominal surgery. JAMA. 2016;315(13):1345.
26. Schönhofer B, Kuhlen R, Neumann P, Westhoff M, Berndt C, Sitter H. Non-Invasive Mechanical Ventilation as Treatment of Acute Respiratory Failure. Dtsch Ärztebl Int. 2008;105(24):424-10000.
27. Carrillo A, Gonzalez-Diaz G, Ferrer M, Martinez-Quintana ME, Lopez-Martinez A, Llamas N, et al. Non-invasive ventilation in community-acquired pneumonia and severe acute respiratory failure. Intensive Care Med. 2012;38(3):458-66.
28. Frat JP, Thille AW, Mercat A, Girault C, Ragot S, Perbet S, et al. High-flow oxygen through nasal cannula in acute hypoxemic respiratory failure. N Engl J Med. 2015;372(23):2185-96.
29. Duan J, Han X, Bai L, Zhou L, Huang S. Assessment of heart rate, acidosis, consciousness, oxygenation, and respiratory rate to predict noninvasive ventilation failure in hypoxemic patients. Intensive Care Med. 2017;43(2): 192-9.
30. Corley A, Caruana LR, Barnett AG, Tronstad O, Fraser JF. Oxygen delivery through high-flow nasal cannulae increase end-expiratory lung volume and reduce respiratory rate in post-cardiac surgical patients. Br J Anaesth. 2011;107(6):998-1004.
31. Baldomero AK, Melzer AC, Greer N, Majeski BN, MacDonald R, Linskens EJ, et al. Effectiveness and harms of high-flow nasal oxygen for acute respiratory failure: an evidence report for a clinical guideline from the American College of Physicians. Ann Intern Med. 2021;174(7):952-66.
32. Lewis SR, Baker PE, Parker R, Smith AF. High-flow nasal cannulae for respiratory support in adult intensive care patients. Cochrane Database Syst Rev. 2021;2021(3): CD010172.
33. Azoulay E, Lemiale V, Mokart D, Nseir S, Argaud L, Pène F, et al. Effect of high-flow nasal oxygen vs standard oxygen on 28-day mortality in immunocompromised patients with acute respiratory failure. JAMA. 2018;320(20):2099.
34. Azoulay E, Pickkers P, Soares M, Perner A, Rello J, Bauer PR, et al. Acute hypoxemic respiratory failure in immunocompromised patients: the Efraim multinational prospective cohort study. Intensive Care Med. 2017;43(12):1808-19.
35. Wilson ME, Mittal A, Dobler CC, Curtis JR, Majzoub AM, Soleimani J, et al. High-flow nasal cannula oxygen in patients with acute respiratory failure and do-not-intubate or do-not-resuscitate orders: a systematic review. J Hospital Med. 2020;15(2):101-6.
36. Fernando SM, Tran A, Sadeghirad B, Burns KEA, Fan E, Brodie D, et al. Noninvasive respiratory support following extubation in critically ill adults: a systematic review and network meta-analysis. Intensive Care Med. 2022;48(2):137-47.
37. Lu Z, Chang W, Meng S, Xue M, Xie J, Xu J, et al. The effect of high-flow nasal oxygen therapy on postoperative pulmonary complications and hospital length of stay in postoperative patients: a systematic review and meta-analysis. J Intensive Care Med. 2020;35(10):1129-40.

38. Ospina-Tascón GA, Calderón-Tapia LE, García AF, Zarama V, Gómez-Álvarez F, Álvarez-Saa T, et al. Effect of high-flow oxygen therapy vs conventional oxygen therapy on invasive mechanical ventilation and clinical recovery in patients with severe COVID-19. JAMA. 2021;326(21):2161.
39. Perkins GD, Ji C, Connolly BA, Couper K, Lall R, Baillie JK, et al. Effect of noninvasive respiratory strategies on intubation or mortality among patients with acute hypoxemic respiratory failure and COVID-19. JAMA. 2022;327(6):546.
40. Grieco DL, Menga LS, Cesarano M, Rosà T, Spadaro S, Bitondo MM, et al. Effect of helmet noninvasive ventilation vs high-flow nasal oxygen on days free of respiratory support in patients with COVID-19 and moderate to severe hypoxemic respiratory failure. JAMA. 2021;325(17):1731.
41. Bouadma L, Mekontso-Dessap A, Burdet C, Merdji H, Poissy J, Dupuis C, et al. High-dose dexamethasone and oxygen support strategies in intensive care unit patients with severe COVID-19 acute hypoxemic respiratory failure. JAMA Intern Med. 2022;182(9):906-16.
42. Cabrini L, Landoni G, Zangrillo A. Minimize nosocomial spread of 2019-nCoV when treating acute respiratory failure. Lancet. 2020;395(10225):685.

CHAPTER 3

Ventilation Strategies to Prevent Postoperative Pulmonary Infection

Mukul Chandra Kapoor

ABSTRACT

Mechanical ventilation is essential to maintain oxygenation and expel carbon dioxide in patients under general anesthesia. Induction of general anesthesia alters pulmonary physiology and causes a reduction in the functional residual capacity. The reduction in the functional capacity promotes atelectasis. Inappropriate mechanical ventilation may cause lung injury. These factors make the patient prone to postoperative pulmonary infections. Conventional mechanical ventilation carries the risk of barotrauma, volutrauma, and biotrauma. To attenuate the risk associated with mechanical ventilation, lung protective ventilation strategies are adopted. Lung protective ventilation involves the use of low tidal volumes along with individualized positive end-expiratory pressure to ensure an open lung at the end of expiration. Lung protective strategies also recommend the use of periodic alveolar recruitment maneuvers to open atelectatic areas of the peripheral and dependent lung units. There is evidence that these strategies in patients with normal lungs during surgery are associated with a significantly lower incidence of postoperative pulmonary infections, improved lung function, and reduced incidence of the need for postoperative mechanical ventilation.

Keywords: Intraoperative mechanical ventilation; Conventional mechanical ventilation; Lung protective ventilation; Alveolar recruitment maneuver; Individualized positive end-expiratory pressure (PEEP); Postoperative pulmonary infections.

KEY POINTS

- Induction of general anesthesia alters pulmonary physiology and causes a reduction in the functional residual capacity.
- Inappropriate mechanical ventilation may cause atelectasis and lung injury making patients prone to postoperative pulmonary infections.
- To attenuate the risk associated with mechanical ventilation, lung protective ventilation strategies are adopted.
- Lung protective ventilation involves the use of low tidal volumes along with individualized positive end-expiratory pressure to ensure an open lung at the end of expiration.

- Lung protective strategies also recommend periodic alveolar recruitment maneuvers to recruit peripheral and dependent lung units.
- There is evidence that these strategies in patients with normal lungs during surgery are associated with a significantly lower incidence of postoperative pulmonary infections, improved lung function, and reduced incidence of the need for postoperative mechanical ventilation.

INTRODUCTION

More than 310 million people globally undergo major surgery yearly. Most major surgeries are performed under general anesthesia (GA).[1] Mechanical ventilation during GA is essential to ventilate the lungs whenever neuromuscular blockade is administered. It is also needed to support the ventilation under GA without muscle relaxants to prevent hypoventilation. Mechanical ventilation; however, can impair lung function, even in healthy individuals.[2] The respiratory drive and muscle function are altered, and lung volumes are reduced with the induction of GA. The ventilatory responses are impaired even at low concentrations of anesthetic agents. The respiratory changes after GA may take up to 6 weeks to normalize.[3]

POSTOPERATIVE PULMONARY INFECTIONS

Postoperative pulmonary complications (PPCs) are the second most common perioperative complication. GA is a significant risk factor for PPC.[4] Postoperative pulmonary complications are associated with higher morbidity, morbidity, length of hospital stay, and increased costs. The incidence of PPCs ranges from 5 to 33%, and it is associated 30-day mortality rate of 20% as compared with 0.2–3% without a PPC.[3-5] Clinicians must identify the risk factors and adopt preventative measures to reduce morbidity and mortality associated with PPCs.

Traditionally, a 10 mL/kg tidal volume (V_T) is set for mechanical ventilation delivery to prevent hypoxemia and atelectasis.[6] Clinical studies have implicated this high V_T for ventilator-induced lung injury due to overinflation of the smaller airways.[7] It is essential to understand the pathophysiology of PPCs to realize the need for intraoperative ventilation strategies.

Pathophysiology of Postoperative Pulmonary Complications

The functional residual capacity (FRC) reduces on induction of anesthesia. This reduction in FRC is accompanied by an altered ventilation distribution during mechanical ventilation and a reduction in cardiac output. This leads to a ventilation-perfusion mismatch causing impaired gas exchange. The factors contributing to the pathophysiology of PPCs is shown in **Flowchart 1**.

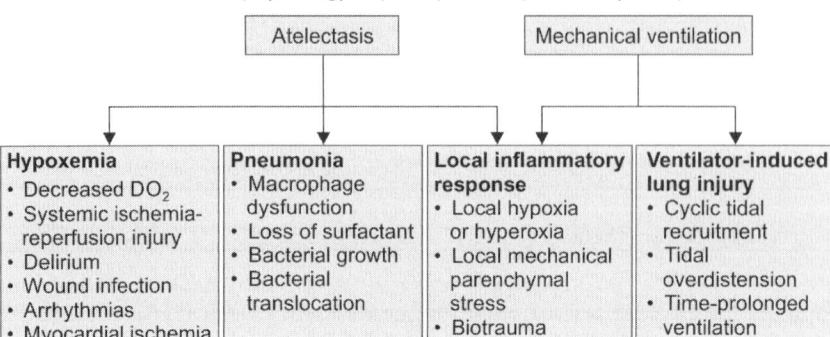

Flowchart 1: Pathophysiology of postoperative pulmonary complications.

Role of Atelectasis in Postoperative Pulmonary Complications

A significant effect of a reduced FRC is the promotion of atelectasis. More than 75% of patients administered a neuromuscular blocker develop atelectasis. Atelectasis occurs in the dependent areas of the lung, independent of the patient's position. Factors contributing to the development of atelectasis include lung tissue compression by the upwardly displaced diaphragm, closure of small airways as FRC becomes lesser than closing volume, and gas absorption from alveoli where the smaller airways that have closed down (absorption atelectasis). GA can cause surfactant alterations and lead to "loss of surfactant atelectasis" in healthy lungs.[8]

Absorption atelectasis is exacerbated by high fractional inspired oxygen (FiO_2) use, particularly at preoxygenation. Atelectasis occurs within a few minutes after induction of GA.[9,10] However, there is no evidence that the use of FiO_2 of 0.8 throughout GA results in more atelectasis after surgery, suggesting that even 20% nitrogen in inspired gas helps prevent absorption atelectasis.[11]

Intraoperative atelectasis contributes to a further decrease in FRC. This alveolar derecruitment makes lung expansion heterogenous, causes cyclic lung over-stress, and increases airway plateau pressures. Atelectasis increases the risk for PPCs.

Moderate positive airway pressure during expiration is adequate to maintain airway patency. If atelectasis occurs, alveolar recruitment maneuvers (ARMs) are required to re-expand the collapsed airways. Ventilation strategies should thus aim to avoid derecruitment and thereby decrease PPCs. They improve oxygenation and respiratory mechanics and reduce oxidative stress, inflammatory response, and lung injury without causing alveolar distension.

A controversial concept of "intraoperative permissive atelectasis" has been proposed for lung protection. This concept recommends low PEEP without using ARMs to reduce static stress in the lungs. This protocol will, however, increase atelectasis in the postoperative period and promote PPCs.[12,13]

Residual Effects of Drugs

Residual effects of neuromuscular blockers may impair respiratory function. Residual effects of neuromuscular blockers cause airway obstruction and increase airway resistance.[14] They also increase the risk of aspiration. Residual NM blockade (TOF ratio <0.9) is associated with significantly low forced vital capacity and peak expiratory flow rate leading to the development of hypoxia and hypercapnia.[15]

Continued sedation from the residual anesthetic and opioid drugs may also cause airway obstruction and central respiratory depression. Low residual anesthetic levels may impair hypoxic response even under normocapnic conditions.[16]

RISK FACTORS FOR POSTOPERATIVE PULMONARY COMPLICATIONS

Studies have reported an association of PPCs with many risk factors. The patient and procedure-related risk factors for developing PPCs can be classified as modifiable and nonmodifiable. The factors are listed in **Table 1**.[3] The details of the role of each of these risk factors and their mitigation are beyond the scope of this chapter.

ROLE OF MECHANICAL VENTILATION IN LUNG INJURY

During mechanical ventilation, there is cyclic overstretching of aerated alveolar areas with high ventilation, from repeated closing at end-expiration and re-opening at the next inspiration with zero end-expiratory pressure (ZEEP). This results in microscopic damage or atelectrauma.[17] Fracture of the alveolar-capillary interface may lead to translocation of protein and edema into the airspace.[18] It may also trigger an inflammatory response in the lungs and initiate the systemic release of inflammatory mediators and thus contributing to systemic organ dysfunction.[17] Other mechanisms described as causing biotrauma are mechanical ventilation-induced cell necrosis, decompartmentalization, mechano-transduction, and direct effects on the vasculature. Biotrauma culminates in decreased pulmonary compliance, increased dead space, hypoxia, and hypercarbia.[17,19]

Conventional Lung Ventilation

Conventional lung ventilation (CLV) is defined as V_T greater than 8 mL/kg of patient body weight with less than 5 cmH_2O positive end-expiratory pressure and without a recruitment maneuver. Traditionally, intraoperative mechanical ventilation is performed with a large V_T (10-15 mL/kg IBW) with no to low levels of PEEP. The lung was exposed to shear stress from recruitment and de-recruitment of small airways (atelectrauma) and

TABLE 1: Patient and procedure-related risk factors for developing postoperative pulmonary complications.[9]

Patient factors		Procedure factors	
Nonmodifiable	**Modifiable**	**Nonmodifiable**	**Modifiable**

• Age
• Male sex
• ASA >2
• Frailty
• Acute respiratory infection (within 1 month)
• Impaired cognition
• Impaired sensorium
• Cerebrovascular accident
• Malignancy
• Weight loss >10% (within 6 months)
• Long-term steroid use
• Prolonged hospitalization
	• Smoking
	• COPD
	• Asthma
	• CHF
	• OSA
	• BMI<18.5 or >40kg
	• BMI >27kg/m^2
	• Hypertension
	• Chronic liver disease
	• Renal failure
	• Ascites
	• Diabetes mellitus
	• Alcohol
	• GERD
	• Preoperative sepsis
	• Preoperative shock
		• *Type of surgery:*
		  – upper abdominal
		  – AAA
		  – Thoracic
		  – Neurosurgery
		  – head and neck
		  – vascular
		• Emergency (vs elective)
		• Duration of procedure
		• Reoperation
		• Multiple GA during admission
			• Mechanical ventilation
			• GA
			• Long-acting NMBDs and TOF ratio <0.7 in PACU
			• Residual neuromuscular block
			• Intermediate-acting NMBDs with surgical time <2 hours (not reversed)
			• Neostigmine
			• Sugammadex with supraglottic airway
			• Failure to use peripheral nerve stimulator
			• Open abdominal surgery (vs laparoscopic)
			• Perioperative nasogastric tube
			• Intraoperative blood transfusion

(AAA: abdominal aortic aneurysm; BMI: Body mass index; CHF: congestive heart failure; COPD: chronic obstructive pulmonary disease; GA: general anaesthesia; GERD: gastroesophageal reflux disease; NMBDs: neuromuscular blocking drugs; PACU: postanesthesia care unit; OSA: obstructive sleep apnea; TOF: train of four)

activation of inflammatory mediators. Excessive inflation pressures cause barotrauma, while excessive lung inflation causes volutrauma. This biotrauma contributes to ventilation-associated lung injury. CLV is associated with a higher incidence of PPCs, hospital length of stay, morbidity, mortality, and high healthcare costs. The effects of inappropriate ventilation settings are shown in **Figure 1**.

Intraoperative Lung Protective Ventilation

Lung protective ventilation (LPV) was initially proposed as the ventilation mode in patients with acute respiratory distress syndrome. The benefit of lung-protective artificial ventilation in acute lung injury is well established.[20]

Ventilation Strategies to Prevent Postoperative Pulmonary Infection

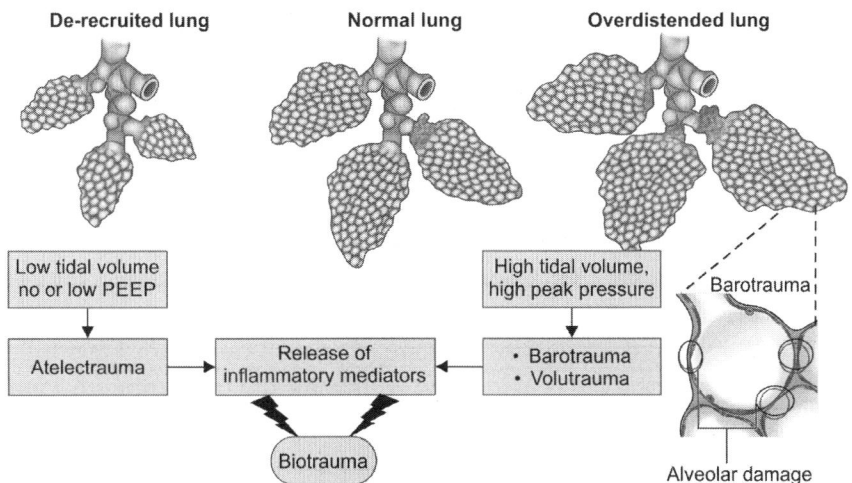

Fig. 1: Effects of inappropriate intraoperative mechanical ventilation.
(PEEP: positive end-expiratory pressure)

Its application to protect healthy lungs during intraoperative mechanical ventilation was described relatively recently. Intraoperative LPV can be defined as the combination of V_T 8 mL/kg or lower and PEEP 5 cmH$_2$O or higher, with or without a recruitment maneuver. LPV is a goal-directed ventilation strategy that is individualized and oriented physiologically.

Increasing evidence suggests that LPV strategies in the operating room offer substantial benefits. High-ventilator driving pressure (DP) is thought to cause lung injury and promote PPCs.[21,22] There is evidence that using protective ventilation strategies in patients with normal lungs during surgery is associated with a significantly lower incidence of PPCs.

Despite the evidence of benefits with LPV, many clinicians continue to use high V_T mechanical ventilation with elevated drive pressures. A study performed on 2,000 patients in France demonstrated that about 20% of patients receive a V_T greater than 10 mL/kg of ideal body weight during GA, and the same percentage underutilized application of PEEP.[23]

Positive end-expiratory pressure is an intensive property of the lung and relates to the expiratory phase. At the same time, ARMs reflect the capacitive property of the lung and are inspiratory phenomena.[24] By maintaining a positive transpulmonary pressure, PEEP opens all pulmonary units to ventilation. Protective ventilation involves using a protocol based on V_T, level of PEEP, and use of ARMs.

Salient Features of the Lung Protective Ventilation Physiology

- *Maintains FRC:* Induction of anesthesia reduces FRC by 1.2–1.5 L, and FRC approaches residual volume. Use of ARM and PEEP restores FRC and combats atelectasis.

- *Combats increased closing pressure:* Alveoli begin to close at about 6–7 cmH_2O in normal-weight healthy patients and about 10–15 cmH_2O in obese patients. This closing pressure increases further with pneumoperitoneum and extreme positions. Individualized PEEP prevents airway closure associated with the increase in the closing pressure.
- *Decreases DP:* During intraoperative mechanical ventilation, a positive pressure is generated by the ventilator to achieve the desired set V_T. The pressure gradient needed to achieve a V_T is defined as the DP. An increasing DP indicates inadequate PEEP, alveolar collapse, and low lung compliance. An increasing DP is also a risk factor for PPCs. Increased DP is associated with volutrauma, barotrauma, and atelectrauma. A lower DP is needed to achieve the set V_T if the smaller airways remain open.

DP is calculated by the formula:
$DP = P_{plat} - PEEP$ (in the volume control mode)
or
$DP = P_{ip} - PEEP$ (in the pressure control mode),
where P_{plat} is the plateau airway pressure and P_{ip} is the peak inspiratory pressure.

Benefits of Intraoperative Lung Protective Ventilation

The benefits of LPV have been very clearly elicited by many studies. They are:
- *Decreased incidence of PPCs:* A randomized multicenter IMPROVE trial found a significantly lower incidence of 10.5% PPCs in the LPV group compared to 27.5% in the CLV group.[25] A meta-analysis of 15 randomized controlled trials (RCT) that included 2,127 patients reported the incidence of PPCs as 8.7% in patients receiving LPV compared to 14.7% in patients receiving CLV.[26]
- *Improved lung function:* Improved intra- and post-operative lung mechanics with improved pulmonary function tests, chest X-ray, arterial oxygenation, and better PaO_2/FiO_2 ratios with a lower modified Clinical Pulmonary Infection Score.[27,28]
- *Decreased need for postoperative ventilation:* A Cochrane analysis of 7 RCTs found a reduced need for invasive/noninvasive postoperative ventilatory support in patients receiving LPV in all the studies considered.[29]
- *Decreased hospital length of stay and mortality:* PPCs are associated with substantial morbidity and mortality, and evidence suggests a reduction of PPCs with intraoperative LPV.[29,30]

EVIDENCE-BASED STRATEGIES FOR INTRAOPERATIVE LUNG PROTECTIVE VENTILATION

Low Tidal Volume

Although conventionally, a V_T of 10 mL/kg of ideal body weight has been used, clinical studies suggest that V_T of 4–5 mL/kg may be more appropriate for lung protection while allowing adequate gas exchange.[31,32] The protective effects against PPCs of low V_T are well established. The use of low V_T ventilation (6–8 mL/kg of ideal body weight) is physiologic as it mimics normal tidal ventilation and prevents barotrauma and volutrauma. Lower V_T decreases intrapulmonary pressure and reduces the risk of ventilation-associated lung injury. However, the possibility of an alveolar collapse of the dependent lung raises the risk of atelectasis and hypercapnia.[33]

A significant reduction in PPCs has been shown in patients ventilated with low (<8 mL/kg) versus conventional (>8 mL/kg) V_T, regardless of the PEEP level used.[26] Reduction of V_T decreases DP until the point alveolar collapse starts, so V_T should not be reduced without prior addition of PEEP. When the level of PEEP is inappropriate, an increase in V_T may reduce the DP by reduction of atelectasis.[21]

Individualized Positive End-expiratory Pressure

A PEEP of 10 cmH_2O is required to prevent atelectasis, improves compliance, promotes more homogenous ventilation, and maintains end-expiratory lung volume (EELV) during mechanical ventilation. It may not, however, improve respiratory function.[13] High PEEP also frequently results in hemodynamic compromise. The ideal level of PEEP to be used along with low V_T is not adequately defined.[13,34] The level of PEEP should be chosen according to the surgical approach and patient positioning.

Individualized PEEP is associated with better respiratory mechanics than fixed PEEP, better respiratory gas distribution to dependent areas, higher oxygenation, and lower DPs. However, hemodynamic depression may be associated with individualized PEEP.[35]

Electrical impedance studies indicate that each patient and each lung region have different lung compliance.[36] Most patients with asthma and chronic obstructive pulmonary disease tend to develop variable auto-PEEPs during mechanical ventilation.[37] Fixed PEEP, whether high or low, is inappropriate, so individualized PEEP based on DP is recommended to protect the lung.[38] Individualized dynamic PEEP, instead of a fixed PEEP, may optimize respiratory mechanics. The aim of individualized PEEP is the maximization of static compliance.

Static compliance is calculated using the equation $V_T/(P_{plat} - PEEP)$, while dynamic compliance is calculated using the equation $VT/(P_{ip} - PEEP)$.

Most modern anesthesia workstations display static compliance.[39] PEEP is most effective when an ARM is performed before the application of PEEP. PEEP is adjusted after an ARM, and PEEP is set at the level where maximal static compliance is achieved.

To set individualized PEEP, Fernandez-Bustamante et al., performed an ARM with an incremental increase of PEEP by 5 cmH_2O stepwise up to 20 cmH_2O. This was followed by a stepwise decrement of 3 cmH_2O. Static compliance was assessed at each step, and PEEP was set at the level corresponding to the maximum static compliance.[39]

A secondary analysis of the PROBESE trial data found that individualized PEEP was associated with improved oxygenation, lower DPs, and homogenous ventilation of dependent lung areas as measured by electrical impedance tomography.[35] To determine individualized PEEP by electric impedance tomography, delay for each pixel is determined after an ARM, and the regional ventilatory delay index is defined. The lower the delay index, the more homogeneous the regional lung ventilation of the lung. The PEEP corresponding to the lowest delay index is set as individualized PEEP.[40]

Individualized PEEP can also be set using esophageal pressure monitoring. A positive end-expiratory transpulmonary pressure ($PEEP_{tp}$) is maintained where $PEEP_{tp}$ is the difference between PEEP and end-expiratory esophageal pressure (EEEP) (a surrogate for pleural pressure).[30]

Another method to titrate an individualized PEEP during GA is based on oxygenation combined with EELV.[41] Individualized PEEP can be clinically set by an easy method based on oxygenation. Following recruitment and initial high PEEP (20 cmH_2O), PEEP is reduced every 2–3 minutes until oxygenation saturation starts to decrease. This PEEP point is called "collapse pressure". Recruitment is repeated, and individualized PEEP is set 1–2 cmH_2O above this "collapse pressure". The oxygen saturation is estimated at a <30% FiO_2.[42]

Alveolar Recruitment Maneuvers

Application of ARMs reopens atelectatic regions and restores EELV. ARMs must be followed by individualized PEEP; otherwise, the benefits are short-lived as atelectasis again sets in within 40 minutes.[43] ARMs have been shown to increase EELV, improve lung compliance, and reduce chest wall elastance.[44,45] ARMs have been shown to improve intraoperative oxygenation in laparoscopic surgery, bariatric surgery, and surgery with Trendelenburg positioning.[46-48]

Classically, for ARMs, hyperinflation of the lung is performed by a one-step method of sustained inspiration with 40 cmH_2O of inspiratory pressure [by setting the adjustable pressure (APL) valve at 40 cmH_2O] for 8–10 seconds **(Fig. 2)**. ARMs are more physiological when performed by the multistep method by gradually increasing the inspiratory pressure by incrementally increasing the APL valve occlusion to 40 cmH_2O and then reducing the occlusion gradually till the desired PEEP **(Fig. 3)**. Periodic "sighs" have also been used for ARM.

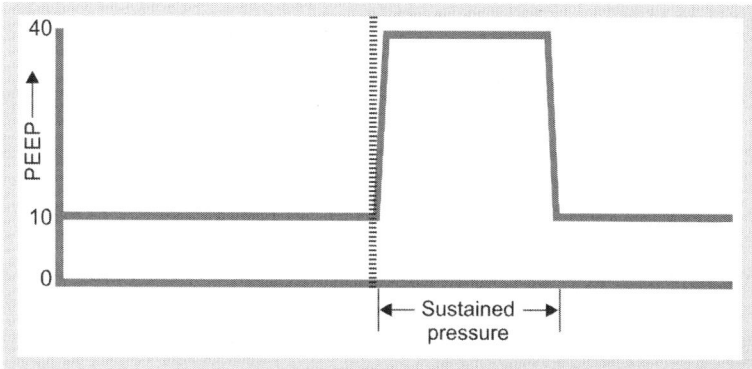

Fig. 2: Single step method for alveolar recruitment with a sustained inspiratory pressure of 40 cmH$_2$O over 8–10 sec. (PEEP: positive end-expiratory pressure)

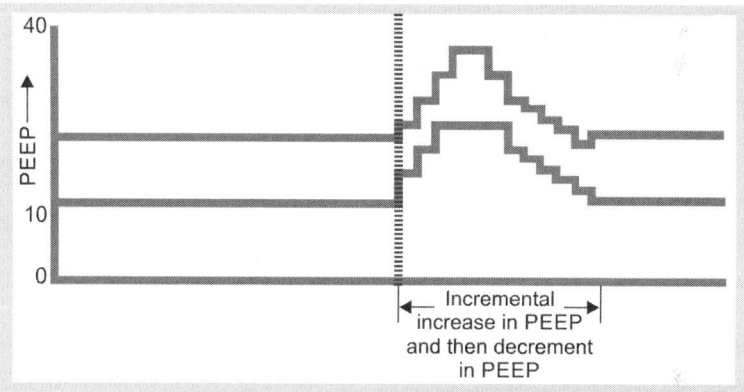

Fig. 3: Multistep method for alveolar recruitment with an incremental increase in PEEP to 40 cmH$_2$O pressure followed by a decrement in PEEP till the desired PEEP level. (PEEP: positive end-expiratory pressure)

Additional Considerations for Lung Protective Ventilation

Inspired Oxygen Concentration

Administration of a high FiO$_2$ before laryngoscopy/tracheal intubation and extubation is commonly practiced. Using FiO$_2$ >80% can cause resorption atelectasis and worsen inflammatory lung injury.[49] Many RCTs have shown that preoxygenation, at induction of anesthesia, performed with 30% oxygen, as opposed to 100% oxygen, is associated with reduced atelectasis.[50] Considering this, the use of a high FiO$_2$ should be restricted to correcting hypoxia and must not be protocoled.

Pressure-Controlled vs. Volume-Controlled Ventilation

Use of pressure-controlled ventilation was proposed for lung protection. Rapid delivery of V$_T$ with a preset maximum inflation pressure was thought to prevent barotrauma. However, investigations have not proved its superiority over volume-controlled ventilation in the intraoperative setting.[51]

LUNG PROTECTIVE VENTILATION DURING DIFFERENT STAGES OF GENERAL ANESTHESIA

Induction of Anesthesia

High FiO_2 or even a FiO_2 of 1.0 is used during preoxygenation and mask ventilation before tracheal intubation to cater for a possible delay in securing the airway in difficult tracheal intubation. Preoxygenation with a FiO_2 of 1.0 is commonly used by most physicians before induction of anesthesia. However, a high FiO_2 before and during anesthesia induction promotes resorption atelectasis. A FiO_2 of 0.8 is safe as it reduces resorption atelectasis and has minimal effects on oxygenation.[52] PEEP should be administered during induction of anesthesia to reduce atelectasis.[53] If PEEP is not applied during the induction, a postintubation ARM must be resorted to. Controlled positive-pressure ventilation or continuous positive airway pressure (CPAP) should be considered during anesthesia induction. Head-up positioning prevents an FRC decrease associated with anesthesia induction.[30]

Maintenance of Anesthesia

Setting the right PEEP level during controlled ventilation is essential as an inappropriate PEEP level may lead to anesthesia-induced atelectasis. This is particularly challenging in obese as they have reduced lung volumes, intrinsic PEEP, low chest wall compliance and are prone to anesthesia-induced atelectasis and ventilation/perfusion mismatch. Alveolar recruitment is recommended before the initiation of intraoperative ventilation. The VT can be maintained using a PEEP that maintains transpulmonary pressure above the "collapse pressure" value.[54] Derecruitment can occur during expiration. PEEP needed to prevent this derecruitment can be estimated from the expiratory limb of the static pressure-volume loop.[55]

Inspiratory/Expiratory Ratio

An inspiratory-expiratory (I:E) ratio of 1:2 ratio is commonly used during mechanical ventilation. Increased lung compliance, better oxygenation, lower alveolar-arterial gradient, and reduced inflammatory markers have been demonstrated by studies using longer inspiratory times.[56] However, a clear benefit of a specific I:E ratio is yet to be established.[30]

Monitoring Ventilation During Anesthesia

The various components of the mechanical breath should be continuously monitored as the lung physiology is dynamic and varies with stages of anesthesia and surgery.[57] Conventionally, monitoring is focused on maintaining oxygenation, and low oxygen saturation is corrected by increasing FiO_2. Increasing the FiO_2 improves oxygenation but fails to correct the ventilation-perfusion mismatch. The lung compliance, DP, and P_{plat} should be monitored on all mechanically ventilated patients, and ventilator settings should be appropriately modified to optimize respiratory mechanics to maintain the V_T.[30]

Emergence from Anesthesia

A high FiO_2 >0.8 during emergence contributes to atelectasis formation. A combination of ARM and low FiO_2 before tracheal extubation decreases atelectasis in the postoperative period. If clinically appropriate, a FiO_2 <0.4 must be used during emergence to reduce atelectasis, but more evidence is needed to recommend this. CPAP maintained while holding a face mask at emergence benefits by reducing the occurrence of postoperative atelectasis and PPC.[58] After extubation, supplemental oxygen should not be administered as a routine but only if the oxygen saturation is <94%.[59]

■ CONCLUSION

General anesthesia is a risk factor for postoperative pulmonary infection. Administration of muscle relaxants makes mechanical ventilation as inescapable requirement to maintain gas exchange. Mechanical ventilation is associated with risks of atelectasis, barotrauma, volutrauma, and biotrauma, which promote postoperative pulmonary infections. Lung protective ventilation helps reduce pulmonary morbidity associated with mechanical ventilation.

■ REFERENCES

1. Weiser TG, Haynes AB, Molina G, Lipsitz SR, Esquivel MM, Uribe-Leitz T, et al. Size and distribution of the global volume of surgery in 2012. Bull World Health Organ. 2016;94(3):201-9F
2. Petrucci N, De Feo C. Lung protective ventilation strategy for the acute respiratory distress syndrome. Cochrane Database Syst Rev. 2013;2:CD003844.
3. Miskovic A, Lumb AB. Postoperative pulmonary complications. Br J Anaesth. 2017;118:317-34.
4. Fernandez-Bustamante A, Frendl G, Sprung J, Kor DJ, Subramaniam B, Ruiz RM, et al. Postoperative pulmonary complications, early mortality, and hospital stay following noncardiothoracic surgery: a multicenter study by the perioperative research network investigators. JAMA Surg. 2017;152:157-66.
5. Canet J, Gallart L, Gomar C, Paluzie G, Vallès J, Castillo J, et al. Prediction of postoperative pulmonary complications in a population based surgical cohort. Anesthesiology. 2010;113:1338-50.

6. Wrigge H, Pelosi P. Tidal volume in patients with normal lungs during general anesthesia: lower the better? Anesthesiology. 2011;114:1011-3.
7. Lellouche F, Dionne S, Simard S, Bussières J, Dagenais F. High tidal volumes in mechanically ventilated patients increase organ dysfunction after cardiac surgery. Anesthesiology. 2012;116:1072-82.
8. Otis DR Jr., Johnson M, Pedley TJ, Kamm RD. Role of pulmonary surfactant in airway closure: a computational study. J Appl Physiol. 1993;75:1323-33.
9. Lundquist H, Hedenstierna G, Strandberg A, Tokics L, Brismar B. CT-assessment of dependent lung densities in man during general anaesthesia. Acta Radiol. 1995;36:626-32.
10. Edmark L, Kostova-Aherdan K, Enlund M, Hedenstierna G. Optimal oxygen concentration during induction of general anesthesia. Anesthesiology. 2003;98:28-33.
11. Hovaguimian F, Lysakowski C, Elia N, Tramer MR. Effect of intraoperative high inspired oxygen fraction on surgical site infection, postoperative nausea and vomiting, and pulmonary function: systematic review and meta-analysis of randomized controlled trials. Anesthesiology. 2013;119:303-16.
12. Cho S, Oh HW, Choi MH, Lee HJ, Woo JH. Effects of intraoperative ventilation strategy on perioperative atelectasis assessed by lung ultrasonography in patients undergoing open abdominal surgery: a prospective randomized controlled study. J Korean Med Sci. 2020;35(39):e327.
13. Güldner A, Kiss T, Neto AS, Hemmes SNT, Canet J, Spieth PM, et al. Intraoperative protective mechanical ventilation for prevention of postoperative pulmonary complications: a comprehensive review of the role of tidal volume, positive end-expiratory pressure, and lung recruitment maneuvers. Anesthesiology. 2015;123:692-713.
14. Herbstreit F, Peters J, Eikermann M. Impaired upper airway integrity by residual neuromuscular blockade. Increased airway collapsibility and blunted genioglossus muscle activity in response to negative pharyngeal pressure. Anesthesiology. 2009;110:1253-60.
15. Kumar GV, Nair AM, Murthy HS, Jalaja KR, Ramachandra K, Parameshwara G. Residual neuromuscular blockade affects postoperative pulmonary function. Anesthesiology. 2012;117:1234-44.
16. Pandit JJ. The variable effect of low-dose volatile anaesthetics on the acute ventilator response to hypoxia in humans: a quantitative review. Anaesthesia. 2002;57:632-43.
17. Plötz FB, Slutsky AS, van Vught AJ, Heijnen CJ. Ventilator-induced lung injury and multiple system organ failure: a critical review of facts and hypotheses. Intensive Care Med. 2004;30:1865-72.
18. Blum JM, Maile M, Park PK, Morris M, Jewell E, Dechert R, et al. A description of intraoperative ventilator management in patients with acute lung injury and the use of lung protective ventilation strategies. Anesthesiology. 2011;115:75-82.
19. Uhlig S. Ventilation-induced lung injury and mechanotransduction: Stretching it too far? Am J Physiol Lung Cell Mol Physiol. 2002;282:L892-6.
20. Acute Respiratory Distress Syndrome Network; Brower RG, Matthay MA, Morris A, Schoenfeld D, Thompson BT, Wheeler A. Ventilation with lower tidal volumes as compared with traditional tidal volumes for acute lung injury and the acute respiratory distress syndrome. N Engl J Med. 2000;342:1301-8.

21. Blank RS, Colquhoun DA, Durieux ME, Kozower BD, McMurry TL, Bender SP, et al. Management of one-lung ventilation: impact of tidal volume on complications after thoracic surgery. Anesthesiology. 2016;124:1286-95.
22. Mathis MR, Duggal NM, Likosky DS, Haft JW, Douville NJ, Vaughn MT, et al. Intraoperative mechanical ventilation and postoperative pulmonary complications after cardiac surgery. Anesthesiology. 2019;131:1046-62.
23. Jaber S, Coisel Y, Chanques G, Futier E, Constantin JM, Michelet P, et al. A multicentre observational study of intraoperative ventilatory management during general anaesthesia: tidal volumes and relation to body weight. Anaesthesia. 2012;67:999-1008.
24. Gattinoni L, Collino F, Maiolo G, Rapetti F, Romitti F, Tonetti T, et al. Positive end-expiratory pressure: how to set it at the individual level. Ann Transl Med. 2017;5(14):288.
25. Futier E, Constantin JM, Paugam-Burtz C, Pascal J, Eurin M, Neuschwander A, et al.; IMPROVE Study Group. A trial of intraoperative low-tidal-volume ventilation in abdominal surgery. N Engl J Med. 2013;369(5):428-37.
26. Neto AS, Hemmes SNT, Barbas CSV, Beiderlinden M, Biehl M, Binnekade JM, et al. The PROVE Network Investigators. Protective versus conventional ventilation for surgery: a systematic review and individual patient data meta-analysis. Anesthesiology. 2015;123:66-78.
27. Severgnini P, Selmo G, Lanza C, Chiesa A, Frigerio A, Bacuzzi A, et al. Protective mechanical ventilation during general anesthesia for open abdominal surgery improves postoperative pulmonary function. Anesthesiology. 2013; 118(6):1307-21.
28. Pi X, Cui Y, Wang C, Guo L, Sun B, Shi J, et al. Low tidal volume with PEEP and recruitment expedite the recovery of pulmonary function. Int J Clin Exp Pathol. 2015;8(11):14305-14.
29. Guay J, Ochroch EA, Kopp S. Intraoperative use of low volume ventilation to decrease postoperative mortality, mechanical ventilation, lengths of stay and lung injury in adults without acute lung injury. Cochrane Database Syst Rev. 2018;7:CD011151.
30. Young CC, Harris EM, Vacchiano C, Bodnar S, Bukowy B, Elliott RRD, et al. Lung-protective ventilation for the surgical patient: international expert panel-based consensus recommendations. Br J Anaesth. 2019;123:898-913.
31. Michelet P, D'Journo XB, Roch A, Doddoli C, Marin V, Papazian L, et al. Protective ventilation influences systemic inflammation after esophagectomy: a randomized controlled study. Anesthesiology. 2006;105:911-9.
32. Shen Y, Zhong M, Wu W, Wang H, Feng M, Tan L, et al. The impact of tidal volume on pulmonary complications following minimally invasive esophagectomy: a randomized and controlled study. J Thorac Cardiovasc Surg. 2013;146:1267-73.
33. Hong CM, Xu DZ, Lu Q, Cheng Y, Pisarenko V, Doucet D, et al. Low tidal volume and high positive end-expiratory pressure mechanical ventilation results in increased inflammation and ventilator-associated lung injury in normal lungs. Anesth Analg. 2010;110:1652-60.
34. Gu W, Wang F, Liu J. Effect of lung-protective ventilation with lower tidal volumes on clinical outcomes among patients undergoing surgery: a meta-analysis of randomized controlled trials. CMAJ. 2015; 187: E101-9.

35. Simon P, Girrbach F, Petroff D, Schliewe N, Hempel G, Lange M, et al.; the PROBESE Investigators of the Protective Ventilation Network; and the Clinical Trial Network of the European Society of Anesthesiology. Individualized versus fixed positive end-expiratory pressure for intraoperative mechanical ventilation in obese patients: a secondary analysis. Anesthesiology. 2021; 134:887-900.
36. Scaramuzzo G, Spadaro S, Waldmann AD, Böhm SH, Ragazzi R, Marangoni E, et al. Heterogeneity of regional inflection points from pressure-volume curves assessed by electrical impedance tomography. Crit Care 2019;23, 119.
37. Reddy VG. Auto-PEEP: How to detect and how to prevent—a review. Middle East J Anaesthesiol. 2005;18(2):293-312.
38. Ahn HJ, MiHye Park M, Kim JA, Yang M, Yoon S, Kim BR, et al. Driving pressure guided ventilation. Korean J Anesthesiol. 2020;73(3):194-204.
39. Fernandez-Bustamante A, Sprung J, Parker RA, Bartels K, Weingarten TN, Kosour C, et al. Individualized PEEP to optimise respiratory mechanics during abdominal surgery: a pilot randomised controlled trial. Br J Anaesth. 2020;125(3):383-92.
40. Karsten J, Luepschen H, Grossherr M, Bruch HP, Leonhardt S, Gehring H, et al. Effect of PEEP on regional ventilation during laparoscopic surgery monitored by electrical impedance tomography. Acta Anaesthesiol Scand. 2011;55:878-86.
41. Reis Miranda D, Gommers D, Struijs A, Dekker R, Mekel J, Feelders R, et al. Ventilation according to the open lung concept attenuates pulmonary inflammatory response in cardiac surgery. Eur J Cardiothorac Surg. 2005; 28:889-95.
42. Tusman G, Bohm SH, Warner DO, Sprung J. Atelectasis and perioperative pulmonary complications in high-risk patients. Curr Opin Anesthesiol. 2012;25:1-10.
43. Rothen HU, Sporre B, Engberg G, Wegenius G, Hedenstierna G. Re-expansion of atelectasis during general anesthesia may have a prolonged effect. Acta Anaesthesiol Scand. 1995;39:118-25.
44. Futier E, Constantin JM, Pelosi P, Chanques G, Kwiatkoskwi F, Jaber S, et al. Intraoperative recruitment maneuver reverses detrimental pneumo-peritoneum-induced respiratory effects in healthy weight and obese patients undergoing laparoscopy. Anesthesiology. 2010;113:1310-9.
45. Cakmakkaya OS, Kaya G, Altintas F, Hayirlioglu M, Ekici B. Restoration of pulmonary compliance after laparoscopic surgery using a simple alveolar recruitment maneuver. J Clin Anesth. 2009;21:422-6.
46. Pang CK, Yap J, Chen PP. The effect of an alveolar recruitment strategy on oxygenation during laparoscopic cholecystectomy. Anaesth Intensive Care. 2003;31:176-80.
47. Whalen FX, Gajic O, Thompson GB, Kendrick ML, Que FL, Williams BA, et al. The effects of the alveolar recruitment maneuver and positive end-expiratory pressure on arterial oxygenation during laparoscopic bariatric surgery. Anesth Analg. 2006;102:298-305.
48. Park HP, Hwang JW, Kim YB, Jeon YT, Park SH, Yun MJ, et al. Effect of pre-emptive alveolar recruitment strategy before pneumoperitoneum on arterial oxygenation during laparoscopic hysterectomy. Anaesth Intensive Care. 2009;37:593-7.

49. Joyce CJ, Baker AB, Kennedy RR. Gas uptake from an unventilated area of lung: computer model of absorption atelectasis. J Appl Physiol (1985). 1993;74: 1107-16.
50. Ferrando C, Suarez-Sipmann F, Tusman G, León I, Romero E, Gracia E, et al. Open lung approach versus standard protective strategies—effects on driving pressure and ventilatory efficiency during anesthesia: a pilot, randomized controlled trial. PLoS One. 2017;12:e0177399.
51. O'Gara B, Talmor D. Perioperative lung protective ventilation. BMJ. 2018; 362:k3030.
52. Edmark L, Auner U, Enlund M, Ostberg E, Hedenstierna G. Oxygen concentration and characteristics of progressive atelectasis formation during anaesthesia. Acta Anaesthesiol Scand. 2011;55:75-81.
53. von Ungern-Sternberg BS, Regli A, Schibler A, Frei FJ, Erb TO. The impact of positive end-expiratory pressure on functional residual capacity and ventilation homogeneity impairment in anesthetized children exposed to high levels of inspired oxygen. Anesth Analg. 2007;104:1364-8.
54. Tusman G, Bohm SH. Prevention and reversal of lung collapse during the intra-operative period. Best Pract Res Clin Anaesthesiol. 2010;24:183-97.
55. Albaiceta GM, Luyando LH, Parra D, Menendez R, Calvo J, Pedreira PR, et al. Inspiratory vs. expiratory pressure-volume curves to set end-expiratory pressure in acute lung injury. Intensive Care Med. 2005;31:1370-8.
56. Kim MS, Kim NY, Lee KY, Choi YD, Hong JH, Bai S-J. The impact of two different inspiratory to expiratory ratios (1: 1 and 1:2) on respiratory mechanics and oxygenation during volume-controlled ventilation in robot-assisted laparoscopic radical prostatectomy: a randomized controlled trial. Can J Anaesth. 2015;62:979-87.
57. Gattinoni L, Marini JJ, Collino F, Maiolo G, Rapetti F, Tonetti T, et al. The future of mechanical ventilation: lessons from the present and the past. Crit Care. 2017;21(1):183.
58. Ireland CJ, Chapman TM, Mathew SF, Herbison GP, Zacharias M. Continuous positive airway pressure (CPAP) during the postoperative period for prevention of post-operative morbidity and mortality following major abdominal surgery. Cochrane Database Syst Rev. 2014; 8:CD008930.
59. Edmark L, Auner U, Lindback J, Enlund M, Hedenstierna G. Post-operative atelectasis a randomized trial investigating a ventilatory strategy and low oxygen fraction during recovery. Acta Anaesthesiol Scand. 2014;58:681-8.

CHAPTER 4

Anesthetic and Intensive Care Management for Lung Transplant

Suresh Rao KG, Santosh V, KR Balakrishnan

ABSTRACT

Lung transplantation is now an accepted treatment modality for lung failure patients, usually with successful outcomes. A thorough preoperative evaluation with a focus on cardiac status is necessary. Intraoperatively communication between surgeon and anesthesiologist is vital for managing hemodynamic instabilities. Postoperatively primary graft dysfunction should be identified early and managed accordingly. Early extracorporeal support is recommended for primary graft dysfunction.

Keywords: Lung transplant; Extracorporeal membrane oxygenation (ECMO); One-lung ventilation; Right ventricular dysfunction; Primary graft dysfunction; Graft Rejection; End-stage lung disease

KEY POINTS

- A lung transplant is the most challenging transplant among all solid organ transplants because of its unique technical, immunogenic, and infectious aspects and carries higher morbidity and mortality.
- Due attention to steroids and anticoagulants in the preoperative period is required.
- Right heart catheterization is required to rule out left ventricular diastolic dysfunction.
- A coronary angiogram is required in patients above the age of 50 years.
- Transesophageal echo is helpful in monitoring the right ventricular function and evaluating pulmonary artery and venous anastomosis for any narrowing.
- Lung isolation is needed, if a transplant is done without cardiopulmonary bypass.
- Protective ventilation with 4–6 mL/kg body weight, optimal PEEP, and least possible FiO_2 to prevent oxygen toxicity is recommended while reperfusing the graft.
- Due precaution is taken to reduce the usage of fluids and vasoconstrictors.
- Venovenous (VV) ECMO may be required in primary graft dysfunction as a bridge to recovery, and VA ECMO in severe pulmonary hypertension.

INTRODUCTION

Lung transplantation has become an increasingly important mode of therapy for patients with a variety of end-stage lung diseases. Several lung transplant procedures are generally available, including single and bilateral lung transplantation, cadaveric lobar transplantation, living-donor lobar lung transplantation, and heart-lung transplantation.[1] The number of lung transplant procedures worldwide is increasing despite persistent donor shortages. Lung transplant remains associated with high perioperative morbidity and mortality and the lowest long-term survival of all the solid organ transplants, notably due to the unique technical, immunological and infectious aspects of transplanting human lungs.[2] In this chapter, perioperative management and postoperative care of lung transplantation will be detailed.

PREOPERATIVE ASSESSMENT

Anesthetic management of a patient undergoing lung transplantation is influenced by the planned surgical approach, urgency of the procedure, patient's preoperative pulmonary status, and clinically significant comorbidities.[3] Besides hematologic and biochemical laboratory assessment, focused cardiac and pulmonary assessment is essential.

Pulmonary Function Assessment

Complete pulmonary function testing, including advanced radiographic imaging like computed tomography (CT) and ventilation-perfusion (V/Q) scan, is done to plan surgical and anesthetic management. The focus should be on the etiology of respiratory failure, current clinical status (any deterioration since assessment), and oxygen requirements. Evaluation of other systemic involvement of connective tissue disorders should be done.

Apart from routine preoperative cardiac assessment as per ACC/AHA guidelines,[4] an echocardiogram and coronary angiogram are performed in individuals over 45 years. A right heart hemodynamic study measures cardiac filling pressures and underlying pulmonary hypertension.

Comorbid Illness: Certain comorbid diseases like diabetes mellitus, hypertension, and renal dysfunction may increase the likelihood of peritransplant complications or adversely affect the outcomes.[5] Dysfunction of other vital organs like renal failure, stroke within 30 days, liver cirrhosis with portal hypertension, recent acute coronary syndrome, and untreatable malignancies are absolute contraindications for lung transplantation.

Frailty related to age or chronic end-organ disease is typically identified and treated, if possible (e.g., physical rehabilitation, nutritional optimization)

Medications: Patients with chronic obstructive pulmonary disease (COPD) and pulmonary arterial hypertension receive regular bronchodilator therapy, inhaled and systemic steroids, and pulmonary vasodilator therapy. It is critically important to continue throughout the perioperative period all chronically administered medications prescribed for pulmonary hypertension.[6] Anticoagulant therapy should be reviewed and modified with drugs with a shorter half life.

Current and historical human leukocyte antigens (HLA) antibody screening tests and the specificity of any preformed HLA antibodies should be reviewed. If the panel reactive antibody titer is high, desensitization should be done.

Adequate blood and blood products should be reserved. Sedative premedication is avoided, especially in those with pulmonary hypertension or supplemental oxygen therapy, and should be administered under strict supervision inside the operating room.

INTRAOPERATIVE MANAGEMENT

The goals of intraoperative management should focus on the preservation of allograft quality, maintenance of cardiovascular stability, and prevention of extrapulmonary complications.[7]

Monitoring and Venous Access

Large bore venous access for rapid volume replacement and invasive monitoring of arterial, central venous, and pulmonary artery pressures via arterial cannula, multilumen central venous line, and pulmonary artery catheter, respectively, is done before induction. Compulsory monitoring includes five-lead electrocardiography, pulse oximetry, urine output, core temperature, capnography, and anesthetic agent gas analysis. Other monitors like depth-of-anesthesia monitoring, cerebral oximetry, arterial blood gas monitoring, continuous cardiac output, and mixed venous oximetry are routinely used during lung transplantation.

Transesophageal Echocardiography

Transesophageal echocardiography (TEE) is essential for continuous cardiac monitoring. It provides real-time analysis of left and right heart preload, left and right ventricular function, regional wall motion abnormalities, pulmonary artery pressures, and intracardiac air, primarily when used in hemodynamic instability. It can detect patent foramen ovale, intracardiac thrombus, and other unanticipated abnormalities. If unexplained or refractory hypoxemia occurs, intracardiac shunting should be suspected. Detailed examination of the pulmonary vein and arterial anastomosis is done to rule out any narrowing.

Induction

Induction of anesthesia is one of the most critical periods, and severe hemodynamic instability should be anticipated. The surgeon and perfusionist must be prepared for emergency initiation of cardiopulmonary bypass if a circulatory collapse occurs. Factors that precipitate cardiac instability include severe hypoxia, hypercarbia, acidosis, blunting of endogenous sympathetic drive, anesthetic drugs causing myocardial depression, vasodilatation, and initiation of positive pressure ventilation. The primary hemodynamic goals of induction are to prevent falls in systemic vascular resistance, maintain myocardial contractility, and avoid any increase in pulmonary vascular resistance.

Rapid sequence intubation with scoline or rocuronium is used. Optimization of hemodynamics may need to be achieved by vasopressor and ionotropic support. A double-lumen tube is preferred in most cases as it allows absolute lung isolation and differential ventilation. Single-lumen ETT with bronchial blockers is an alternative. The double-lumen tube is exchanged for a single-lumen ETT at the end of the surgery; tube exchanger is preferred during this.

Broad-spectrum antibiotics are given as prophylaxis before incision. For patients with suppurative lung disease or a current chest infection, the choice of antibiotics is determined by microbiological culture. The microbiological burden of the donor should also be taken into account.

Ventilation

Specific ventilation strategies like low-inspiratory pressures and minimal tidal volume to avoid dynamic hyperinflation, high-airway pressures, and high positive end-expiratory pressure (PEEP) should be employed.[8] One should focus primarily on arterial pH rather than arterial PCO_2 since most patients are adapted to chronic hypercapnia.

■ MAINTENANCE OF ANESTHESIA

Inhalation anesthesia with sevoflurane/isoflurane is the preferred choice. A total intravenous anesthetic technique has also been described. Inhalational agents have bronchodilatory effects in patients with obstructive airway disease.

One-lung ventilation (OLV) is better tolerated in the lung with greater perfusion. Strategies that decrease the shunt fraction in one lung ventilation should be employed. If severe respiratory acidosis or hypoxemia occurs, mechanical circulatory support should be initiated.

Reduction of pulmonary hypertension and vascular resistance is a principal goal of intraoperative management at every stage of the operation.[9] Vasoactive agents most commonly used are milrinone, noradrenaline, and adrenaline. Inhaled pulmonary vasodilators are used to reduce pulmonary vascular resistance (PVR) selectively. Inhaled nitric oxide is the first choice inside the operating room in patients at risk of right ventricular failure.

MECHANICAL CIRCULATORY SUPPORT

Intraoperative extracorporeal membrane oxygenation (ECMO) [Venovenous (VV) or venoarterial (VA)] should be considered in case of refractory hypoxemia, supra-systemic pulmonary artery pressures, and impossible lung protective ventilation strategy. TEE is essential in this decision-making.[10]

Warm beating heart cardiopulmonary bypass (CPB) is also routinely used for lung transplantation based on institutional experience. CPB is also employed when the recipient requires plasmapheresis due to HLA mismatch and HLA antibodies against the donor. Bypass times are often prolonged, so a centrifugal pump offers an advantage over a continuous flow roller pump. An ECMO oxygenator is routinely used.

Venous drainage is generally affected by surgical manipulation of the heart and hilum therefore, strict vigilance is required. Bicaval-cannulation is preferred. The advantages of CPB are hemodynamic stability and allow controlled reperfusion of each graft. Disadvantages of CPB are hemolysis and activation of proinflammatory mediators that can cause lung injury. It also increases the need for blood product transfusion due to haemodilution, coagulopathy, and platelet dysfunction. The use of CPB has been associated with a more extended period of postoperative mechanical ventilation, more pulmonary edema, and increased early morbidity, although this is controversial.

SURGICAL CONSIDERATIONS AND ANASTAMOSIS

In redo surgeries, restrictive or supportive lung disease, extensive pleural adhesions may complicate surgical explantation and need massive blood transfusions.

For bilateral sequential single-lung transplantation performed without CPB, if there is a significant perfusion mismatch between the two lungs, transplantation is done for the lung with lower perfusion. Bronchial anastomosis is initially followed by pulmonary artery and finally pulmonary venous anastomosis. Thorough bronchial toileting using a flexible bronchoscope is done after the bronchial anastomosis. Pulmonary venous anastomosis is done by grafting an island off the donor atrium containing the upper and lower pulmonary veins onto the recipient's left atrium. During this stage, the application of an atrial clamp can cause arrhythmias, decreased left atrial preload, or coronary artery occlusion. Surgical retraction on the heart causes intermittent periods of hypotension and low cardiac output. Hence, regular communication between the anesthetist and surgeon is essential.

Vasoactive drugs and fluids are required to maintain hemodynamic stability. Caution should be exercised as low-pressure pulmonary edema in the grafts may occur, if an excessive fluid has been given. Before tying the final stitch of the atrial anastomosis, the graft is entirely desired. This is done by inflating the lung to a sustained pressure of 15–20 cmH$_2$O and partially releasing the pulmonary artery clamp. The atrial clamp is then released to deair the atrial cuff before the final knot is tied. At this point, hypotension may occur due to several causes.

Sometimes leaks in the vascular anastomosis may need to be controlled by placing additional sutures. A significant amount of blood loss may rapidly occur in the interim requiring prompt intravascular volume replacement. Temporary myocardial stunning occurs as the initial venous return to the left atrium is cold, contains ischemic metabolites, and is acellular. Treatment with a small bolus of adrenaline or calcium is often required to improve myocardial contractility. Coronary artery air embolism may also occur. This is usually seen in the right coronary artery as it is uppermost in the supine position. ST depression or elevation may be seen in the inferior leads and, if treated with vasopressors, is usually transient.

The pulmonary artery clamp is slowly released, limiting initial flows to the vascular bed of the graft, which has been shown to reduce primary graft dysfunction (PGD). To reduce lung injury, initial ventilation to the graft should be with a low FiO$_2$ tolerated, low-peak inspiratory pressures of 15–20 cmH$_2$O, and PEEP of 5 cmH$_2$O. The respiratory rate is initially set to 8–10 breaths per minute. Once the pulmonary artery clamp is fully released, ventilation settings must be adjusted to ensure adequate minute ventilation and CO$_2$ removal and the FiO$_2$ titrated to a safe oxygen saturation level.

■ POSTOPERATIVE ANALGESIA

Multimodal analgesia with intravenous opioids and regional anesthesia techniques are essential in reducing morbidity. Nonsteroidal anti-inflammatory drugs (NSAIDs) like ibuprofen, ketorolac, and other nephrotoxic drugs should be avoided due to their synergistic action with calcineurin inhibitors.

Epidural Analgesia

Adequate postoperative analgesia is essential to facilitate tracheal extubation. Thoracic epidural analgesia (TEA) provides superior analgesia compared with systemic opioids.[11] However, unique risks associated with preoperative epidural catheter placement must be considered in the lung transplant population. First, in the event of a bloody tap, the risk of an epidural hematoma is magnified after full heparinization for CPB. Timely decompression may be delayed due to prolonged surgery and the inability to elicit clinical signs in patients under general anesthesia. Second, the benefit of TEA is shortened or lost, if tracheal extubation is delayed due to other complications. An alternative is to insert the epidural postoperatively in an awake or lightly sedated patient before extubation or only if systemic multimodal analgesics are inadequate. For single-sided surgery, paravertebral catheter insertion is an alternative to TEA.

Immunosuppressants

One primary strategy of immunosuppressant induction agents is to suppress the potentially robust T cell immune response to the allograft in the immediate postoperative period after lung transplantation. All lung transplant programs use high-dose steroids like methyl-prednisolone for immunosuppression before implantation of the donor organ. Available induction agents are adjuncts to steroids and deplete existing T cells and/or interrupt T cell activation and proliferation. These induction strategies can be classified into two groups: Monoclonal and polyclonal agents. The decision to use induction therapy and its type must be made based upon comorbidities to balance the effects of immunosuppression on both risks of infection and rejection.

The most common monoclonal induction agent utilized in lung transplantation is basiliximab or alemtuzumab. Induction with alemtuzumab has been associated with greater freedom from developing acute and chronic rejection in lung transplant recipients. Antithymocyte/lymphocyte globulin (ATG) is a polyclonal antibody preparation that nonspecifically binds to antigens on the surface of T cells, resulting in lymphocyte depletion.

The most common complication of these immunosuppressive drugs is acute renal injury. Though transient, renal dysfunction can be exacerbated by associated comorbid illness. Calcineurin inhibitors like cyclosporine and tacrolimus cause vasoconstriction of the renal arteriole, thereby reducing renal blood flow and glomerular filtration rate.

Triple drug maintenance immunosuppression therapy is considered the standard of care after lung transplantation and consists of steroids, calcineurin inhibitors, and antimetabolites. It is not uncommon for patients to require a switch to alternative immunosuppressive regimens based on individual tolerability. These drugs have a narrow therapeutic index, so levels should be frequently monitored. There can also be significant interpatient and intrapatient variability. This variability is due to genetic polymorphisms of cytochrome P450 3A enzymes and the transport protein P-glycoprotein, age, clinical status (time after transplant, liver function, and gut function), disease states (i.e., cystic fibrosis), and presence of interacting medications.

Ventilatory Management

The primary goals of ventilatory strategies are to provide adequate minute ventilation and to avoid ventilator-induced lung injuries like volutrauma, barotrauma, and oxygen toxicity.[12] From the time of bronchial anastomosis, lung protective ventilation is initiated [low tidal volume (4–6 mL/kg ideal body weight) and low driving pressures to limit the plateau pressure below 30 cmH$_2$O].[8] During reperfusion, the lowest acceptable FiO$_2$ is used to maintain oxygen saturations >92%. A FiO$_2$ 40% is ideal for preventing acute lung injury. No particular ventilation mode is proven beneficial in the early postoperative period, though the pressure control mode with pressure control set below 15 and optimal PEEP is commonly used.[13]

The management should be individualized to achieve set target goals. Sudden deterioration in oxygenation and a decrease in lung compliance are early indicators of graft dysfunction. The differential diagnosis for postoperative hypoxemia includes PGD, anastomotic issues, pneumothorax, atelectasis, fluid overload, cardiac failure, etc. Frequent desaturations may indicate pulmonary hypertensive episodes, which should be managed with inhaled nitric oxide or pulmonary vasodilators, sedation, and muscle relaxation.[14] In many instances, sudden hypoxemia and hypercapnia require emergency bronchoscopic removal of secretions and mucous plugs.

Single-lung transplantation, as for emphysema, pose different challenges. The native and donor lungs will have other respiratory mechanics depending on the native lung disease. In COPD patients, there is a high risk of hyperinflation and auto-PEEP in the native lungs, so lower PEEP is generally employed.

Primary Graft Dysfunction

It is a syndrome of acute severe lung injury, which occurs within 72 hours postlung allograft transplant without any major identifiable cause.[15] It is one of the significant causes of morbidity and mortality in the early postoperative period, with a reported incidence of about 10–25%.[16] It is characterized by progressive hypoxemia, and diffuse alveolar infiltrates in a chest X-ray.

In 2016, the International Society for Heart and Lung Transplantation (ISHLT) consensus statement of the working group on PGD,[17] standardized the definition of PGD **(Table 1)**. Assessment is carried out at specific time points after reperfusion; within the first 6 hours (T0), post 24 hours (T24), 48 hours (T48), and 72 hours (T72). Ideally, the P/F ratio is measured on a FiO$_2$ of 1.0 and PEEP of 5 cmH$_2$O.

TABLE 1: Grading of primary graft dysfunction.

Grade	Pulmonary edema on chest radiograph	PaO$_2$/FiO$_2$ ratio
0	No	Any
1	Yes	>300
2	Yes	200–300
3	Yes	<200

ECMO POSTLUNG TRANSPLANT

Early initiation of ECMO is advised in patients with refractory hypoxemia, ideally within 24 hours after transplantation.[18,19]

Venovenous ECMO with ultra-lung protective ventilation (3 mL/kg) may limit ventilator-induced lung injury and improve graft survival. Oxygen supply to the graft via pulmonary arteries is crucial as bronchial arterial blood supply to the implanted lung is lacking.

Venoarterial ECMO is established in case of severe hemodynamic instability or a severe pulmonary hypertensive crisis. As VA ECMO shunts blood away from the lung, maintaining normal pulmonary artery pressure and pulsatility is essential to prevent graft hypoxia.

In certain situations, VVA ECMO, which combines both VV and VA ECMO techniques, can be utilized to regulate adequate pulmonary perfusion and systemic oxygenation.

WEANING OF MECHANICAL VENTILATION

Chest X-ray is done daily in the initial week. Malposition of invasive lines, diaphragmatic position, atelectasis, and evidence of rejection like infiltrates/opacities, pleural abnormalities, and pneumonia should be examined. Bedside lung ultrasound also is beneficial. In case of unclear findings, CT without contrast is warranted.

Early tracheal extubation is ideal for postlung transplantation. Inhaled nitric oxide at 10–20 PPM, when used to manage pulmonary hypertension post-transplant, is generally weaned in 24–48 hours. PEEP is then weaned, followed by FiO_2 according to serial blood gases and hemodynamics.

Early tracheostomy should be considered in patients requiring prolonged mechanical ventilation. Flexible fiber-optic bronchoscopy is performed in all patients for better trachea bronchial toileting and to evaluate the integrity of the airways. Post-tracheal extubation, aggressive respiratory physiotherapy with incentive spirometry and early mobilization is initiated.

HEMODYNAMIC MANAGEMENT

Invasive cardiovascular monitoring is essential, as early postoperative hemodynamics can be very labile. In high-risk cases like elevated pulmonary arterial pressures at the time of transplant or an underlying diagnosis of pulmonary arterial hypertension, Pulmonary artery catheters with continuous cardiac output and TEE are used to aid management.[20]

An obstruction to the pulmonary vein flow (due to clot, kinking, or narrow anastomosis) may present with hypoxia. TEE becomes a powerful tool in differentiating this condition from other causes, such as acute graft rejection or reperfusion injury. The turbulence of flow, pulmonary vein diameter of <0.5 cm, peak systolic flow velocity >1 m/s, and pulmonary vein-left atrial pressure gradient (PVLAG) ≥10-12 mm Hg support the diagnosis of pulmonary vein stenosis.[21]

Hemodynamic goals are to maintain adequate systemic perfusion and oxygen delivery by avoiding hypotension and pulmonary hypertension. Sudden increases in pulmonary vascular resistance can lead to right heart failure and should be monitored continuously. Pulmonary vasodilators like nitric oxide, inhaled prostacyclin, and milrinone reduce the right ventricular afterload and help the right ventricle recover. A cardiac index of 2.2-2.5 is ideal. Vasopressors and ionotropic agents may be required to support hemodynamics.[22] Caution should be used if high-dose vasopressors are used as they may compromise airway mucosal circulation. Serial lactate levels and mixed venous saturations are measured and guided by clinical status.

Arrhythmias, generally supraventricular in origin, are commonly seen, with a reported incidence of 34-74%.[23] Hemodynamically significant arrhythmias should be cardioverted immediately.

■ FLUID MANAGEMENT

Reperfusion pulmonary edema is common after lung transplantation due to leaky capillaries, and loss of lymphatic drainage should be managed aggressively. Diuretic infusion is required to maintain a total negative balance.

Volume replacement with colloid (5% albumin) rather than crystalloids should be considered. Hematocrit in the range of 25-30% is maintained. Point of care testing of coagulation like thromboelastogram (TEG) should guide blood product replacement.

■ INFECTION AND SEPSIS MANAGEMENT

Infectious complications contribute substantially to increased postoperative morbidity and mortality following lung transplant. Data suggest that more than 25% of postoperative deaths are due to infectious causes.[24] Postoperative lung complications after lung transplant are listed in **Table 2**.

Lung transplant recipients are uniquely high risk for bacterial and fungal infections. A high level of immunosuppression is maintained. Allograft denervation leads to decreased mucociliary clearance and absent cough reflex. There is also continuous exposure to environmental pathogens and colonizing organisms from the upper respiratory tract.

Bronchoscopy with bronchoalveolar lavage (BAL) is the most sensitive test to rule out infections. Bacterial pneumonia is the most common infection postlung transplant.[25] Viral infections in the early postoperative period are uncommon. Empirical broad-spectrum antibiotics should be initiated intraoperatively before incision, followed by targeted antibiotics for the BAL cultures of the explanted lung from the donor. Antifungal prophylaxis, *Pneumocystis carinii* prophylaxis, and cytomegalovirus prophylaxis are started from postoperative day 2.

TABLE 2: Postoperative complications after lung transplantation.

Respiratory	Cardiovascular	Surgical
• Primary graft dysfunction • Pulmonary embolism • Pleural effusions • Transfusion related acute lung injury (TRALI)	• Right heart dysfunction • Arrythmias • Myocardial ischemia	• Bleeding • Pulmonary arterial stenosis • Pulmonary venous thrombosis • Bronchial anastomotic dehiscence
Immunological	**Renal**	**Infectious**
• Hyperacute rejection • Acute rejection • Side effects of drugs	Acute kidney injury	• Bacterial pneumonia • Fungal infections • Viral infections (CMV, EBV)

(CMV: cytomegalovirus; EBV: Epstein-Barr virus)

CONCLUSION

The perioperative and postoperative care of lung transplant recipients requires meticulous attention to detail with a multidisciplinary team approach. Anesthesiologists should have knowledge about transplant immunology, intensive care, TEE, thoracic, and cardiac anesthesia to manage these patients successfully.

REFERENCES

1. Weill D. Lung transplantation: indications and contraindications. J Thorac Dis. 2018;10(7):4574-87.
2. Thabut G, Mal H. Outcomes after lung transplantation. J Thorac Dis. 2017;9(8):2684-91.
3. Buckwell E, Vickery B, Sidebotham D. Anaesthesia for lung transplantation. BJA Educ. 2020;20(11):368-76.
4. Fleisher LA, Fleischmann KE, Auerbach AD, Barnason SA, Beckman JA, Bozkurt B, et al. 2014 ACC/AHA guideline on perioperative cardiovascular evaluation and management of patients undergoing noncardiac surgery: executive summary: a report of the American College of Cardiology/American Heart Association Task Force on Practice Guidelines. Circulation. 2014;130(24):2215-45.
5. Schulze PC, Jiang J, Yang J, Cheema FH, Schaeffle K, Kato TS, et al. Preoperative assessment of high-risk candidates to predict survival after heart transplantation. Circ Heart Fail. 2013;6(3):527-34.
6. Gille J, Seyfarth HJ, Gerlach S, Malcharek M, Czeslick E, Sablotzki A. Perioperative anesthesiological management of patients with pulmonary hypertension. Anesthesiol Res Pract. 2012;2012:356982.
7. Buckwell E, Vickery B, Sidebotham D. Anaesthesia for lung transplantation. BJA Educ. 2020;20(11):368-76.
8. Barnes L, Reed RM, Parekh KR, Bhama JK, Pena T, Rajagopal S, et al. Mechanical ventilation for the lung transplant recipient. Curr Pulmonol Rep. 2015;4(2):88-96.
9. Tomasi R, Betz D, Schlager S, Kammerer T, Hoechter DJ, Weig T, et al. Intraoperative anesthetic management of lung transplantation: center-specific

practices and geographic and centers size differences. J Cardiothorac Vasc Anesth. 2018;32(1):62-9.
10. Lus F, Sommer W, Tudorache I, Avsar M, Siemeni T, Salman J, et al. Five-year experience with intraoperative extracorporeal membrane oxygenation in lung transplantation: Indications and midterm results. J Heart Lung Transplant Off Publ Int Soc Heart Transplant. 2016;35(1):49-58.
11. Feltracco P, Barbieri S, Milevoj M, Serra E, Michieletto E, Carollo C, et al. Thoracic epidural analgesia in lung transplantation. Transplant Proc. 2010;42(4):1265-9.
12. Lau CL, Patterson GA, Palmer SM. Critical care aspects of lung transplantation. J Intensive Care Med. 2004;19(2):83-104.
13. King CS, Valentine V, Cattamanchi A, Franco-Palacios D, Shlobin OA, Brown AW, et al. Early postoperative management after lung transplantation: results of an international survey. Clin Transplant. 2017;31(7).
14. Kao CC, Parulekar AD. Postoperative management of lung transplant recipients. J Thorac Dis. 2019;11(Suppl 14):S1782-88.
15. Altun GT, Arslantaş MK, Cinel İ. Primary graft dysfunction after lung transplantation. Turk J Anaesthesiol Reanim. 2015;43(6):418-23.
16. Christie JD, Kotloff RM, Ahya VN, Tino G, Pochettino A, Gaughan C, et al. The effect of primary graft dysfunction on survival after lung transplantation. Am J Respir Crit Care Med. 2005;171(11):1312-6.
17. Snell GI, Yusen RD, Weill D, Strueber M, Garrity E, Reed A, et al. Report of the ISHLT Working Group on primary lung graft dysfunction, part I: definition and grading-A 2016 Consensus Group statement of the International Society for Heart and Lung Transplantation. J Heart Lung Transplant Off Publ Int Soc Heart Transplant. 2017;36(10):1097-103.
18. Fischer S, Bohn D, Rycus P, Pierre AF, de Perrot M, Waddell TK, et al. Extracorporeal membrane oxygenation for primary graft dysfunction after lung transplantation: analysis of the Extracorporeal Life Support Organization (ELSO) registry. J Heart Lung Transplant Off Publ Int Soc Heart Transplant. 2007;26(5):472-7.
19. Wigfield CH, Lindsey JD, Steffens TG, Edwards NM, Love RB. Early institution of extracorporeal membrane oxygenation for primary graft dysfunction after lung transplantation improves outcome. J Heart Lung Transplant Off Publ Int Soc Heart Transplant. 2007;26(4):331-8.
20. Kim SY, Jeong SJ, Lee JG, Park MS, Paik HC, Na S, et al. Critical care after lung transplantation. Acute Crit Care. 2018;33(4):206-15.
21. Kachulis B, Mitrev L, Jordan D. Intraoperative anesthetic management of lung transplantation patients. Best Pract Res Clin Anaesthesiol. 2017;31(2):261-72.
22. Castillo M. Anesthetic management for lung transplantation. Curr Opin Anaesthesiol. 2011;24(1):32-6.
23. Lazaro MT, Ussetti P, Merino JL. Atrial fibrillation, atrial flutter, or both after pulmonary transplantation. Chest. 2005;127(4):1461-2; author reply 1462.
24. Yusen RD, Edwards LB, Kucheryavaya AY, Benden C, Dipchand AI, Dobbels F, et al. The registry of the International Society for Heart and Lung Transplantation: thirty-first adult lung and heart-lung transplant report--2014; focus theme: retransplantation. J Heart Lung Transplant Off Publ Int Soc Heart Transplant. 2014;33(10):1009-24.
25. Remund KF, Best M, Egan JJ. Infections relevant to lung transplantation. Proc Am Thorac Soc. 2009;6(1):94-100.

CHAPTER

5

Pediatric Obstructive Sleep Apnea: A Comprehensive Review

Arvind Chandrakantan, Adam C Adler

ABSTRACT

Pediatric obstructive sleep apnea (OSA) is present in up to 7% of children and presents with everything from nasal turbulence to cessation in gas exchange. The brain has neurocognitive morbidity associated with persistent pediatric OSA. Up-to-date knowledge and cooperative planning are required to ensure optimal outcomes in children with OSA. This comprehensive review covers the major perioperative concerns with OSA, including preoperative polysomnography, PK/PD, drug-induced sleep endoscopy (DISE), postoperative risk stratification, and the role for consumer sleep technology.

Keywords: Pediatrics; Obstructive sleep apnea; Polysomnography; Sleep disordered breathing.

KEY POINTS

- Pediatric OSA is a common disease with numerous end-organ sequelae. The reversibility of the neurocognitive symptomatology is unknown.
- Certain high-risk populations have a high incidence of residual OSA even after surgical therapy. DISE may be of use in identifying further sites of obstruction in these patients.
- There is greater heterogeneity in pharmacodynamic phenotypes, so precision medicine remains unavailable currently to guide pharmacotherapeutic decisions.

INTRODUCTION

Untreated obstructive sleep apnea (OSA) has numerous and systemic consequences **(Fig. 1)**. Sleep apnea is often under or misdiagnosed in children owing to the vastly different risk factors, clinical presentations, and underlying etiology in children when compared with adults.[1] In children, prolonged and untreated OSA may present neurocognitive manifestations such as poor school performance, impulsivity, memory, and learning impairments.[2] In contrast, adult symptoms often include daytime hypersomnolence, fatigue, and headache, among others.

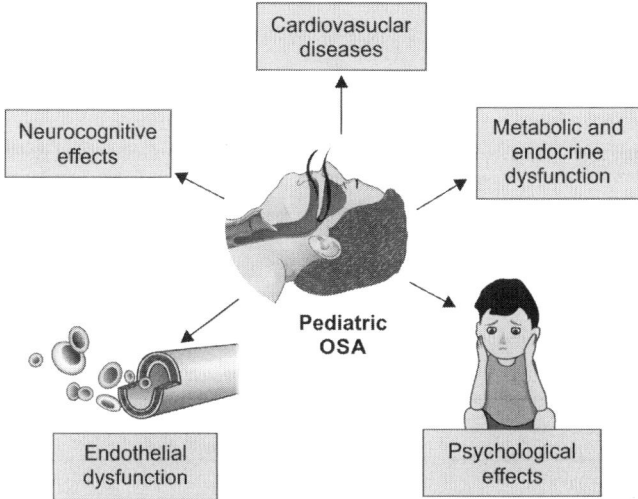

Fig. 1: Graphic abstract. Conceptualizing the sequelae of pediatric obstructive sleep apnea (OSA). This abstract diagram relays the various biopsychosocial systems affected by pediatric OSA.
Source: With permission under Creative Commons. Thomas et al., 2022 Children.

In adults with OSA, treatment is multifaceted focused on lifestyle modification (diet), weight loss, and continuous positive airway pressure (CPAP), with surgical intervention being the exception. This may change in coming years with larger number of adults being treated with the inspire device; however, this is out of the scope of this review. In children, adenotonsillar hypertrophy is the primary etiology of OSA, with adenotonsillectomy (AT) serving as the primary treatment. Despite the incidence of OSA, at least in the USA, the number of children undergoing AT is low compared to disease incidence **(Table 1)**.

Despite surgical intervention, a number of children, especially those with severe or very severe disease, morbidly obese patients, and those with syndromic OSA, continue to have residual symptoms of OSA, suggesting other sites of obstruction, which necessitates follow up diagnostic studies and interventional airway procedures.

▪ PEDIATRIC OSA

Nonsyndromic pediatric OSA can be described by three distinct phenotypes based on the primary etiology, including the early-onset neonatal type, which is mostly centrally mediated apnea, the early childhood phenotype (discussed here), and the adolescent phenotype (often related to obesity). The typical age of presentation of pediatric OSA is between 2 and 14 years.[3] Adolescent OSA is considered a separate disease phenotype with variable progression and overlap with adult OSA, particularly related to obesity.[4]

TABLE 1: Number of children undergoing adenotonsillectomy.

Year of data reported	Procedure(s)	Setting	Age Range (years)	Estimated cases (unique patients)	Estimated rate (per 1,000)	Data source	Reference	Notes
2010	• Tonsillectomy • Adenotonsillectomy • Adenoidectomy	Ambulatory	<15	358,000	—	2010 National Hospital Ambulatory Medical Care Survey (NHAMCS)	Hall MJ, Schwartzman A, Zhang J, et al. Ambulatory surgery data from hospitals and ambulatory surgery centers: United States, 2010. Natl Health Stat Report 2017;102:1-15.	2010 NHAMCS a nationally representative survey of hospitals and ASCs conducted by the National Center for Health Statistics (NCHS). This survey has provided data on ambulatory medical care services provided in hospital emergency and outpatient departments since 1992.
2006b	Tonsillectomy	Ambulatory	<18	583,000	7.91	2006 National Survey of Ambulatory Surgery (NSAS)	Boss EF, Marsteller JA, Simon AE. Outpatient tonsillectomy in children: demographic and geographic variation in the United States, 2006. J Pediatrics 2012;160(5):814-9.	The NSAS is a nationally representative sample of visits to freestanding and hospital-based ambulatory surgery centers in the US conducted by the National Center for Health Statistics (NCHS), CDC. The NSAS includes data from ~52,000 ambulatory surgery encounters obtained from 142 hospital-based and 295 freestanding ASCs (74.4% unweighted response rate) by using a multistage probability design

Contd...

Contd...

Year of data reported	Procedure(s)	Setting	Age Range (years)	Estimated cases (unique patients)	Estimated rate (per 1,000)	Data source	Reference	Notes
2006a	• Tonsillectomy • Adenotonsillectomy • Adenoidectomy	Inpatient and Ambulatory	<18	695,029	9.43	National Hospital Discharge Survey (NHDS) and NSAS	Bhattacharyya N, Lin HW. Changes and consistencies in the epidemiology of pediatric adenotonsillar surgery, 1996–2006. Otolaryngology-Head and Neck Surgery 2010;143: 680-4.	Data for calendar year 1996 were obtained from both the NSAS and the NHDS 1996 releases
1996	• Tonsillectomy • Adenotonsillectomy • Adenoidectomy	Inpatient and Ambulatory	<18	441,870	6.4	National Hospital Discharge Survey (NHDS) and NSAS	Bhattacharyya N, Lin HW. Changes and consistencies in the epidemiology of pediatric adenotonsillar surgery, 1996–2006. Otdaryngology-Head and Neck Surgery 2010;143: 680-4.	Data for calendar year 2006 were obtained from both the NSAS and NHDS data sets, 2006 releases

Neonatal OSA is largely a result of prematurity and is treated with transient positive airway pressure (PAP) therapy and caffeine.[5] While obesity has been identified as a causative factor in some pediatric OSA patients,[6,7] there are two distinct and different parts of the clinical phenotype, with a significant number of children being overweight, and another group being normal or even underweight.[8] Pediatric OSA can be diagnosed from birth through adolescence with tremendous heterogeneity in clinical phenotypes.[9]

Neurological and Behavioral Manifestations of Pediatric OSA

There have been several papers that have reviewed the effect of intermittent hypoxia on the developing brain.[10,11] This includes two detailed reviews we have published previously.[12,13] The major clinical manifestations of pediatric OSA are daytime hypersomnolence and inattention, which results in behavioral disturbances, as well as learning and memory difficulties.

Anesthetic Considerations in Children with OSA

The Role of Preoperative Polysomnography

Polysomnography (PSG) testing remains the gold standard for diagnosing OSA, although it is not routinely performed. The American Academy of Otolaryngology/Head and Neck Surgery (AAO/HNS) guidelines differ from the American Academy of Pediatrics' recommendation that all children with OSA symptoms receive PSG before AT.[14] The 2019 AAO/HNS tonsillectomy guidelines state that children with OSA should be referred for preoperative PSG, if they are (1) <2 years of age or if they exhibit any of the following: (2) obesity, (3) down syndrome, (4) craniofacial abnormalities, (5) neuromuscular disorders, (6) sickle cell disease, or (7) mucopolysaccharidoses.

The severity of OSA has traditionally been stratified delineated on the apnea-hypopnea index (AHI) derived from a PSG with pediatric classification including 1-5 events/hour as mild, 5-10 as moderate, and >10 as severe sleep apnea. At Texas Children's Hospital, most patients are otherwise healthy and present with symptoms of obstructive sleep-disordered breathing and are presumed to have mild-to-moderate disease. Following AT, all patients are observed for a minimum of 2 hours to ensure adequate hydration, analgesia, and maintenance of oxygen saturation before discharge from the postanesthesia recovery. Those with severe OSA, either presumed or by PSG, patients <3 years of age, and those with significant comorbidities (i.e., craniofacial anomalies, cardiopulmonary disease, syndromic OSA, and history of severe prematurity) are often admitted for overnight observation with continuous oximetry. Nationally, in the USA, there is wide variability in practice; however, there seems to be a wider margin of safety in children with mild-moderate OSA.[15] PSG results are also used to determine suitability for case performance at ambulatory surgical centers and postoperative discharge versus inpatient admission (ICU vs. surgical floor).[16] The preoperative PSG therefore has the potential to influence perioperative care, specifically with regards to appropriating surgical location and same-day discharge decisions. In the absence of formal PSG testing, providers should discuss the severity of OSA with the surgeon to determine the appropriate plan for postoperative disposition. However, the presence of OSA alone has been correlated with difficulty during anesthetic induction. A number of children with the OSA phenotype are obese,[17] and obesity is correlated with difficult intubation.[18] This may at least partially explain this finding. Furthermore, PSG indices are not robust indicators of end-organ sequelae from the primary disease. In a retrospective analysis, the authors studied whether PSG indices could be applied to predict neurocognitive symptomatology. PSG parameters alone were not able to predict neurocognitive symptoms[19] suggests that there are other factors, such as temporality or other insults, which contribute to this disease consequence.

Residual OSA and Implementation of Drug-Induced Sleep Endoscopy

Despite treatment with AT, many pediatric patients experience postoperative residual OSA. In nonsyndromic children, the prevalence of residual disease can be around 38%, with the incidence varying based on age, OSA severity, and obesity.[20-22] Those with craniofacial anomalies and syndromic OSA have a greater incidence of continued disease burden. This observation of continued disease suggests an alternate site of obstruction within the upper airway necessitating additional evaluation.[23]

Drug-induced sleep endoscopy (DISE) is a common technique used by otorhinolaryngologists (ORL) to inspect the airway for sites of anatomical obstruction. The ORL surgeon uses a nasopharyngoscopy of short video fiber-optic scope, most commonly using the VOTE and SERS scores and including inspection of the nasal airway, nasopharynx, velum, oropharynx, hypopharynx, arytenoids, tongue base, and epiglottis.[24,25] The airway is scored based on the degree of anterolateral or circumferential collapse observed. The major issue with anesthetic management of DISE is that most anesthetics uniformly create some degree of airway collapse, whether intravenous or inhalational.[26-29] However, the degree to which the airway is affected is based on the drug used and often the concentration used. Given that commonly used anesthetic agents can affect the findings of these studies, the authors have published a very simple regimen that is useful in these patients **(Box 1)**.[30]

Additionally, a swivel adapter on the anesthesia mask can provide varying levels of CPAP under direct observation of the airway to observe the dynamic effect on the airway itself.[31] The anesthetic conduct can

> **BOX 1:** Texas children protocol: Drug-induced sleep endoscopy.
>
> **Texas children's protocol: Drug-induced sleep endoscopy**
> - Inhalational induction with maintenance of spontaneous ventilation
> - Intravenous line placement
> - Once deep sedation achieved, reduce sevoflurane concentration to minimal concentration needed to perform DISE, (approx. 0.7–1.2 MAC). Consider passing nasal suction prior to DISE to assess anesthetic depth
> - If patient is insufficiently sedated, deepen anesthetic using sevoflurane then reduce concentration to minimal concentration needed to perform DISE
> - Continue endoscopy—if insufficiently sedated; administer 0.1 mg/kg of midazolam (maximum 2 mg)
> - Continue endoscopy—if insufficiently sedated; administer dexmedetomidine 0.25 µg/kg—titrated slowly
> - Continue endoscopy—if insufficiently sedated; administer additional dexmedetomidine 0,25 µg/kg boluses titrated to effect while watching HR/NIBP
> - Use glycopyrrolate are 0.02 mg/kg for bradycardia that may occur
> - Continue endoscopy—if insufficiently sedated; administer 1 mg/kg of ketamine—may repeat as needed
>
> **General considerations**
> - Consider oxygen blow-by using mask or orally placed endotracheal tube
> - Patient should be supine with neck in neutral position. Airway maneuvers should be minimized
> - Use of oral/nasal airway, continuous positive pressure (if using swivel adapter) should not be performed as this may result in false negative findings
> - Perform jaw thrust when instructed by surgeon, to evaluate obstruction with and without law thrust maneuver
> - Consult preoperative polysomnography study for the SpO_2 nadir which should be the lower boundary of desaturation tolerated during the procedure

highly impact DISE findings with oversedation resulting in false-positive findings of airway obstruction that does not occur during normal sleep versus accidental support of the airway with jaw thrust or a neck roll that may result in false-negative findings due to the support that is not present during normal sleep.

General anesthesia is architecturally dissimilar to mammalian sleep, as demonstrated by EEG.[32] There have been numerous radiological assays, which have been advanced to recapitulate sleeping airway dynamics.[33,34] There has been a trend toward presurgical airway evaluation using a DISE, especially in high-risk patients (e.g., obese or syndromic).[35,36] Additionally, postAT DISE has been used to identify residual areas of obstruction for high-risk patients or those with residual OSA. DISE has been proposed by several investigators to preoperatively to guide surgical therapy as well as to manage postoperative expectations regarding residual disease (or none).[24,37,38] Comparing preoperative PSG CPAP values and PEEP intraoperatively from

DISE demonstrated significant disparities.[31] This suggests that laboratory PSG studies underestimate the CPAP needed to maintain airway patency during sleep.

Anesthetic Pharmacology for Children with OSA

Several drugs have been studied in AT in children. Dexamethasone has been evaluated in several studies and reduces several postoperative sequelae, including pain, nausea, and vomiting, without increasing the rate of postoperative hemorrhage.[39-42] Dexmedetomidine is a commonly utilized adjunct for patients with OSA undergoing AT. Dexmedetomidine confers some analgesia and also helps reduce anesthetic requirements without increasing postoperative respiratory complications. Dexmedetomidine reduces emergence agitation/delirium incidence after sevoflurane-based anesthesia.[43,44] A randomized trial of dose-related effects (0.5 µg/kg vs. 1.0 µg/kg) demonstrated equal efficacy between both groups.[45]

Dexmedetomidine does not increase postoperative bradycardia.[46] Furthermore, the intraoperative hemodynamic profile of patients who received even a single dose of dexmedetomidine was quite favorable.[47] When compared against tramadol, dexmedetomidine was associated with a longer time to tracheal extubation. However, it had fewer respiratory complications on tracheal extubation and in the immediate postoperative period.[48] There also is one study demonstrating that early administration of dexmedetomidine is more beneficial at preventing emergence agitation compared to late administration.[49] However, dexmedetomidine does not change overall opioid consumption.[50]

Ketamine has also been shown in several studies to decrease opioid usage and facilitate postoperative pain relief. A meta-analysis found that ketamine administered during tonsillectomy provided some postoperative pain relief. There was clinical trial heterogeneity,[51] making it difficult to extrapolate these studies into practice. A comparison of ropivacaine alone versus ketamine/ropivacaine injected directly into the tonsillar fossa. While there was an immediate analgesic benefit, at 24 hour postoperatively, the ketamine/ropivacaine group utilized more postoperative analgesia.[52] However, the ketamine has to be administered intravenously rather than by direct infiltration.[53] A similar effect was found in a study comparing intravenous ketamine alone versus intravenous ketamine/acetaminophen with decreased pain scores 6 hours after surgery. However, the groups converged with regards to analgesic use at 12 hours.[54]

Nonsteroidal anti-inflammatory drugs (NSAIDs) have been long used for pediatric AT surgery, and the ones commonly used (paracetamol and ibuprofen) appear to be safe in conventional dosages. Opioids in addition to NSAIDs seem to confer no additional benefit, as demonstrated by parental surverys.[55] The combination of ibuprofen and paracetamol has been demonstrated to be equianalgesic to morphin;[56,57] however, increased doses of ibuprofen seem to confer little additional benefit.[58] Ibuprofen seems to be superior to paracetamol as a standalone analgesic.[59]

Morphine use has been associated with a prolonged length of stay following AT in children with OSA.[60] Furthermore, the metabolism of morphine is altered with both obesity and the presence of OSA,[61] and since these often overlap this makes morphine pharmacokinetics somewhat unpredictable. Specific genotypes, including the OCT1 and ABCC3 genotypes, may play a significant role in morphine pharmacokinetics, but their overall effects are far from clear now and further pharmacogenomic work is necessary.[62-64]

Codeine has raised concern following a number of postoperative pediatric mortalities.[65] Codeine is a prodrug converted by the cytochrome P450-2D6 system to an analog of morphine that provides analgesia. A small but unknown percentage of the population has a 2D6 genetic polymorphism resulting in faster conversion of codeine to morphine **(Fig. 2)**, some of them being labeled as "ultra-rapid metabolizers." This resulted in a black box

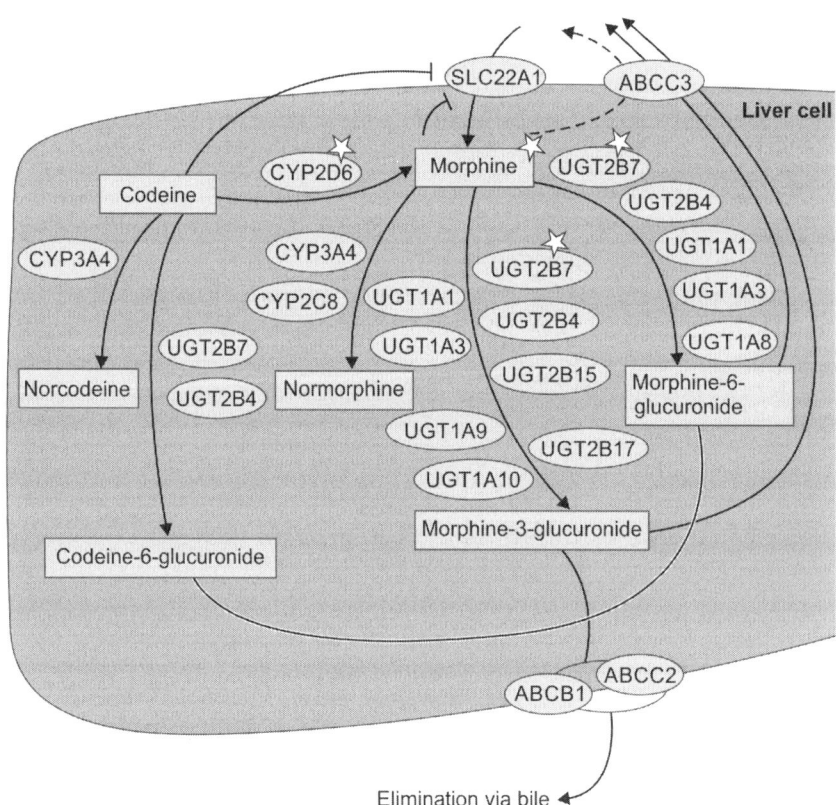

Fig. 2: Conversion of codeine to morphine.
Source: With permission under Creative Commons. Pharm GKB.

warning from the United States Food and Drug Administration on codeine and drastically reduced postoperative opioid prescriptions.[66] The ultrarapid polymorphism of CYP2D6 affects most oral opioids (including oxycodone, hydrocodone, and tramadol) in children.[67] However, to date, we could not locate specific studies in Indian children on the effect of polymorphisms on opioid pharmacokinetics. However, given the severe impact of codeine on children with this polymorphism, we recommend against its use in children.

Perioperative Complications in Children with OSA

Obstructive sleep apnea severity has direct bearing on the perioperative course in children undoing AT. However, this does not seem to be true with an NSQIP study of laryngeal surgery patients with OSA,[68] suggesting that surgery type has a significant effect on postoperative outcomes. OSA severity has been shown to lead to an increase in postoperative respiratory complications, particularly for children with an AHI ≥5 events/hour and oxygen saturation nadir ≤80% on preoperative polysomnography.[69] This effect has been substantiated in more recent studies of extreme or severe OSA, demonstrating a higher incidence of postoperative adverse events.[70] These patients are generally admitted, as postoperative oxygen desaturations require continuous overnight pulse oximetry.[71] Statham et al., examined 3,404 patients under 6 years of age with clinically diagnosed OSA undergoing AT. They identified a two-fold increased risk of postoperative respiratory complications after AT in patients younger than 3 years compared with patients aged 3–5 years (9.8 vs. 4.9%).[72] Furthermore, the diagnosis of severe OSA (AHI >10) has been associated with more difficult induction of anesthesia.[73] While perioperative mortality from AT is still rare, children less than 14 kg are at greater risk for significant perioperative respiratory complications.[74] This was further demonstrated by a recent single-center study demonstrating that a higher AHI in young children required greater postoperative respiratory intervention, although the number was still low.[75]

While the immediate postoperative complication rate remains low, there can be events after the 2-hour window.[76] Postoperative disposition notwithstanding, the rates of both major and minor pulmonary complications are greater in children with severe OSA[77,78] and require deliberate patient evaluation in the context of comorbidities. Furthermore, concomitant cardiac disease and other airway anomalies are independent predictors of perioperative respiratory adverse events.[69]

■ CONCLUSION

Pediatric OSA is very different from its adult phenotype in presentation, heterogeneity, and therapy. Variations in pharmacological dosing of common medications require judicious planning, as medication effects may vary greatly across different pediatric populations and OSA types. However, there is much work to be done on this front. DISE is being increasingly adopted to guide therapy, particularly in high-risk children with multiple sites of obstruction.

REFERENCES

1. Yuen KM, Pelayo R. Socioeconomic impact of pediatric sleep disorders. Sleep Med Clin. 2017;12:23-30.
2. Chandrakantan A, Musso MF, Floyd T, Adler AC. Pediatric obstructive sleep apnea: preoperative and neurocognitive considerations for perioperative management. Paediatr Anaesth. 2020;30(5):529-36.
3. Don DM, Geller KA, Koempel JA, Ward SD. Age specific differences in pediatric obstructive sleep apnea. Int J Pediatr Otorhinolaryngol. 2009;73:1025-8.
4. Chan KC, Au CT, Hui LL, Ng SK, Wing YK, Li AM. How OSA evolves from childhood to young adulthood: natural history from a 10-year follow-up study. Chest. 2019;156:120-30.
5. Chandrasekar I, Tablizo MA, Witmans M, Cruz JM, Cummins M, Estrellado-Cruz W. Obstructive sleep apnea in neonates. Children (Basel). 2022;9(3):419.
6. Patinkin ZW, Feinn R, Santos M. Metabolic consequences of obstructive sleep apnea in adolescents with obesity: a systematic literature review and meta-analysis. Child Obes 2017;13:102-10.
7. Bin-Hasan S, Katz S, Nugent Z, Nehme J, Lu Z, Khayat A, et al. Prevalence of obstructive sleep apnea among obese toddlers and preschool children. Sleep Breath. 2018;22:511-5.
8. Keefe KR, Patel PN, Levi JR. The shifting relationship between weight and pediatric obstructive sleep apnea: a historical review. Laryngoscope. 2018;129(10):2414-19.
9. Tan HL, Kheirandish-Gozal L, Gozal D. Obstructive sleep apnea in children: update on the recognition, treatment and management of persistent disease. Expert Rev Respir Med. 2016;10:431-9.
10. Feng J, Wu Q, Zhang D, Chen BY. Hippocampal impairments are associated with intermittent hypoxia of obstructive sleep apnea. Chin Med J (Engl). 2012;125:696-701.
11. Lambert HK, Peverill M, Sambrook KA, Rosen ML, Sheridan MA, McLaughlin KA. Altered development of hippocampus-dependent associative learning following early-life adversity. Dev Cogn Neurosci. 2019;38:100666.
12. Chandrakantan A, Adler AC, Tohsun M, Kheradamand F, Ray RS, Roth S. Intermittent hypoxia and effects on early learning/memory: exploring the hippocampal cellular effects of pediatric obstructive sleep apnea. Anesth Analg. 2020;133(1):93-103.
13. Chandrakantan A, Adler AC. Pediatric obstructive sleep apnea and neurocognition. Anesthesiol Clin. 2020;38:693-707.
14. Roland PS, Rosenfeld RM, Brooks LJ, Friedman NR, Jones J, Kim TW, et al., American Academy of O-H, Neck Surgery F. Clinical practice guideline: polysomnography for sleep-disordered breathing prior to tonsillectomy in children. Otolaryngol Head Neck Surg. 2011;145:S1-15.

15. Alsuhebani M, Walia H, Miller R, Elmaraghy C, Tumin D, Tobias JD, et al. Overnight inpatient admission and revisit rates after pediatric adenotonsillectomy. Ther Clin Risk Manag. 2019;15:689-99.
16. Adler AC, Leung S, Lee BH, Dubow SR. Preparing your pediatric patients and their families for the operating room: reducing fear of the unknown. Pediatr Rev. 2018;39:13-26.
17. Kang KT, Weng WC, Lee PL, Hsu WC. Age- and gender-related characteristics in pediatric obstructive sleep apnea. Pediatr Pulmonol. 2022;57(6):1520-26.
18. Yakushiji H, Goto T, Shirasaka W, Hagiwara Y, Watase H, Okamoto H, et al., Japanese Emergency Medicine Network i. Associations of obesity with tracheal intubation success on first attempt and adverse events in the emergency department: An analysis of the multicenter prospective observational study in Japan. PLoS One. 2018;13:e0195938.
19. Chandrakantan A, Patel D, Glaun M, Mehta D, Musso MF, Patel A, Adler AC. Polysomnography in children with obstructive sleep apnoea and neurocognitive disorders. Clin Otolaryngol. 2020;45(6):885-88.
20. Coutras SW, Limjuco A, Davis KE, Carr MM. Sleep endoscopy findings in children with persistent obstructive sleep apnea after adenotonsillectomy. Int J Pediatr Otorhinolaryngol. 2018;107:190-3.
21. Lee CH, Hsu WC, Chang WH, Lin MT, Kang KT. Polysomnographic findings after adenotonsillectomy for obstructive sleep apnoea in obese and non-obese children: a systematic review and meta-analysis. Clin Otolaryngol. 2016;41:498-510.
22. Imanguli M, Ulualp SO. Risk factors for residual obstructive sleep apnea after adenotonsillectomy in children. Laryngoscope. 2016;126:2624-9.
23. Wilcox LJ, Bergeron M, Reghunathan S, Ishman SL. An updated review of pediatric drug-induced sleep endoscopy. Laryngoscope Investig Otolaryngol. 2017;2:423-31.
24. Lam DJ, Weaver EM, Macarthur CJ, Milczuk HA, O'Neill E, Smith TL, et al. Assessment of pediatric obstructive sleep apnea using a drug-induced sleep endoscopy rating scale. Laryngoscope. 2016;126:1492-8.
25. Kezirian EJ, Hohenhorst W, de Vries N. Drug-induced sleep endoscopy: the VOTE classification. Eur Arch Otorhinolaryngol. 2011;268:1233-6.
26. Mishima G, Sanuki T, Sato S, Kobayashi M, Kurata S, Ayuse T. Upper-airway collapsibility and compensatory responses under moderate sedation with ketamine, dexmedetomidine, and propofol in healthy volunteers. Physiol Rep. 2020;8:e14439.
27. Crawford MW, Arrica M, Macgowan CK, Yoo SJ. Extent and localization of changes in upper airway caliber with varying concentrations of sevoflurane in children. Anesthesiology. 2006;105:1147-52; discussion 5A.
28. Eastwood PR, Platt PR, Shepherd K, Maddison K, Hillman DR. Collapsibility of the upper airway at different concentrations of propofol anesthesia. Anesthesiology. 2005;103:470-7.
29. Eastwood PR, Szollosi I, Platt PR, Hillman DR. Collapsibility of the upper airway during anesthesia with isoflurane. Anesthesiology. 2002;97:786-93.
30. Adler AC, Musso MF, Mehta DK, Chandrakantan A. Pediatric drug induced sleep endoscopy: a simple sedation recipe. Ann Otol Rhinol Laryngol. 2019:3489419892292.

31. Adler AC, Chandrakantan A, Musso MF. Continuous positive airway pressure titration during pediatric drug induced sleep endoscopy. Ann Otol Rhinol Laryngol. 2021:34894211055527.
32. Akeju O, Brown EN. Neural oscillations demonstrate that general anesthesia and sedative states are neurophysiologically distinct from sleep. Curr Opin Neurobiol. 2017;44:178-85.
33. Kreuzer I, Osthaus WA, Schultz A, Schultz B. Influence of the sevoflurane concentration on the occurrence of epileptiform EEG patterns. PLoS One. 2014;9:e89191.
34. von Ungern-Sternberg BS, Saudan S, Petak F, Hantos Z, Habre W. Desflurane but not sevoflurane impairs airway and respiratory tissue mechanics in children with susceptible airways. Anesthesiology. 2008;108:216-24.
35. Lennon CJ, Wang RY, Wallace A, Chinnadurai S. Risk of failure of adenotonsillectomy for obstructive sleep apnea in obese pediatric patients. Int J Pediatr Otorhinolaryngol. 2017;92:7-10.
36. Chan DK, Jan TA, Koltai PJ. Effect of obesity and medical comorbidities on outcomes after adjunct surgery for obstructive sleep apnea in cases of adenotonsillectomy failure. Arch Otolaryngol Head Neck Surg. 2012;138:891-6.
37. Lam DJ, Krane NA, Mitchell RB. Relationship between drug-induced sleep endoscopy findings, tonsil size, and polysomnographic outcomes of adenotonsillectomy in children. Otolaryngol Head Neck Surg. 2019;161:507-13.
38. He S, Peddireddy NS, Smith DF, Duggins AL, Heubi C, Shott SR, et al. Outcomes of drug-induced sleep endoscopy-directed surgery for pediatric obstructive sleep apnea. Otolaryngol Head Neck Surg. 2018;158:559-65.
39. Yiu Y, Mahida JB, Cooper JN, Elsey NM, Deans KJ, Minneci PC, et al. The effect of perioperative dexamethasone dosing on post-tonsillectomy hemorrhage risk. Int J Pediatr Otorhinolaryngol. 2017;98:19-24.
40. Bellis JR, Pirmohamed M, Nunn AJ, Loke YK, De S, Golder S, et al. Dexamethasone and haemorrhage risk in paediatric tonsillectomy: a systematic review and meta-analysis. Br J Anaesth. 2014;113:23-42.
41. Gallagher TQ, Hill C, Ojha S, Ference E, Keamy DG, Williams M, et al. Perioperative dexamethasone administration and risk of bleeding following tonsillectomy in children: a randomized controlled trial. JAMA. 2012;308:1221-6.
42. Windfuhr JP, Chen YS, Propst EJ, Guldner C. The effect of dexamethasone on post-tonsillectomy nausea, vomiting and bleeding. Braz J Otorhinolaryngol. 2011;77:373-9.
43. Shi M, Miao S, Gu T, Wang D, Zhang H, Liu J. Dexmedetomidine for the prevention of emergence delirium and postoperative behavioral changes in pediatric patients with sevoflurane anesthesia: a double-blind, randomized trial. Drug Des Devel Ther. 2019;13:897-905.
44. Zhang YZ, Wang X, Wu JM, Song CY, Cui XG. Optimal dexmedetomidine dose to prevent emergence agitation under sevoflurane and remifentanil anesthesia during pediatric tonsillectomy and adenoidectomy. Front Pharmacol. 2019;10:1091.
45. Yi W, Li J, Zhuang Y, Wan L, Li W, Jia J. The effect of two different doses of dexmedetomidine to prevent emergence agitation in children undergoing adenotonsillectomy: a randomized controlled trial. Braz J Anesthesiol. 2022;72:63-8.

46. Bush B, Tobias JD, Lin C, Ruda J, Jatana KR, Essig G, et al. Postoperative bradycardia following adenotonsillectomy in children: Does intraoperative administration of dexmedetomidine play a role? Int J Pediatr Otorhinolaryngol. 2018;104:210-5.
47. Sharma K, Kumar M, Gandhi R. Effect of single-dose dexmedetomidine on intraoperative hemodynamics and postoperative recovery during pediatric adenotonsillectomy. Anesth Essays Res. 2019;13:63-7.
48. Koceroglu I, Devrim S, Bingol Tanriverdi T, Gura Celik M. The effects of dexmedetomidine and tramadol on post-operative pain and agitation, and extubation quality in paediatric patients undergoing adenotonsillectomy surgery: a randomized trial. J Clin Pharm Ther. 2020;45:340-6.
49. Sadeghi A, Sajad Razavi S, Eghbali A, Alireza Mahdavi S, Kimia F, Panah A. The comparison of the efficacy of early versus late administration of dexmedetomidine on postoperative emergence agitation in children undergoing oral surgeries: a randomized clinical trial. Iran J Med Sci. 2022;47:25-32.
50. Adler AC, Daszkowski A, Tan JC, Poliner AD, Wei EZ, Nathanson BH, et al. The association of dexmedetomidine on perioperative opioid consumption in children undergoing adenotonsillectomy with and without obstructive sleep apnea. Anesth Analg. 2021;133:1260-8.
51. Cho HK, Kim KW, Jeong YM, Lee HS, Lee YJ, Hwang SH. Efficacy of ketamine in improving pain after tonsillectomy in children: meta-analysis. PLoS One. 2014;9:e101259.
52. Hong B, Lim CS, Kim YH, Lee JU, Kim YM, Jung C, et al. Comparison of topical ropivacaine with and without ketamine on post-surgical pain in children undergoing tonsillectomy: a randomized controlled double-blind study. J Anesth. 2017;31:559-64.
53. Caixeta JAS, Sampaio JCS, da Costa PSS, Avelino MAG. Analgesia for adenotonsillectomy in children: a comparison between peritonsillar infiltration of tramadol, ketamine, and placebo. Eur Arch Otorhinolaryngol. 2020;277:1815-22.
54. Kimiaei Asadi H, Nikooseresht M, Noori L, Behnoud F. The effect of administration of ketamine and paracetamol versus paracetamol singly on postoperative pain, nausea and vomiting after pediatric adenotonsillectomy. Anesth Pain Med. 2016;6:e31210.
55. Adler AC, Mehta DK, Messner AH, Salemi JL, Chandrakantan A. Parental assessment of pain control following pediatric adenotonsillectomy: do opioids make a difference? Int J Pediatr Otorhinolaryngol. 2020;134:110045.
56. Kelly LE, Sommer DD, Ramakrishna J, Hoffbauer S, Arbab-Tafti S, Reid D, et al. Morphine or Ibuprofen for post-tonsillectomy analgesia: a randomized trial. Pediatrics. 2015;135:307-13.
57. Playne R, Anderson BJ, Frampton C, Stanescu I, Atkinson HC. Analgesic effectiveness, pharmacokinetics, and safety of a paracetamol/ibuprofen fixed-dose combination in children undergoing adenotonsillectomy: a randomized, single-blind, parallel group trial. Paediatr Anaesth. 2018;28:1087-95.
58. Hannam JA, Anderson BJ, Potts A. Acetaminophen, ibuprofen, and tramadol analgesic interactions after adenotonsillectomy. Paediatr Anaesth. 2018;28:841-51.

59. Mirashrafi F, Tavakolnejad F, Amirzargar B, Abasi A, Amali A. Effect of paracetamol versus ibuprofen in adenotonsillectomy. Iran J Otorhinolaryngol. 2021;33:355-9.
60. O'Brien DC, Desai Y, Schubart J, Swanson RT, Chung S, Parekh U, et al. Effect of intra-op morphine on children with OSA undergoing tonsillectomy. Int J Pediatr Otorhinolaryngol 2019;125:141-6.
61. Dalesio NM, Lee CKK, Hendrix CW, Kerns N, Hsu A, Clarke W, et al. Effects of Obstructive sleep apnea and obesity on morphine pharmacokinetics in children. Anesth Analg. 2019.
62. Hahn D, Fukuda T, Euteneuer JC, Mizuno T, Vinks AA, Sadhasivam S, et al. Influence of MRP3 genetics and hepatic expression ontogeny for morphine disposition in neonatal and pediatric patients. J Clin Pharmacol. 2020;60: 992-8.
63. Hahn D, Emoto C, Euteneuer JC, Mizuno T, Vinks AA, Fukuda T. Influence of OCT1 ontogeny and genetic variation on morphine disposition in critically ill neonates: lessons from PBPK modeling and clinical study. Clin Pharmacol Ther. 2019;105:761-8.
64. Emoto C, Johnson TN, Neuhoff S, Hahn D, Vinks AA, Fukuda T. PBPK model of morphine incorporating developmental changes in hepatic OCT1 and UGT2B7 proteins to explain the variability in clearances in neonates and small infants. CPT Pharmacometrics Syst Pharmacol. 2018;7:464-73.
65. Kelly LE, Rieder M, van den Anker J, Malkin B, Ross C, Neely MN, et al. More codeine fatalities after tonsillectomy in North American children. Pediatrics. 2012;129:e1343-7.
66. Goldman JL, Ziegler C, Burckardt EM. Otolaryngology practice patterns in pediatric tonsillectomy: the impact of the codeine boxed warning. Laryngoscope. 2018;128:264-8.
67. Balyan R, Mecoli M, Venkatasubramanian R, Chidambaran V, Kamos N, Clay S, et al. CYP2D6 pharmacogenetic and oxycodone pharmacokinetic association study in pediatric surgical patients. Pharmacogenomics. 2017;18:337-48.
68. Kuo CC, Elrakhawy M, Carr MM. Children undergoing laryngeal surgery for obstructive sleep apnea: NSQIP analysis of length of stay, readmissions, and reoperations. Ann Otol Rhinol Laryngol. 2022:34894221078366.
69. Katz SL, Monsour A, Barrowman N, Hoey L, Bromwich M, Momoli F, et al. Predictors of postoperative respiratory complications in children undergoing adenotonsillectomy. J Clin Sleep Med. 2020;16:41-8.
70. Mills TG, Bhattacharjee R, Nation J, Ewing E, Lesser DJ. Management and outcome of extreme pediatric obstructive sleep apnea. Sleep Med. 2021;87:138-42.
71. Keamy DG, Chhabra KR, Hartnick CJ. Predictors of complications following adenotonsillectomy in children with severe obstructive sleep apnea. Int J Pediatr Otorhinolaryngol. 2015;79:1838-41.
72. Statham MM, Elluru RG, Buncher R, Kalra M. Adenotonsillectomy for obstructive sleep apnea syndrome in young children: prevalence of pulmonary complications. Arch Otolaryngol Head Neck Surg. 2006;132:476-80.
73. Kang KT, Chang IS, Tseng CC, Weng WC, Hsiao TY, Lee PL, et al. Impacts of disease severity on postoperative complications in children with sleep-disordered breathing. Laryngoscope. 2017;127:2646-52.

74. Baijal RG, Bidani SA, Minard CG, Watcha MF. Perioperative respiratory complications following awake and deep extubation in children undergoing adenotonsillectomy. Paediatr Anaesth. 2015;25:392-9.
75. Billings KR, Somani SN, Lavin J, Bhushan B. Polysomnography variables associated with postoperative respiratory issues in children <3 years of age undergoing adenotonsillectomy for obstructive sleep apnea. Int J Pediatr Otorhinolaryngol. 2020;137:110215.
76. Ekstein M, Zac L, Schvartz R, Goren O, Weiniger CF, DeRowe A, et al. Respiratory complications after adenotonsillectomy in high-risk children with obstructive sleep apnea: a retrospective cohort study. Acta Anaesthesiol Scand. 2020;64:292-300.
77. Cote CJ, Posner KL, Domino KB. Death or neurologic injury after tonsillectomy in children with a focus on obstructive sleep apnea: Houston, we have a problem! Anesth Analg. 2014;118:1276-83.
78. Hill CA, Litvak A, Canapari C, Cummings B, Collins C, Keamy DG, et al. A pilot study to identify pre- and peri-operative risk factors for airway complications following adenotonsillectomy for treatment of severe pediatric OSA. Int J Pediatr Otorhinolaryngol. 2011;75:1385-90.

CHAPTER 6

Assessment of Functional Capacity

Gautam Khanna

ABSTRACT

Assessing functional capacity or exercise tolerance is an essential component of risk determination for a patient undergoing surgery. Patients with poor functional capacity have high perioperative morbidity and mortality. Identifying such patients allows referring them for additional cardiovascular testing and optimization of their comorbidities before intermediate or high-risk surgery. This helps mitigate their perioperative risk.

There are a variety of tests, both objective and subjective, which help us to identify patients and categorize them into various risk categories. This helps them make an informed decision regarding their care.

The aim of this chapter is to familiarize the reader with the advantages and pitfalls of the tests available.

Keywords: Metabolic equivalents (METs); Maximal oxygen uptake (VO_2 max); Peak oxygen uptake (VO_2 peak); Anaerobic threshold (AT); VE/VCO_2.

KEY POINTS

- Unstructured assessment of patient functional status through history taking of activities of daily living poorly correlates with functional capacity and postoperative outcomes.
- Dukes activity severity index score of <34 can predict poor surgical outcomes with good sensitivity but poor specificity.
- A 6-minute walk test is a poor predictor of surgical outcomes due to its limited use and lack of clearly defined endpoints.
- An incremental shuttle walk distance <250 m can point toward high 30-day mortality after major colorectal surgery, and hence warrants further evaluation.
- Cardiopulmonary Exercise Testing remains the gold standard for assessment of functional capacity, and a VO_2 peak >14–15 mL/kg/min, anaerobic threshold (AT) >11 mL/kg/min, and VE/VCO_2 at AT 41–42 mL/kg/min predicts good functional capacity.

INTRODUCTION

The main aim of a functional capacity assessment is to assess whether a patient has the physiological reserve capacity to undergo a surgical procedure safely without any untoward complications. Functional capacity reflects responses of cardiovascular, circulatory, pulmonary, neuromuscular, and hematological systems to standard stress.

Functional capacity is the maximum physical activity an individual can undertake, defined by maximal oxygen uptake (VO_2 max). Maximal oxygen uptake is the point at which the oxygen uptake reaches a plateau despite increasing the workload. However, the VO_2 plateau, which occurs at maximal exercise, may not always be seen (on the graph) hence instead, the VO_2 peak is used. VO_2 peak is the oxygen uptake at the best effort.[1]

One standard method of assessing functional capacity is metabolic equivalents (METs) quantification. The higher the METs, the higher the functional capacity. One MET is defined as resting metabolic rate, i.e., the amount of oxygen consumed at rest (3.5 mL O_2/kg/min, 1.2 Kcal/min for a 70-kg person).[2] Guidelines recommend using METs to measure exercise intensities (light, <3.0 METs; moderate, 3.0–5.9 METs; vigorous, ≥6.0 METs).[3]

The routine use of METs in preoperative assessments has enabled us to predict and risk stratify patients at an increased risk of perioperative complications. It is well-known that patients with low METs are at an increased risk of perioperative morbidity and mortality. It is imperative to perform an accurate assessment of METs in our routine preoperative checkups. Patients who cannot perform 4 METs should be thoroughly evaluated with a multidisciplinary approach, and risks of poor surgical outcomes need to be discussed with the patient.[4]

The most common way of assessing functional capacity in routine clinical practice is by taking a history of a patient's general activity. Based on the history, the interviewer makes a subjective assessment of the patient's functional capacity. The challenge faced in this approach is that the subjective assessment does not accurately estimate the patient's actual exercise capacity. A multicenter, international, and prospective cohort study of patients undergoing major noncardiac surgery and subjective assessment (estimation of METs by history taking) reported a very poor correlation between it and postoperative death and myocardial infarction (MI). Instead, Duke activity status index (DASI) score is currently the recommended questionnaire to assess functional capacity before noncardiac surgery. It is known to have better reliability in predicting perioperative outcomes.[5,6]

Dukes Activity Severity Index

Dukes activity severity index score involves following a 12-item questionnaire in which patients report their ability to perform everyday physical tasks or exercises that have been described below. Each of the tasks is given points and the sum of the points. Points from the "YES" answers give the final DASI score. The DASI score ranges from 0 to 58.2 points.

Each question in the DASI questionnaire is assigned a weighting based on the known metabolic cost of that activity.

- Can you take care of yourself (eating, dressing, bathing, or using the toilet)? (2.75)
- Can you walk indoors, such as around your house? (1.75)
- Can you walk a block or two on level ground? (2.75)
- Can you climb a flight of stairs or walk up a hill? (5.50)
- Can you run a short distance? (8.00)
- Can you do light work around the house, such as dusting or washing dishes? (2.70)
- Can you do moderate work around the house, such as vacuuming, sweeping floors, or carrying groceries? (3.50)
- Can you do yard work such as raking leaves, weeding, or pushing a power mower? (4.50)
- Can you have sexual relations? (5.25)
- Can you participate in moderate recreational activities such as golf, bowling, dancing, doubles tennis, or throwing a baseball or football? (6.00)
- Can you participate in strenuous sports such as swimming, singles tennis, football, basketball, or skiing? (7.50)
- The DASI score equals the sum of weightings from "YES" replies.

A formula converts the final DASI score to estimate the VO_2 peak and then METs.

$$VO_2 \text{ peak (mL/kg/min)} = (0.43 \times \text{DASI score}) + 9.6$$
$$\text{Estimated METs} = (0.43 \times \text{DASI score}) + 9.6$$

Studies have attempted to establish a threshold for DASI. It has been shown that self-reported functional capacity with DASI scores of 34 or higher were associated with:

- Reduced chances of 30-day death or myocardial injury.
- Reduced odds of 1-year death or new disability.

Self-reported DASI scores of below 34 were associated with:

- Increased odds of 30-day death or MI
- Moderate-to-severe complications.[7]

The problem with the DASI score is that the formula that uses the DASI score to estimate METs is inaccurate. The METs study found that patients with a DASI score of 34 had an overestimation of METs by a factor of 2.[8]

The American Heart Association (AHA) uses the DASI-based formula to calculate METs (less than METs) for further cardiac evaluation of patients undergoing noncardiac surgery. This would erroneously lead to patients with poor functional capacity being classified as fit for surgery without further cardiac evaluation.

Six-minute Walk Test

The six-minute walking test (6MWT) was developed by the American Thoracic Society, and it was officially introduced in 2002.[9]

The 6MWT is an exercise test used to assess the functional capacity. In this test, the patient is expected to walk for 6 minutes, and the distance covered over 6 minutes is used to assess the functional capacity. Variables observed in 6MWT include distance covered, oxygen saturation, heart rate, modified Borg dyspnea scale, and leg fatigue. Leg fatigue is also rated using a scale similar to the Borg scale (where 0 is no fatigue, 3 is moderate fatigue, 5 is severe fatigue, 7 is extreme fatigue, and 10 is maximal fatigue). The median 6MWT distance for healthy individuals is between 500 and 600 m **(Box 1)**.[10]

The test had gained popularity due to its ease of use and low cost. Still, the lack of standardization and inability to define cut-off points has limited its use in routine clinical practice in preoperative assessment.

Stair Climbing Test (SCT)

Stair climbing test (SCT) is a first-line functional screening test to select patients who can undergo surgery safely. During the preoperative assessment, patients are asked about their ability to climb two flights of stairs without stopping or experiencing shortness of breath or chest pain. There is a lack of standardization in this test in terms of duration of stair climbing, speed of ascent, number of steps per flight, the height of each step, and the criteria for stopping the test are variable. There are significant inconsistencies over the

---

BOX 1: Modified BORG scale.[10]

0 – No shortness of breath. No oxygen use.
1 – Very slight shortness of breath.
2 – Slight shortness of breath.
3 – Moderate shortness of breath. Able to accomplish MOST OF the normal activities.
4 – Somewhat severe shortness of breath. Able to accomplish normal activities with frequent rest periods.
5 – Severe shortness of breath. Able to accomplish normal activities with frequent rest periods.
6 – Difficulty with normal activities including the use of a bathroom.
7 – Very severe shortness of breath.
8 – UNABLE to do basic activities. Unable to ambulate.
Notify the physician immediately, if:
9 – Very, very severe shortness of breath.
10 – Maximal breathlessness. Oxygen requirement >50%. Acute Respiratory failure.

number of stairs, which correlate to 4 METs in surgical patients; as a result, it is only accepted as a surrogate marker.

However, a study on patients undergoing major abdominal surgery predicted that patients who could climb 12 stairs in 26.5 seconds or more had an increased risk of perioperative complications.[11]

Incremental Shuttle Walk Test (ISWT)

In this test, the patient walks back and forth between two markers set 10 m apart, and the walking speed is increased by 0.17 m/s each minute in a graded fashion, paced by an audio signal. Measurements include the incremental shuttle walk distance (ISWD), heart rate, oxygen saturation, noninvasive systolic and diastolic blood pressures, and modified Borg dyspnea scale. Typical values for the ISWD vary with age but are usually between 560 and 820 m in healthy individuals.[12]

If the patient is too breathless to maintain speed or cannot maintain the pace, or there is any drop in oxygen saturation to less than or equal to 85%, the test is discontinued. A patient unable to complete 25 shuttles (250 m) twice shows a reduced VO_2 max of <10 mL/kg/min.[13] If a patient can complete 400 m on ISWT, then the patient is fit to undergo surgery.[14]

The cut-off points for predicting postoperative complications vary according to the surgery. For example, the threshold for poor surgical outcomes in major colorectal surgery has been quoted as <250.[15] Currently, due to the lack of evidence and limited studies recommending the use of ISWT cut-off points for defining a high-risk surgical patient scheduled for noncardiac surgery, it is suggested that individuals who are unable to achieve >250 m on ISWT should undergo formal functional testing [Cardiopulmonary Exercise Testing (CPET)] to quantify functional capacity.

Stress Testing

Using either exercise stress echocardiography (ESE) or dobutamine stress echocardiography (DSE) may indicate the presence of significant coronary artery disease (CAD) by changing ventricular regional wall motion under stressful conditions. Unlike ESE, DSE is the only surrogate marker of functional capacity. It involves a graded increase in dobutamine infusion to achieve an 85% target heart rate. It provides an assessment of cardiac contractility and left ventricular wall motion abnormalities. It is limited in providing information on respiratory reserve.

These tests have excellent sensitivity in excluding patients with CAD and identify individuals at low risk of postoperative cardiac complications.[15] ESE and DSE (despite being indirect indicators of function status) have a modest ability to predict 30-day perioperative morbidity and mortality.[16]

Cardiopulmonary Exercise Testing

The gold standard method for measuring functional capacity is the maximal rate of oxygen uptake (also known as VO_2 max). VO_2 max is measured during CPET. Maximal oxygen uptake is the point at which the oxygen uptake reaches a plateau despite increasing the workload. Sometimes, the patient suffers fatigue before the plateau is reached. This point is labeled as VO_2 peak and is defined as oxygen uptake at the best effort.[17]

The anaerobic threshold is where oxygen-independent (or "anaerobic") metabolism is required in addition to aerobic metabolism to sustain exercise performance. The anaerobic threshold is where the energy or the ATP is produced via oxygen-independent pathways leading to the generation of pyruvic acid and lactate. The anaerobic thresholds are usually measured by lactate or ventilator thresholds (VT).

There are two defined VTs measured during CPET testing VT1 and VT2. VT1 is also called the first ventilatory threshold. It is a marker of intensity observed in a person's breathing at a point where lactate accumulates in the blood. As the exercise intensity increases, VT1 can be identified when the breathing rate increases. A person at VT1 can no longer talk comfortably—but can still string together a few words—while exercising. Also observed in a person's breathing during exercise is VT2 or the second ventilatory threshold. It is a higher marker of intensity than VT1. At VT2, lactate has accumulated in the blood, and the person needs to breathe heavily. At this rapid rate of breathing, the exerciser can no longer speak. The exercise duration will necessarily decrease due to the intensity level. VT2 can also be called the respiratory compensation threshold (RCT) and the onset of blood lactate accumulation (OBLA).

The ventilatory efficiency at the anaerobic threshold is measured by the ratio of minute ventilation and carbon dioxide production VE/VCO_2 ratio. It is the ratio of the volume of air needed to ventilate 1 L of carbon dioxide in a unit of time. This measures an increase in the respiratory drive as workload increases. A ratio of less than 34 indicates ventilatory inefficiency.[18]

During CPET, the patient must perform an incremental exercise on an upright cycle ergometer while breathing through a mouthpiece. The patient follows a standardized protocol up to limitation by symptoms. The test assesses the integrative exercise responses involving the cardiovascular, pulmonary, and musculoskeletal systems. Data obtained during CPET include heart rate, noninvasive blood pressure, 12-lead ECG, oxygen uptake (VO_2), carbon dioxide production (VCO_2), oxygen saturation, gas flow rates, and work rate.

The CPET testing involves using an exercise machine (static bicycle or a treadmill), and the patient exercises against increasing resistance based on Bruce protocol. Values measured during exercise include peak oxygen

TABLE 1: Absolute and relative contraindications of CPET.

Absolute	Relative
Acute MI (3–5 days)	Left or right main coronary stenosis
Angina at rest	Stenotic valvular heart disease (Moderate)
Symptomatic (chest pain, low BP, dizziness, sweating) uncontrolled arrhythmias	Severe untreated arterial hypertension at rest BP >220
Poorly controlled asthma	Asymptomatic arrhythmias
Syncope	Conduction blocks
Active valvular endocarditis	Hypertrophic cardiomyopathy
Acute myocarditis or pericarditis	Significant pulmonary hypertension
Symptomatic severe aortic stenosis	Advanced or complicated pregnancy
Poorly controlled heart failure	Electrolyte abnormalities
Pulmonary embolus or pulmonary infarction	Orthopedic impairment that compromises exercise performance
Thrombosis of lower extremities	
Dissecting aneurysm	
Respiratory failure	
Room air desaturation at rest SpO_2 ≤85%	
Pulmonary edema	
Acute noncardiopulmonary disorder that may affect exercise performance or be aggravated by exercise (i.e., infection, renal failure, thyrotoxicosis)	

Source: Adapted from ATS/ACCS statement.[8]

consumption (VO_2 peak), power, heart rate, anaerobic threshold (AT), ventilatory thresholds, O_2 uptake slope, O_2 pulse, and heart rate recovery. The three most widely used variables are AT and VO_2 peak and VE/VCO_2 ratio at AT. It is widely accepted that the VO_2 peak of <15 mL/kg/min and an AT of <11 mL/kg/min are associated with a high risk of morbidity and mortality **(Table 1)**.[19] The indications to stop CPET are given in **Box 2**.

■ CONCLUSION

The measures of assessing functional capacity have their benefits and limitations. As a result, assessing functional capacity should involve using more than one method. CPET testing remains the gold standard for assessing functional capacity, but its use is limited by the lack of expertise in interpreting the graph and the equipment needed.

> **BOX 2:** Indications for terminating CPET.
> - Angina pain
> - Ischemic ECG changes (Acute ST changes)
> - Complex ectopic beats
> - Appearance of high degree A-V block (2nd or 3rd)
> - Fall in systolic pressure >20 mm Hg from the highest value of blood pressure taken during the test
> - Hypertension (>250/120 mm Hg)
> - Symptomatic oxygen desaturation (SpO_2 ≤80%)
> - Appearance of pallor
> - Loss of motor coordination
> - Development of an acute confusion also state
> - Feeling of dizziness or faintness
> - Respiratory failure
>
> *Source:* Adapted from ATS/ACC statement.[8]

REFERENCES

1. Older P, Hall A, Hader R. Cardiopulmonary exercise testing as a screening test for perioperative management of major surgery in the elderly. Chest. 1999;116(2):355-62.
2. Jette M, Sidney K. Metabolic Equivalents (METS) in exercise testing, exercise prescription, and evaluation of functional capacity. Clin Cardio. 1990;13:555-56.
3. Haskell WL, Lee IM, Pate RR, Powell KE, Blair SN, Franklin BA, et al. Physical activity and public health: updated recommendation for adults from the American College of Sports Medicine and the American Heart Association. Med Sci Sports Exerc. 2007;39(8):1423-34.
4. Weinstein AS, Sigurdsson MI, Bader AM. Comparison of preoperative assessment of patient's metabolic equivalents (METs) estimated from history versus measured by exercise cardiac stress testing. Anesthesiol Res Pract. 2018;2018:5912726.
5. Wijeysundera DN, Pearse RM, Shulman MA, Abbott TEF, Torres E, Ambosta A, et al., METS study investigators. Assessment of functional capacity before major non-cardiac surgery: an international, prospective cohort study. Lancet. 2018;391(10140):2631-40.
6. Wijeysundera DN, Beattie WS, Hillis GS, Abbott TEF, Shulman MA, Ackland GL, et al. Integration of the Duke Activity Status Index into preoperative risk evaluation: a multicentre prospective cohort study. Br J Anaesth. 2020;124(3):261-70.
7. Riedel B, Li MH, Lee CHA, Ismail H, Cuthbertson BH, Wijeysundera DN, et al., METS Study Investigators. A simplified (modified) Duke Activity Status Index (M-DASI) to characterize functional capacity: a secondary analysis of the Measurement of Exercise Tolerance before Surgery (METS) study. Br J Anaesth. 2021;126:181-90.
8. ATS Committee on Proficiency Standards for Clinical Pulmonary Function Laboratories. ATS statement: guidelines for the six-minute walk test. Am J Respir Crit Care Med. 2002;166(1):111-7.
9. Crisafulli E, Clini E. Measures of dyspnea in pulmonary rehabilitation. Multidiscip Respir Med. 2010;5:202-10.

10. Borg E, Borg G, Larsson K, Letzter M, Sundblad BM. An index for breathlessness and leg fatigue. Scand J Med Sci Sports. 2010;20(4):644-50.
11. Baker S, Waldrop M, Swords J, Wang T, Heslin M, Contreras C, et al. Timed stair-climbing as a surrogate marker for sarcopenia measurements in predicting surgical outcomes. J Gastrointest Surg. 2019;23:2459-65.
12. Harrison SL, Greening N, Houchen-Wolloff L, Bankart J, Morgan MDL, Steiner MC, et al. Age-specific normal values for the incremental shuttle walk test in a healthy British population. J Cardiopulm Rehabil Prev. 2013;33:309-13.
13. Wang J, Olak J, Ultmann RE, Ferguson MK. Assessment of pulmonary complications after lung resection. Ann Thorac Surg. 1999;67:1444-7.
14. Charloux A, Brunelli A, Bolliger CT, Rocco G, Sculier JP, Varela G, et al. Lung function evaluation before surgery in lung cancer patients: How are recent advances put into practice? A survey among members of the European Society of Thoracic Surgeons (ESTS) and of the Thoracic Oncology Section of the European Respiratory Society (ERS) Interact. Cardiovasc Thorac Surg. 2009;9:925-31.
15. Silvapulle E, Darvall J. Subjective methods for preoperative assessment of functional capacity. BJA Educ. 2022;22(7):249-57.
16. Garner K, Pomeroy W, Arnold J. Exercise stress testing: indications and common questions. Am Fam Physician. 2017;96:293-99.
17. Loewen G, Watson D, Kohman L, Herndon JE 2nd, Shennib H, Kernstine K, et al. Preoperative exercise VO_2 measurement for lung resection candidates: Results of Cancer and Leukemia Group B Protocol 9238. J Thorac Oncol. 2007;2:619-25.
18. Mezzani A. Cardiopulmonary exercise testing: basics of methodology and measurements. Ann Am Thorac Soc. 2017;14:S3-11.
19. Colson M, Baglin J, Bolsin S, Grocott M. Cardiopulmonary exercise testing predicts 5 year survival after major surgery. Br J Anaesth. 2012;109:735-41.

CHAPTER

7

Role of Adjuncts for Regional and Neuraxial Anesthesia

Balavenkata Subramanian Jagannathan,
Madhanmohan Chandramohan, Vipin Kumar Goel

ABSTRACT

Ever since local anesthetics were used for regional blocks, the pursuit for finding the ideal local anesthetic drug started, which should have properties such as immediate onset, differential blockade, better safety profile, prolonged analgesia, and anti-inflammatory action. To date, none of the local anesthetic drugs in practice has all the abovesaid properties. These shortcomings of the local anesthetic's pharmacokinetics and pharmacodynamics are managed by various regional anesthetic techniques and the incorporation of a few other classes of drugs. A regional anesthetic technique such as perineural catheter placement is used to prolong the analgesia but placing the catheter and maintenance of drug infusion might not be feasible all the time due to various reasons, and also the possibility of local anesthetic toxicity is a concern. To overcome all these issues, adjuvants are introduced into the clinical practice of regional anesthesia. Adjuvants/additives to local anesthetics are drugs that per se do not have any action akin to local anesthetics but, when administered either systemically or perineurally, prolong the analgesic effect and or reduce the adverse effects. As we come across the literature, many drugs have been tried to improve the safety profile of local anesthetics and also to prolong the analgesia in the postoperative period. We discuss the various adjuvants used in regional anesthesia, their mechanism of action, synergistic effects, adverse effects, and clinical usage in present-day practice.

Keywords: Adjuncts; Adjuvants; Additives; Local anesthetics; Postoperative analgesia.

KEY POINTS

- An ideal local anesthetic (LA) should have differential blockade with prolonged analgesia, devoid of adverse effects, and high therapeutic index.
- Adjuncts/adjuvants to local anesthetic are drugs belonging to various classes with various receptors of action, but clinically used to reduce the LA dose and provide prolonged analgesia.

- Though many classes of drugs are used as adjuncts to LA, their usage is off-label, and none of the adjunct drugs is approved by US Food and Drug Administration (FDA).
- Few adjuvants are used both perineurally as well as intravascularly depending on the class of drug used with clinically comparable efficacy.
- Adjuvants are added to LA in the central neuraxial blocks and peripheral compartment/nerve blocks, depending upon the target structures and effect required.
- Adjuvants to LA can be broadly classified as opioid and non-opioid based on pharmacology; also as adjuvants to neuraxial blockade and adjuvants for a peripheral blockade.
- The discovery of opioid receptors in the peripheral nervous system paved the way to include opioids as an adjunct to LA for peripheral nerve blocks.
- Vasoconstrictors, mainly adrenaline, are used with LA as adjuvant as it causes local vasoconstriction, thereby improving the safety profile of LA and also its toxic doses.
- Alpha-2 agonists, which are mainly used as sedatives, analgesics, and perioperative sympatholytics, are being used as adjuvants to LA with promising prolongation of postoperative analgesia.
- N-methyl-D-aspartate (NMDA) antagonist drugs—ketamine and magnesium—have also been tried as adjuncts to LA as they can reduce peripheral nerve excitability. Still, very limited studies are available to support their efficacy as adjuncts.
- Dexamethasone is a glucocorticoid steroid drug having anti-inflammatory, antiemetic, and analgesic properties, and it is a commonly used additive to LA for its safety profile with prolonged action of nerve blockade.
- Miscellaneous drugs such as midazolam, neostigmine, sodium bicarbonate, and non-steroidal anti-inflammatory drugs (NSAIDs) are used as adjuvants to LA to reduce the onset of action, sedation, and to reduce local inflammatory responses.
- Recently the concept of multimodal perineural adjuvants (MMPNA) has been practiced where more than one adjuvant drug, with different receptors of action, produces more favorable effects.

INTRODUCTION

Regional anesthesia (RA) has evolved in the recent past mainly because of the introduction of equipment such as ultrasound and peripheral nerve stimulators, which have improved the success rates and also relatively reduced the complications of landmark-based procedures. The introduction of newer long-acting local anesthetics (LA) led to the usage of RA not only for the intraoperative period, but also in the postoperative period for analgesia.

We are in such an era that almost any surgical procedure can be provided with some form of regional blocks. So it is very prudent to learn the intricacies of the RA techniques, equipment, and pharmacology of the drugs used in blocks. The best form of analgesia that can be given to a patient during the postoperative period will be regional blocks. To provide that safely and effectively, all the RA providers must know about different LAs, the safety profile of blocks, continuous block techniques, and usage of non-LA drugs to provide regional analgesia. A regional anesthetic technique such as perineural catheter placement is used to prolong the analgesia, but placing the catheter and maintenance of drug infusion might not be feasible all the time due to various reasons. The possibility of local anesthetic toxicity is also a concern.[1] Non-LA drug, which is co-administered as adjuncts in the regional blocks either perineurally or intravenously, acts synergistically with LA to enhance the safety, quality, and efficacy of the blockade.[2] Many different classes of drugs are used as adjuncts to LA in RA for their properties of reducing the onset of the blockade, improving the therapeutic index of the drug, duration, and quality of analgesia. Adjuvant drugs play an important role in postoperative analgesia by increasing the duration significantly, making the primary block provide good pain relief compared to continuous peripheral regional analgesia. Though many drugs have been in wide practice as adjuvants to LA at present, all of them are used off-label and are not Food and Drug Administration (FDA) recommended.[3] We elaborate on adjuvant drugs in the modern practice of RA with their pharmacology and clinical efficacy for providing safe anesthesia and analgesia.

■ CLASSIFICATION

Available Adjuvant drugs can be broadly classified in **Table 1**.

Opioid Adjuvants

Opioid receptors are abundant in the central nervous system, but the peripheral nervous system is devoid of the receptors, and they are transported to the periphery only when inflammation occurs. Opioid receptors and neuropeptides (e.g., substance P) are synthesized in the dorsal root ganglion and transported along intra-axonal microtubules into central and peripheral processes of the primary afferent neuron. The opioid drugs administered will

TABLE 1: Available adjuvant drugs.

Opioid	Nonopioid
Morphine, diamorphine, fentanyl, buprenorphine, tramadol, butorphanol, etc.	α-2 agonists, vasoconstrictor, steroids, non-steroidal anti-inflammatory drugs (NSAIDs), N-methyl-D-aspartate (NMDA) antagonists, midazolam, sodium bicarbonate, and neostigmine.

act both locally and centrally depending upon the route as well as the dose of administration. Peripherally administered opioid drugs produce prolonged analgesia by directly binding at opioid receptors and also by producing centrally mediated action post-systemic absorption.[4] Opioid drugs such as morphine, diamorphine, fentanyl, buprenorphine, and tramadol are used as LA adjuvants mainly in the central neuraxial blockades (CNB). Though they may not prolong the motor blockade of the RA, they may prolong the duration of analgesia by directly inhibiting the receptors in the substantia gelatinosa dorsal horn of the spinal cord.[5]

Morphine

Morphine is a long-acting hydrophilic opioid and has been used as an additive to LA in both CNB and peripheral blocks. Several mechanisms such as central action after absorption, opioid receptors in the peripheral nerves, and impairing sodium and potassium conduction on the nerves have been attributed to morphine.[6] Morphine produces excellent analgesia postcentral neuraxial administration as an LA adjuvant.[7] It is the first opioid drug to be used intrathecally as an adjuvant. The recommended dosage for intrathecal and epidural administration is 50–200 μg[8] and 1–3 mg,[9,10] respectively. When morphine is added to intrathecal bupivacaine, the duration of postoperative analgesia is prolonged by >8 hours compared with bupivacaine alone. It reduces cumulative 24-hour opioid consumption and the number of patients requiring morphine as a rescue analgesic and decreases pain intensity up to 12 hours postoperatively.[11] Morphine is not routinely used in peripheral nerve blocks due to negative results in the past. Recently few studies[12,13] used morphine in the dose of 5 mg as an adjuvant to LA in brachial plexus block and found moderate to good prolongation of analgesia. Though prolonged effective analgesia is provided by morphine as an adjuvant to LA, it also produces adverse effects such as respiratory depression, pruritus, nausea, and vomiting.[14]

Fentanyl

Fentanyl, a short-acting lipophilic opioid drug, is easily available and extensively used for perioperative analgesia. It is also a commonly used opioid as an adjuvant to LA in central neuraxial blocks, where it acts in the receptors present in the dorsal horn. Intrathecal fentanyl as an LA adjuvant is used in a dose ranging from 7.5–50 μg[15,16] but most literature shows 25 μg as a routine dose. The meta-analysis[11] of single-shot intrathecal opioids with LA concluded that intrathecal fentanyl with bupivacaine prolonged postoperative analgesia for about 2 hours. Fentanyl is also routinely administered along with LA in epidural infusions with a loading dose of 50–100 μg followed by 1–2 μg/mL of LA. Fentanyl is also tried in peripheral nerve blocks as an adjuvant to LA, where prolongation of the duration of analgesia is noted.[17,18] Compared to morphine, respiratory depression is minimal, whereas pruritus is a frequent adverse effect of intrathecal fentanyl with a risk of 27.3%.[11]

Buprenorphine

Buprenorphine is a centrally acting highly lipid soluble partial opioid agonist. It exhibits analgesic properties both at spinal and supraspinal levels. It has more receptor affinity than morphine (50 times) and fentanyl (24 times). Leffler A et al.[19] found that buprenorphine has local anesthetic-like properties and can inhibit voltage-gated Na channels, thereby prolonging the anesthesia. Its metabolite acts in κ and δ opioid receptors, producing antihyperalgesic effects. Of all the available opioids, buprenorphine seems to be the most effective adjuvant for LA.[20] It is more lipid soluble than morphine and fentanyl. Buprenorphine has also been used in intrathecal (75–150 µg) and epidural routes (150–300 µg) with reasonable efficacy.[21,22] Buprenorphine is also studied as an adjuvant in peripheral nerve block at a dose of 300 µg and found to prolong the analgesia duration significantly.[23]

Tramadol

Tramadol is a weak M-opioid receptor agonist and has properties of serotonin release, inhibition of norepinephrine reuptake, and inhibition of sodium channels.[24] Tramadol has been used as an adjuvant to LA in doses ranging from 10–50 mg intrathecally, with the success rate differing from minimal to good.[25] Like morphine and fentanyl, tramadol is also used as an adjuvant in epidural anesthesia with a dose of 1–2 mg/kg. Though the efficacy is lesser than morphine, the incidences of respiratory depression were the least. The major disadvantage of epidural tramadol is the incidence of nausea and vomiting while using a dose >50 mg. Tramadol has been studied in peripheral nerve blocks as an adjuvant to LA to prolong the analgesia, but the majority of the studies showed unsatisfactory results.[26,27]

Vasoactive Drugs

Epinephrine

Local anesthetic drugs have intrinsic vasodilatory properties except for cocaine and ropivacaine. This local vasodilatory action leads to faster systemic absorption, thereby decreasing the duration of action and possibilities of local anesthetic systemic toxicity (LAST). Adding a vasoconstrictor to LA decreases the systemic absorption, prolongs the duration of action, reduces the incidence of LAST, and also a vascular mark to identify intravascular drug injection.[28] Epinephrine is the routinely used additive to LA for vasoconstriction, and its addition increases the toxic dose of LA.

Epinephrine is used as an adjunct to LA in doses of 0.2–0.3 mg in spinal anesthesia.[29] However, due to its severe vasoconstricting property, adrenaline is not advised as an additive to LA in spinal anesthesia. Lignocaine premixed with adrenaline (5 µg/mL) is commonly used in regional blocks and epidural anesthesia. Epinephrine improves the duration of action of short and intermediate LA, whereas similar prolongation is not observed with long-acting such as ropivacaine and bupivacaine. Epinephrine causes increased neurotoxicity, especially in diabetic neuropathy patients, where neural damage can occur due to poor vascular supply.[30]

Alpha 2 Agonists

Alpha 2 agonists are non-selective imidazoline derivatives used perioperatively as antihypertensives and for procedural sedation. They are extensively used as an adjunct to LA owing to prolonging the sensory blockade in both central neuraxial and peripheral nerve blocks. Clonidine and dexmedetomidine (dexmed) are the two commonly used Alpha 2 agonists as additives to LA in regional blocks. When administered intrathecally, it acts by binding to postsynaptic alpha-2 receptors in the dorsal horn of the spinal cord and preventing the nociceptive transmission by inhibiting the presynaptic release of excitatory neurotransmitters. Alpha-2 agonists reduce preganglionic sympathetic outflow, causing a fall in blood pressure at the spinal dorsal horn level, and the sedative effect is mediated supraspinally.[31] Clonidine has a specificity of 220:1 (a-2:a1), whereas dexmed exhibits a specificity of 1620:1.[32]

Clonidine

Clonidine is used as an additive to LA, producing an increase in the duration of analgesia and sensory and motor blockade.[33] Clonidine acts by hyperpolarizing dorsal horn neurons through increased pK conductance. Clonidine is believed to increase potassium conduction, thus blocking the conduction of the pain fibers and prolonging the duration of the local anesthetic action.[3] It also produces local vasoconstriction, thereby reducing the systemic absorption of LA. Clonidine is an adjuvant to LA both intrathecally and epidurally. The intrathecal dose ranges between 15–50 µg though a dose higher than 30 µg produces adverse effects such as bradycardia, hypotension, and possibly excessive sedation. Epidural administration of clonidine is usually with a dose of 50–100 µg, and a continuous infusion is not usually preferred. Neuraxial clonidine is also used to provide hypotensive anesthesia for a bloodless surgical field. Clonidine is also utilized in peripheral nerve block as an adjunct to LA in the dose and is found to decrease the block onset and increase the duration of analgesia.[33] The dose in peripheral blocks such as brachial plexus blocks ranges from 1.5–2 µg/kg body weight.[34,35]

Dexmedetomidine

Dexmedetomidine possesses anxiolytic, sedative, and analgesic properties, causing no respiratory impairment.[36] Many studies have proven that perineural administered dexmed produces an extended duration of analgesia and sensory and motor blockade. Unlike clonidine, dexmed can prolong the sensory blockade without prolonging the motor blockade; this is because of a greater inhibitory effect on A-delta and C-nerve fibers relative to motor neurons. Animal studies have shown that perineural dexmed does not cause histopathological changes and is neuroprotective with reduced perineural inflammation.[37] Dexmed is used in central neuraxial blocks, especially in intrathecal blocks, and found to increase the mean duration of postoperative analgesia by 7 hours.[38] The dosage of intrathecal dexmed is 5 µg with LA in many of the studies available in the literature. Dexmed is also extensively studied as an adjuvant to LA in peripheral nerve blocks such as brachial plexus blocks. The optimal dose of perineural dexmed with a maximum duration of sensory block and minimum hemodynamic adverse effects is 50–60 µg.[39]

The most common side effects are bradycardia, arterial and orthostatic hypotension, sedation, rebound hypertension, and syncope. Bradycardia, due to dexmed, is resistant to atropine and might require higher doses. Meta-analyses have shown that perineural dexmed when compared to clonidine, is superior in terms of block characteristics, but inferior to dexamethasone.[40,41]

Midazolam

Midazolam is a short-acting benzodiazepine that acts on γ-aminobutyric acid type A (GABA-A) receptors, producing sedation, anti-anxiety, and anterograde amnesia. Midazolam as an adjunct to LA is not a commonly practiced technique though few recent studies show its efficacy in providing prolonged analgesia and procedural sedation.[42,43] It is believed to potentiate LA and also produce antinociception without any adverse effects.[44] Initially, it was proposed that the analgesic adjuvant action of midazolam with LA was due to peripherally present GABA-A receptors. However, a recent study by Yilmaz et al.[45] identified that the mechanism for midazolam-induced nerve block involves acting at the 18-kd translocator protein (TSPO). Midazolam (preservative free) is used in a dosage of 2 mg intrathecally with bupivacaine as an adjunct producing an increase in the duration of analgesia without many hemodynamic variations and adverse effects.[43,46] Midazolam is also tried as an adjuvant to LA in peripheral nerve block at a dose of 50 µg/kg and shortens the block onset and improves postoperative analgesia. However, there is no supportive meta-analysis available in the literature to prove its effectiveness as an adjuvant to LA in peripheral nerve blocks. There is a fear that neurotoxicity prevails while using midazolam perineurally[47] though no proper human study is available to substantiate this adverse effect.

N-methyl-D-aspartate Antagonists

N-methyl-D-aspartate receptor plays a significant role in pain modulation and contributes to developing a wind-up phenomenon, central sensitization, and peripheral sensitization.[48]

Ketamine

Ketamine is a non-competitive NMDA antagonist with local anesthetic-like properties.[49] Ketamine produces dissociative anesthesia and excellent analgesia, but many undesirable adverse effects are associated. Ketamine as an adjuvant to LA can be used for postoperative analgesia or to reduce exogenous opioid-induced hyperalgesia. It has two optical isomers: the S-(+) and the R-(-) isomer having different pharmacologic actions. The S(+) isomer is preservative free and used as adjuvants in neuraxial blockades. The primary mechanism of action of the spinal anesthetic ketamine is non-competitive blocking of the NMDA ionophore. The commonly used intrathecal ketamine dose is 25 mg.[50] Preservative-free ketamine administered epidurally in doses of 0.5–1 mg/kg reduces intraoperative and postoperative analgesic requirements.[29] Ketamine as an LA adjunct in caudal blocks in pediatric patients is very beneficial by providing an extended duration of analgesia without significant adverse effects.[51] Intravenous ketamine given in patients administered with neuraxial blockade had shown an increase in the duration of analgesia as quoted by a few studies.

Magnesium

Magnesium is a non-competitive NMDA and calcium receptor antagonist potentiating anesthetic action, thereby reducing the requirement. It has been observed that when used along with LA, it prolongs the duration of anesthesia and analgesia.[52] Magnesium decreases peripheral nerve excitability and enhances the ability of lidocaine to raise the excitation threshold of A-beta fibers. It has been studied as an adjunct to LA in intrathecal, epidural, and peripheral nerve blocks. Few studies have used intrathecal magnesium in doses of 50–100 mg, and the preferred concentration is 50% magnesium. A meta-analysis concluded it might offer a little extension of postoperative analgesia with LA.[53] Epidural magnesium is used in smaller doses such as 50–100 mg in labor analgesia,[54] whereas doses up to 500 mg are used for postoperative analgesia.[55] Magnesium is utilized as an adjunct to LA in various peripheral blocks such as brachial plexus, paravertebral, and femoral nerve blocks in doses ranging from 150–200 mg. The meta-analysis on magnesium as an adjunct to LA in peripheral blocks concluded that it provides a superior analgesic efficacy. It prolongs the postoperative motor, sensory, and analgesic duration.[56]

Dexamethasone

Dexamethasone is a corticosteroid drug most commonly and widely used as an adjuvant to LA in regional anesthesia. Dexamethasone decreases pain and increases the duration of analgesia when administered perineural and/or intravenous.[57] Various mechanisms were proposed for prolonging the analgesia, and reducing the release of inflammatory mediators from the site of insult is one of the most accepted actions. Other proposed mechanisms of action are inhibiting potassium channel-mediated discharge of nociceptive C-fibers, reducing ectopic neuronal discharge,[58] and local vasoconstriction by acting in glucocorticoid receptors.[59] Dexamethasone, as an adjuvant to LA in regional anesthesia, is mainly used to prolong the duration of analgesia. Still, it may reduce shivering and postoperative nausea, and vomiting.[60] Dexamethasone 8 mg, used in epidural blocks[61] is found to prolong the duration of analgesia without any significant adverse effects. Perineural dexamethasone is extensively studied in peripheral nerve blocks for its ability to prolong the duration of motor and sensory blockade. It is used in doses 4, 5, 7.5, 8, and 10 mg in various peripheral nerve block studies along with LA. The Cochrane Database review by Pehora et al. concluded that perineural dexamethasone prolongs the sensory and motor blockade for approximately 6 hours.[62] The cumulative 24-hour opioid consumption was significantly reduced for the perineural and intravenous dexamethasone (19.25 mg reduction and 6.58 mg reduction, respectively).[62] Intravenous dexamethasone, as an adjuvant to LA, prolonged the duration of sensory and motor blockade comparable to perineural dexamethasone. At present, there is no human study or case report available to show that perineural dexamethasone can be neurotoxic. No literature is available analyzing its long-term adverse effects. The only adverse effect of perioperative dexamethasone use is the incidences of hyperglycemia. Though the incidence is more in diabetic individuals and with a dose of >8 mg, it is preferred to reduce the dose and try any other adjuvant, which does not produce any glycemic alteration.

Miscellaneous Drugs

Many other drugs such as sodium bicarbonate, neostigmine, NSAIDs, etc., are tried as adjuvants to LA either to shorten the onset of blockade or to improve the perioperative anesthesia and analgesia. Due to non-convincing results, many of them are rarely used or used only in a few situations.

Sodium Bicarbonate

Sodium bicarbonate is added to LA, especially lignocaine, to shorten the onset-time of the blockade in epidural and peripheral nerve blocks.[63] It is a well-known fact that when the pKa of LA is close to the pH of the site of drug administration, the onset is quicker. Alkalization of LA by adding sodium bicarbonate reduces the pKa of the LA and brings it closer to the tissue potential of hydrogen (pH). Though it is proven that sodium bicarbonate hastens the blockade, clinically, it does create much difference as the time reduced is clinically insignificant. Apart from reducing the onset of LA action, it does not improve the quality of blockade or its duration of action.

Non-steroidal Anti-inflammatory Drugs

Non-steroidal anti-inflammatory drugs play an important role in multimodal analgesia in the perioperative period due to their properties as anti-inflammatory and antipyretic. It is also devoid of respiratory complications caused mainly by opioids. NSAIDs block cyclooxygenase 1 and 2 leading to prostaglandin synthesis inhibition. Though they produce effective analgesia when administered intravenously, their usage perineurally is not much studied and advised. They are used as adjuvant to LA in intravenous regional anesthesia (IVRA), intra-articular, and skin infiltration alone. These routes of administration also do not offer any added benefits compared to the intravenous route. Currently, the intravenous route alone is preferred for NSAIDs as an adjuvant to LA rather than the perineural route.[3]

Other Drugs

Adenosine, neostigmine, dextran, hyaluronidase, potassium chloride, droperidol, phenylephrine, verapamil, etc., have been used as adjuvants to LA in various regional blocks with varying results. These drugs are rarely used due to non-proven benefits from their inclusion in RA as adjuncts.

MULTIMODAL PERINEURAL ADJUVANT

Multimodal perineural adjuvant is a novel technique where more than one adjuvant drug from a different class is added to LA in regional blocks. Drugs that are used in this technique are clonidine, buprenorphine, and dexamethasone.[64] Though this technique done in vivo in rat sciatic nerve was devoid of any neurotoxicity, no randomized clinical trials in humans are available at present to prove its safety in the human nervous system. Recent observational analysis in pediatric peripheral nerve blocks done by Tafoya et al.[65] has used dexmed, dexamethasone, and buprenorphine as adjuvants. MMPNA technique needs much more effective analysis in the future to bring out the best possible combination to provide maximum benefit from each of the drugs.

CONCLUSION

Regional anesthesia techniques such as central neuraxial, peripheral nerve, and compartment blocks have revolutionized how anesthesia is provided for surgery. The inclusion of adjuvants in RA shortens the onset of blocks, can provide dense blockade, improves the safety profile of the LA, and most importantly, increases the duration of postoperative analgesia. It provides an option to tackle postoperative pain when the continuous perineural block is impossible. Perineural catheter-related complications such as secondary block failure, local infection, and catheter kinking/knotting can be avoided when long-acting LA is used with adjuvants such as dexamethasone, Alpha 2 agonists, and a few opioid drugs. Yet another major advantage of using adjuvants in RA is their ability to reduce postoperative opioid consumption, thereby preventing dreaded complications such as respiratory depression. Many high-quality randomized control trials should study the adjuvants' different doses, their safety profile, and significant added advantages to provide safe regional anesthesia.

REFERENCES

1. Yang S, Abrahams MS, Hurn PD, Grafe MR, Kirsch JR. Local anesthetic Schwann cell toxicity is time and concentration dependent. Reg Anesth Pain Med. 2011;36(5):444-51.
2. Swain A, Nag DS, Sahu S, Samaddar DP. Adjuvants to local anesthetics: current understanding and future trends. World J Clin Cases. 2017;5(8):307-23.
3. Prabhakar A, Lambert T, Kaye RJ, Gaignard SM, Ragusa J, Wheat S, et al. Adjuvants in clinical regional anesthesia practice: a comprehensive review. Best Pract Res Clin Anaesthesiol. 2019;33(4):415-23. Erratum in: Best Pract Res Clin Anaesthesiol. 2021;35(4):E3-4.
4. Wajima Z, Shitara T, Nakajima Y, Kim C, Kobayashi N, Kadotani H, et al. Comparison of continuous brachial plexus infusion of butorphanol, mepivacaine and mepivacaine-butorphanol mixtures for post-operative analgesia. Br J Anaesth. 1995;75(5):548-51.
5. Dhaliwal A, Gupta M. Physiology, Opioid Receptor. [Updated 2021 Jul 26]. In: StatPearls [Internet]. Treasure Island (FL): StatPearls Publishing; 2022.
6. Bazin JE, Massoni C, Bruelle P, Fenies V, Groslier D, Schoeffler P. The addition of opioids to local anaesthetics in brachial plexus block: The comparative effects of morphine, buprenorphine and sufentanil. Anaesthesia. 1997;52(9):858-62.
7. Liu SS, Block BM, Wu CL. Effects of perioperative central neuraxial analgesia on outcome after coronary artery bypass surgery: a meta-analysis. Anesthesiology. 2004;101(1):153-161.
8. Karaman S, Kocabas S, Uyar M, Hayzaran S, Firat V. The effects of sufentanil or morphine added to hyperbaric bupivacaine in spinal anesthesia for caesarean section. Eur J Anaesthesiol. 2006;23(4):285-91.
9. Bonnet MP, Mignon A, Mazoit JX, Ozier Y, Marret E. Analgesic efficacy and adverse effects of epidural morphine compared to parenteral opioids after elective caesarean section: a systematic review. Eur J Pain. 2010;14(9):894.e1-9.
10. Singh SI, Rehou S, Marmai KL, Jones APM. The efficacy of 2 doses of epidural morphine for postcesarean delivery analgesia: a randomized noninferiority trial. Anesth Analg. 2013;117(3):677-85.
11. Pöpping DM, Elia N, Marret E, Wenk M, Tramèr MR. Opioids added to local anesthetics for single-shot intrathecal anesthesia in patients undergoing minor surgery: a meta-analysis of randomized trials. Pain. 2012;153(4):784-93.

12. Mohamed KH, Abdelrahman KA, Elameer AN, Ali IH. Morphine as an adjuvant to local anesthetics in axillary brachial plexus block in forearm and hand surgery. J Curr Med Res Pract. 2019;4:131-6.
13. Venkatraman R, Pushparani A, Karthik K, Nandhini P. Comparison of morphine, dexmedetomidine and dexamethasone as an adjuvant to ropivacaine in ultrasound-guided supraclavicular brachial plexus block for postoperative analgesia-a randomized controlled trial. J Anaesthesiol Clin Pharmacol. 2021;37(1):102-7.
14. Yurashevich M, Habib AS. Monitoring, prevention and treatment of side effects of long-acting neuraxial opioids for post-cesarean analgesia. Int J Obstet Anesth. 2019;39:117-28.
15. Ferrarezi WPP, Braga AFA, Ferreira VB, Mendes SQ, Brandão MJN, Braga FSDS, et al. Spinal anesthesia for elective cesarean section. Bupivacaine associated with different doses of fentanyl: randomized clinical trial. Braz J Anesthesiol, 2021;71(6): 642-8.
16. Özmen S, Yavuz L, Eroglu F. The effect of anesthesia and postoperative analgesia of saddle block during perianal operations. Turk J Anaesthesiol Reanim. 2000;28(2):100-4.
17. Hamed MA, Ghaber S, Reda A. Dexmedetomidine and Fentanyl as an adjunct to Bupivacaine 0.5% in supraclavicular nerve block: a randomized controlled study. Anesth Essays Res. 2018;12(2):475-9.
18. Rajkhowa T, Das N, Parua S. Fentanyl as an adjuvant for brachial plexus block: a randomized comparative study. Int J Clin Trials. 2016;3:64-7.
19. Leffler A, Frank G, Kishner K, Niedermirtl F, Koppert W, Reeh PW, et al. Local anesthetic-like inhibition of voltage-gated Na(+) channels by the partial μ-opioid receptor agonist buprenorphine. Anesthesiology. 2012;116(6):1335-46.
20. Bailard NS, Ortiz J, Flores RA. Additives to local anesthetics for peripheral nerve blocks: Evidence, limitations, and recommendations. Am J Health Syst Pharm. 2014;71(5):373-85.
21. Anderson CTM. Adjuvants in Regional and Neuraxial Anesthesia: An Update. In: Paediatric Anaesthesiology. Las Vegas, NV: Society for Pediatric Anesthesia and the American Academy of Pediatrics Section on Anesthesiology and Pain Medicine; 2013.
22. Shaikh SI, Kiran M. Intrathecal buprenorphine for post-operative analgesia: A prospective randomised double blind study. J Anaesth Clin Pharmacol. 2010;26(1):35-8.
23. Jain N, Khare A, Khandelwal S, Mathur P, Singh M, Mathur V. Buprenorphine as an adjuvant to 0.5% ropivacaine for ultrasound-guided supraclavicular brachial plexus block: a randomized, double-blind, prospective study. Indian J Pain. 2017;31:112-8.
24. Haeseler G, Foadi N, Ahrens J, Dengler R, Hecker H, Leuwer M. Tramadol, fentanyl and sufentanil but not morphine block voltage-operated sodium channels. Pain. 2006;126(1-3):234-44.
25. Subedi A, Biswas BK, Tripathi M, Bhattarai BK, Pokharel K. Analgesic effects of intrathecal tramadol in patients undergoing caesarean section: a randomised, double-blind study. Int J Obstet Anesth. 2013;22(4):316-21.
26. Sarsu S, Mizrak A, Karakurum G. Tramadol use for axillary brachial plexus blockade. J Surg Res. 2011;165(1):e23-7.

27. Robaux S, Blunt C, Viel E, Cuvillon P, Nouguier P, Dautel G, et al. Tramadol added to 1.5% mepivacaine for axillary brachial plexus block improves postoperative analgesia dose-dependently. Anesth Analg. 2004;98(4):1172-7.
28. Dogru K, Duygulu F, Yildiz K, Kotanoglu MS, Madenoglu H, Boyaci A. Hemodynamic and blockage effects of high/low epinephrine doses during axillary brachial plexus blockade with lidocaine 1.5%: a randomized, double-blinded study. Reg Anesth Pain Med. 2003;28(5):401-5.
29. Abdalla IA. Additives for spinal anesthesia. Sudan Med J. 2016;52(3):109-13.
30. Kroin JS, Buvanendran A, Williams DK, Wagenaar B, Moric M, Tuman KJ, et al. Local anesthetic sciatic nerve block and nerve fiber damage in diabetic rats. Reg Anesth Pain Med. 2010;35:343-50.
31. Yaksh TL, Hua XY, Kalcheva I, Nozaki-Taguchi N, Marsala M. The spinal biology in humans and animals of pain states generated by persistent small afferent input. Proc Natl Acad Sci U S A. 1999;96(14):7680-6.
32. Gertler R, Brown HC, Mitchell DH, Silvius EN. Dexmedetomidine: a novel sedative-analgesic agent. Proc (Bayl Univ Med Cent). 2001;14(1):13-21.
33. Pöpping DM, Elia N, Marret E, Wenk M, Tramèr MR. Clonidine as an adjuvant to local anesthetics for peripheral nerve and plexus blocks: a meta-analysis of randomized trials. Anesthesiology. 2009;111(2):406-15.
34. Kelika, P, Arun JM. (2017). Evaluation of clonidine as an adjuvant to brachial plexus block and its comparison with tramadol. J Anaesthesiol Clin Pharmacol. 2017;33(2):197-202.
35. Bedi V, Petkar J, Dindor BK, Narang A, Tungaria H, Petkar KS. Perineural versus intravenous clonidine as an adjuvant to Bupivacaine in supraclavicular Brachial plexus block. Egyptian J Anaesth. 2017;33(3):257-61.
36. Mantz J, Josserand J, Hamada S, Dexmedetomidine: new insights. Eur J Anaesthesiol. 2011;28:3-6.
37. Brummett CM, Norat MA, Palmisano JM, Lydic R. Perineural administration of dexmedetomidine in combination with bupivacaine enhances sensory and motor blockade in sciatic nerve block without inducing neurotoxicity in rat. Anesthesiology. 2008;109(3):502-11.
38. Wu HH, Wang HT, Jin JJ, Cui GB, Zhou KC, Chen Y, et al. Does dexmedetomidine as a neuraxial adjuvant facilitate better anesthesia and analgesia? A systematic review and meta-analysis. PloS One. 2014;9(3):e93114.
39. Vorobeichik L, Brull R, Abdallah FW. Evidence basis for using perineural dexmedetomidine to enhance the quality of brachial plexus nerve blocks: a systematic review and meta-analysis of randomized controlled trials. Br J Anaesth. 2017;118(2):167-81.
40. El-Boghdadly K, Brull R, Sehmbi H, Abdallah FW. Perineural Dexmedetomidine is more effective than clonidine when added to local anesthetic for supraclavicular brachial plexus block: a systematic review and meta-analysis. Anesth Analg. 2017;124(6):2008-20.
41. Albrecht E, Vorobeichik L, Jacot-Guillarmod A, Fournier N, Abdallah FW. Dexamethasone is superior to Dexmedetomidine as a perineural adjunct for supraclavicular brachial plexus block: systematic review and indirect meta-analysis. Anesth Analg. 2019;128(3):543-54.
42. Nanjegowda N, Nataraj MS, Kavaranganahalli DM, Kini G. The effects of intrathecal midazolam on the duration of analgesia in patients undergoing knee arthroscopy. South Afr J Anaesth Analg. 2011;17(3):255-9.

43. Kapdi M, Desai S. Comparative study of intrathecal preservative-free midazolam versus nalbuphine as an adjuvant to intrathecal bupivacaine (0.5%) in patients undergoing elective lower-segment caesarean section. Ain-Shams J Anesthesiol. 2021;13:33.
44. Han MA, Kim MJ. The effects of intrathecal midazolam added to bupivacaine on duration of sensory block and BIS sedation score. Korean J Anesthesiol. 2006;50:408-12.
45. Yilmaz E, Hough KA, Gebhart GF, Williams BA, Gold MS. Mechanisms underlying midazolam-induced peripheral nerve block and neurotoxicity. Reg Anesth Pain Med. 2014;39(6):525-33.
46. Shukla U, Prabhakar T, Malhotra K, Srivastava D. Dexmedetomidine versus midazolam as adjuvants to intrathecal bupivacaine. J Anaesthesiol Clin Pharmacol. 2016;32(2):214-9.
47. Kirksey MA, Haskins SC, Cheng J, Liu SS. Local anesthetic peripheral nerve block adjuvants for prolongation of analgesia: a systematic qualitative review. PLoS One. 2015;10(9):e0137312.
48. Kreutzwiser D, Tawfic QA. Expanding role of NMDA receptor antagonists in the management of pain. CNS Drugs. 2019;33(4):347-74.
49. Weber WV, Jawalekar KS, Jawalekar SR. The effect of ketamine on nerve conduction in isolated sciatic nerves of the toad. Neurosci Lett. 1975;1(2):115-120.
50. Shrestha SK, Bhattarai B, Shah R. Comparative study of hyperbaric bupivacaine plus ketamine vs bupivacaine plus fentanyl for spinal anesthesia during caeserean section. Kathmandu Univ Med J. 2013;11(44):287-91.
51. Schnabel A, Poepping DM, Kranke P, Zahn PK, Pogatzki-Zahn EM. Efficacy and adverse effects of ketamine as an additive for paediatric caudal anesthesia: a quantitative systematic review of randomized controlled trials. Br J Anaesth. 2011;107(4):601-11.
52. Koinig H, Wallner T, Marhofer P, Andel H, Hörauf K, Mayer N. Magnesium sulfate reduces intra- and postoperative analgesic requirements. Anesth Analg. 1998;87(1):206-10.
53. Pascual-Ramírez J, Gil-Trujillo S, Alcantarilla C. Intrathecal magnesium as analgesic adjuvant for spinal anesthesia: a meta-analysis of randomized trials. Minerva Anestesiol. 2013;79(6):667-78.
54. Hasanein R, El-Sayed W, Khalil M. The value of epidural magnesium sulfate as an adjuvant to bupivacaine and fentanyl for labor analgesia. Egyptian J Anaesth. 2013;29(3):219-24.
55. Elsharkawy RA, Farahat TE, Abdelhafez MS. Analgesic effect of adding magnesium sulfate to epidural levobupivacaine in patients with pre-eclampsia undergoing elective cesarean section. J Anaesthesiol Clin Pharmacol. 2018; 34(3):328-34.
56. Li M, Jin S, Zhao X, Xu Z, Ni X, Zhang L, et al. Does magnesium sulfate as an adjuvant of local anesthetics facilitate better effect of perineural nerve blocks? Clin J Pain. 2016;32(12):1053-61.
57. Fredrickson Franzca MJ, Danesh-Clough TK, White R. Adjuvant dexamethasone for bupivacaine sciatic and ankle blocks: results from 2 randomized-controlled trials. Reg Anesth Pain Med. 2013;38(4):300-7.
58. Johansson A, Hao J, Sjölund B. Local corticosteroid application blocks transmission in normal nociceptive C-fibres. Acta Anesthesiol Scand. 1990;34(5):335-8.

59. Wang PH, Tsai CL, Lee JS, Wu KC, Cheng KI, Jou IM. Effects of topical corticosteroids on the sciatic nerve: an experimental study to adduce the safety in treating carpel tunnel syndrome. J Hand Surg Eur Vol. 2011;36(3):236-43.
60. Ismaiel MAMAN, El Safty OMT, El-Agamy AES, Mohamed OMZ, Ali MMMM. A comparative study between dexmedetomidine and dexamethasone as an intrathecal adjuvant for prevention of perioperative shivering in cesarean section. Ain-Shams J Anesthesiol. 2020;12:53.
61. Adel-Aziz MR, Abdelrahim MG, Nagiub GM. The effects of adding dexamethasone to epidural bupivacaine for lower limb orthopedic surgery. J Curr Med Res Pract 2019;4(2):192-5.
62. Pehora C, Pearson AM, Kaushal A, Crawford MW, Johnston B. Dexamethasone as an adjuvant to peripheral nerve block. Cochrane Database Syst Rev. 2017;11(11):CD011770.
63. Benzon HT, Toleikis JR, Dixit P, Goodman I, Hill JA. Onset, intensity of blockade and somatosensory evoked potential changes of the lumbosacral dermatomes after epidural anesthesia with alkalinized lidocaine. Anesth Analg. 1993;76(2):328-32.
64. Williams BA, Butt MT, Zeller JR, Coffee S, Pippi MA. Multimodal perineural analgesia with combined bupivacaine-clonidine-buprenorphine-dexamethasone: safe in vivo and chemically compatible in solution. Pain Med. 2015;16(1):186-98.
65. Tafoya SP, Tumber SS. The use of multimodal perineural adjuvants in pediatric peripheral nerve blocks: technique and experiences. Cureus. 2022;14(3): e23186.

CHAPTER

8

Myocardial Injury after Non-cardiac Surgery

Alok Kumar, Jayakrishnan S

▪ ABSTRACT

Myocardial injury after noncardiac surgery (MINS) encompasses a range of myocardial injuries due to surgical stress that does not classically fit the definition of myocardial infarction (MI). Preoperative cardiovascular risk assessment is paramount as recognizing patients at increased risk of MINS helps plan and guide the line of treatment during and after surgery. Maintaining a minimum perfusion pressure [mean arterial pressure (MAP)] > 65 mmHg is shown to lower the risk of MI/MINS, acute kidney injury, central nervous system (CNS) ischemic events, and mortality. Using arterial catheters for invasive blood pressure monitoring and serial cardiac troponin (cTn) measurements in high-risk patients aids in early identification and prompt correction of hypotensive episodes and ischemic injuries, thus avoiding potential adverse outcomes. Stress testing (exercise or pharmacological), Single-photon emission computed tomography/positron emission tomography-computed tomography (SPECT/PET-CT), and myocardial perfusion scan are some of the noninvasive cardiac imaging modalities that may be considered. Routine coronary angiography is only advised in patients with high-risk factors for MINS. Antithrombotic therapy with aspirin has been associated with an increased chance of survival in patients with perioperative MI.

Patients already on long-term β-blockers should continue in the perioperative period. β-blockers are not mandated to prevent perioperative MI in a new patient. Similarly, neither aspirin nor clonidine is advised de novo to reduce perioperative MINS. Temporary preoperative withholding of angiotensin-converting enzyme (ACE) inhibitors/angiotensin receptor blockers (ARBs) may reduce MINS. The use of statins is thought to benefit and is recommended in patients with MINS. Initiating or intensifying cardiovascular risk prevention therapy for a presumed atherosclerotic disease reduces the cardiac event-free survival period and should be strongly considered.

Keywords: Myocardial infarction; Perioperative MI; Myocardial injury; Surgical stress; Noncardiac surgery.

KEY POINTS

- Myocardial injury after noncardiac surgery (MINS) encompasses a range of myocardial injuries due to surgical stress that does not classically fit the definition of MI. Perioperative MI (PMI) is a spectrum of MINS.
- Preoperative cardiovascular risk assessment is paramount as recognizing patients at increased risk of MINS helps plan and guide the line of treatment during and after surgery.
- Maintaining a minimum perfusion pressure >65 mm Hg is shown to lower the risk of MI/MINS, acute kidney injury, CNS ischemic events, and mortality.
- Patients already on long-term β-blockers should continue in the perioperative period. β-blockers are not mandated to prevent perioperative MI in a new patient.
- Initiating or intensifying cardiovascular risk prevention therapy for a presumed atherosclerotic disease reduces the cardiac event-free survival period and should be strongly considered.

INTRODUCTION

Myocardial infarction is the leading cause of morbidity and mortality worldwide. Acute myocardial infarction (AMI) is a significant perioperative cardiovascular complication in patients who undergo noncardiac surgery, especially in patients with comorbidities or a history of heart disease. The magnitude of the problem can be better conceived considering that a large number of noncardiac surgeries are performed each year and also the prevalence of comorbidities and cardiac conditions.[1] Thus, early detection and treatment of perioperative myocardial infarction (PMI) leading to better outcomes can provide significant health benefits to the patient. More than one-third of perioperative deaths are caused due to cardiac complications, which may also be the cause of significant morbidity, the increased length of stays in hospital, and the overall prognosis of the patient. With pharmacological and technological advancement, management and prevention of cardiovascular complications in the perioperative period have resulted in development of many cardiovascular risk prediction models. However, there still is a lack of clarity on the prevention strategies and optimal management of perioperative MI.

DEFINITIONS

Myocardial infarction is categorized into five classes **(Table 1)**.[2] The fourth universal definition of myocardial infarction (2018)[3] lays out the criteria for myocardial injury and MI **(Table 1)**. The universal definition excludes damage due to causes like myocarditis/trauma.

However, defining and diagnosing PMI is difficult as it mostly manifests without chest pain and physiological signs and symptoms consistent with myocardial ischemia in patients under general anesthesia or sedation.[4,5]

TABLE 1: Classification of myocardial infarction (MI).

Myocardial infarction	*Myocardial injury*
• *Myocardial infarction:* Ischemia due to inadequate oxygen supply to the cardiac tissue leading to damage to the myocardium • It is classified on basis of causes of ischemia • *Type 1 MI:* Primary coronary event (plaque erosion and/or rupture, fissuring, or dissection) • *Type 2 MI:* Secondary to oxygen demand-supply mismatch causing ischemia (e.g., coronary artery spasm, coronary embolism, anemia, arrhythmias, and hyper- or hypotension) • *Type 3 MI:* Sudden unexpected cardiac death • *Type 4 MI:* Percutaneous coronary intervention (PCI)/stent thrombosis • *Type 5 MI:* Associated with coronary artery bypass graft surgery	• *Myocardial injury:* Evidence of elevated cardiac troponin (cTn) without ischemia • At least one value should be above the 99th percentile upper reference limit • Rise and/or fall of cTn indicates acute myocardial injury

Electrocardiogram (ECG) changes associated are subtle/transient. This results in their late recognition leading to considerable morbidity and mortality.

A new, improved concept of PMI, called MINS was introduced by the Vascular Events in Noncardiac Surgery Patients Cohort Evaluation (VISION) investigators. It included a spectrum of myocardial injuries, including MI that does not satisfy the accepted definition of MI.

The MINS has been defined as at least one serum cardiac troponin (cTn) level exceeding the 99th percentile of the upper limit in the postoperative period, possibly due to an ischemic mechanism. The increase in the serum assay and subsequent fall is supposedly indicative of acute myocardial injury. However, it is mandatory to rule out any other nonischemic causes. Also rise in cTn levels must be within the first 30 days of the surgery (typically within 72 hours). It has been observed that such a rise happens within 48 hours of the insult in most cases.[6] Absence of overt clinical signs and symptoms relating to MI does not rule out a diagnosis of MINS. Such clinical symptoms may not be evident because of the anesthesia given during the surgery. Therefore, a preoperative baseline cTn measurement followed by another measurement within 48–72 hours is highly recommended for high-risk patients. Elderly aged (>65 years) or age >45 years with a history of atherosclerotic disease are at high risk for such cardiovascular events. Such repeat cTn assays establish the rise and fall pattern necessary to clinch the diagnosis of MINS. In such high-risk patients, a postoperative cTn value of >20% of a baseline cTn concentration raises the suspicion of MINS.[3]

Serum cTn levels have been associated with adverse prognosis in patients diagnosed with MINS in the perioperative period. In the MINS setting, even in the absence of clinical signs and symptoms of ischemia, serum cTn levels associated with adverse prognosis are ≥65 ng/L; 20–65 ng/L with a rise of ≥5 ng/L; or any increase of ≥14 ng/L.

■ ETIOPATHOGENESIS

Myocardial injury after noncardiac surgery is primarily an ischemic disease. Factors contributing to MINS are anesthesia and surgical trauma, perioperative hemodynamic fluctuations, vascular inflammation and/or endothelial dysfunction, and increased platelet activation with hypercoagulability.

Two mechanisms can lead to MINS **(Flowchart 1)**. First, anesthesia and surgical stress (along with pain, anemia, and hypothermia) cause the release of catecholamines and cortisol resulting in hyperdynamic circulation and thus exerting a shear leading to plaque rupture. A procoagulant state due to increased platelet aggregation and elevated coagulation factors or severe coronary vasospasm may lead to the formation of an occlusive or nonocclusive thrombus and MI. This is type 1 PMI. The second mechanism is the myocardial oxygen supply-demand mismatch in patients with significant and obstructive coronary artery disease (CAD), which could be triggered

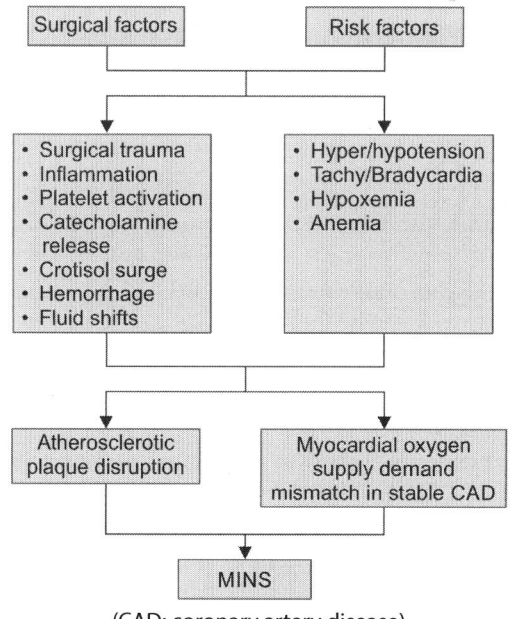

Flowchart 1: Mechanisms of myocardial injury after noncardiac surgery (MINS).

(CAD: coronary artery disease)

due to perioperative factors such as intraoperative and postoperative hypotension, hypertension, tachycardia, anemia, hypoxemia, hypercarbia, and hypothermia. This is defined as type 2 PMI.

RISK FACTORS AND ASSESSMENT

Preoperative cardiovascular risk assessment is paramount as identifying patients with an increased risk of MINS helps plan and guide the line of treatment during and after surgery. Patients with increased risk of MINS require vigilant cTn surveillance in the perioperative period. Apart from it, case-specific alterations in intraoperative care are required, like invasive monitoring and measures, to avoid hemodynamic fluctuations.[6]

Various risk factors have been identified for identifying patients at high risk for MINS. These are demographic factors such as elderly age (≥75 years) and male gender; the functional capacity of the patient; comorbidities such as hypertension, diabetes, CAD, peripheral artery disease, cerebrovascular disease, chronic kidney disease, and untreated severe obstructive sleep apnea (OSA); preexisting cardiovascular ailments such as atrial fibrillation and heart failure; poor cardiac risk indices like the Revised Cardiac Risk Index (RCRI); and type of surgery. Apart from this, various preoperative testing suggests a high risk for MINS and may be used to identify the at-risk population **(Box 1)**.

Although men are more likely to develop MINS, both male and female patients, once diagnosed with MINS, have a similar association with mortality.[6,7] A Duke Activity Status Index (DASI) score ≤ 34 has been associated with a higher risk of MINS, whereas subjective assessment by anesthesiologists and exercise testing has little or no association with the risk of MINS.[8] Cardiovascular comorbidities such as CAD, cerebrovascular disease, peripheral artery occlusive disease, heart failure, atrial fibrillation, and hypertension are strong predictors of MINS. Also, other noncardiovascular conditions such as severe OSA, diabetes, and impaired kidney function are independent predictors of MINS.[6] Risk scoring systems which include individual cardiovascular and noncardiovascular comorbidities such as the RCRI, National Surgical

---

BOX 1: Tests indicating an increased risk of myocardial injury after noncardiac surgery (MINS).

- Elevated brain natriuretic peptide (BNP) or N-terminal pro-BNP (NT-proBNP)
- Neutrophil-lymphocyte ratio >4
- Elevated blood glucose concentration
- Elevated reticulated platelet concentration
- Reversibility of myocardial perfusion testing

Quality Improvement Program (NSQIP), and STOP-Bang are shown to be predictive of MINS.[9,10]

Preoperative laboratory investigations can also be used to estimate the risk of MINS. The natriuretic peptides [brain natriuretic peptide (BNP) or N-terminal pro-BNP (NT-pro BNP)] are found to have a strong association with vascular death and MINS within 30 days after noncardiac surgery. It has been established that BNP values <92 ng/L were associated with a reduced risk of perioperative adverse cardiac events. In contrast, higher values have been associated with increased all-cause mortality, including fatal MI.[11] A NT-proBNP <200 pg/mL had ≤3% risk for MI or death, whereas patients with NT-proBNP values between 200 and 1,500 pg/mL showed a 7.9% risk of MI or death.[12] Further, in cardiopulmonary exercise testing, impaired heart rate recovery (≤12 bpm during the first minute) after exercise and reversible defects in stress myocardial perfusion imaging (MPI) is associated with MINS.

The type of procedure a patient undergoes is an important determinant of whether a patient would develop myocardial injury in the perioperative period **(Table 2)**. Moreover, patients undergoing urgent or emergency procedures have two to three times increased risk of developing MINS. The surgical estimated risk of fatal and nonfatal myocardial injury has been classified into low risk (<1%), intermediate risk (1–5%), and high risk (>5%) procedures in the European Society of Cardiology/European Society of Anaesthesiology (ESC/ESA) guidelines **(Table 3)**.[13]

TABLE 2: Surgeries with highest incidence of myocardial injury.[6]

Type of surgery	Incidence of myocardial injury
Vascular	19%
Orthopedic	12%
Thoracic	9%
General	9%

TABLE 3: A 30-day risk for a cardiovascular event in the perioperative setting.

Low risk (<1%)	Intermediate risk (1–5%)	High risk (>5%)
• Superficial surgery • Breast • Dental • Reconstructive • Eye/ear, nose, and throat (ENT) • Minor gynecologic/orthopedic/urologic procedures	• Intraperitoneal • Major orthopedic/neurologic/gynecologic/urologic procedures • Renal transplant • Head and neck surgery • Endovascular aneurysm repair/peripheral arterial angioplasty	• Heart/lung/liver transplant • Major vascular surgery • Esophagectomy • Adrenal abscission • Right or left lung resection • Duodenopancreatic surgery

MANAGEMENT

Preoperative Medical Management

Currently, we face a lack of understanding on effective and prudent ways of preventing perioperative myocardial injury. MINS is a novel concept, and how various interventions affect MI may not be relevant on the general outcome of MINS even though MINS encompasses MI also. Trials with MINS as the primary outcome are underway and are yet to be published.

However, recommendations based on available evidence are as follows:
- Starting β-blockers is not advised to prevent perioperative myocardial injury.
- For patients already on long-term β-blockers, it is advised to continue the same β-blockers in the perioperative period.[14] However, dose adjustments might be needed to avoid the risks of hemodynamic instability.

Based on observational studies, there is no clinical benefit of β-blockers in preventing MINS.
- Neither aspirin nor clonidine should be introduced to lower the incidence of perioperative MI and MINS.[6]
- Temporary preoperative withholding of angiotensin-converting enzyme (ACE) inhibitors/angiotensin receptor blockers (ARBs) may reduce MINS.
- Statins have been used previously in the perioperative period with the idea that they would decrease the risk of MINS. However, currently, the benefits of statin in preventing MINS are considered uncertain.
- Remote ischemic preconditioning (RIPC) is a process of inducing short cycles of ischemia at a distant organ (mostly limbs). It is supposed to increase the ischemic tolerance of a distant organ (myocardium) to subsequent ischemic insult. RIPC, as an effective strategy, has been tried to reduce the risk of MINS. However, the current literature does not support any reduction in the incidence of MINS using RIPC.[15]

There is no clear evidence of the beneficial or harmful effects of nitrous oxide, sevoflurane volatile anesthesia, and intravenous general anesthesia.

Intraoperative Hypotension and Tachycardia

Anesthetic drugs, techniques, patient comorbidities, and surgical handling are all known to cause hemodynamic perturbations. The primary aim of hemodynamic management is the maintenance of end-organ perfusion. However, the risk of anesthesia is not devoid of moments of hypotension. Such moments of intraoperative hypotension (IOH) pose a risk of fatal and nonfatal myocardial injury apart from other organ dysfunction. The reduction in blood pressure resulting in organ hypoperfusion and damage depends on the product of severity and duration of hypotension.[16] The relation between

IOH and end-organ injury and further mortality is essential as the occurrence is common during surgeries. Also, unlike patient factors, it is a modifiable risk factor mainly under our control. Maintaining a minimum target MAP >65 mm Hg is shown to lower the risk of MI/MINS, acute kidney injury (AKI), CNS ischemic events, and mortality.[6,16,17] It is still unclear which specific component of blood pressure (systolic, diastolic, or MAP) is the most appropriate for treatment. Continuous intraoperative blood pressure monitoring helps respond quickly to IOH, thereby decreasing the chances and severity of IOH. Using arterial catheters for invasive blood pressure monitoring aids in early identification and prompt correction of hypotensive episodes, thus avoiding potential adverse outcomes. Postoperative control of blood pressure may be equally important in reducing perioperative adverse events.

Heart rate is the most oxygen-consuming determinant for the heart among preload, afterload, and heart rate. Any amount of tachycardia causes myocardial oxygen supply-demand mismatch as it increases myocardial oxygen demand and limits diastolic coronary perfusion time. Heart rates of >100 beats per minute induce myocardial injury in high-risk patients.

Postoperative Surveillance

In a nonsurgical setting, myocardial ischemia/infarction diagnosis can be made when the patients present with symptoms and meet the diagnostic criteria. However, diagnosis of MI in a perioperative setting is precluded by sedatives, analgesics, and other anesthetic drugs. Most established symptoms to diagnose MI are masked as the patient is under anesthesia. Also, the electrocardiographic abnormalities are transient and difficult to interpret on the monitor. Therefore, serial measurement of cTn levels is considered imperative for identifying the myocardial injury. To avoid missing prognostically critical myocardial injury, the recent American Heart Association (AHA) and ESA scientific statement on MINS[6,18] recommends serial cTn measurements in the initial 48–72 hours after noncardiac surgery in patients at increased risk of developing MINS. To see a rise in cTn level, it is mandatory to have a baseline cTn measurement before surgery in such a cohort to prevent any cardiovascular event.

The Canadian Cardiovascular Society guidelines have identified patients with increased risk (>5%) of a fatal and nonfatal cardiovascular event in the postoperative period based on various parameters. These are high baseline NT-proBNP/BNP levels or RCRI score ≥1, and age >65 years or age 45–64 years with significant cardiovascular disease.[19]

Postoperative Management

Optimal postoperative management of MINS is filled with uncertainties owing to the lack of trials with MINS as the endpoint. Thus, management should be individualized based on the likely etiology of the cardiovascular event. Specific incidents such as acute pulmonary embolism, acute decompensation due to preexisting valvular heart disease, or heart failure causing MINS should be considered and managed as primary lesions and not MINS per se. Thus, cardiovascular testing may be considered to ascertain the cause of myocardial injury.

Lifestyle changes such as stress management, diet modification, smoking discontinuation, any form of physical activity, and optimization of the cardiovascular risk factors are presumed to be beneficial owing to their benefits in secondary prevention of cardiovascular diseases.

Antithrombotic therapy with aspirin is beneficial and is found to be associated with reduced 30-day mortality in patients with perioperative MI. Intensifying anticoagulation therapy using dabigatran is shown to lower the long-term incidence of cardiovascular events without causing a significant increase in major bleeding risks.[20] However, currently, dabigatran is not used in patients with perioperative myocardial injury.

Statins are presumed to be beneficial and are recommended in patients with MINS. The recommendation is based on consensus and observational data due to the lack of trials. Risk prevention for any adverse cardiovascular event should be initiated and pursued aggressively in high-risk cases. It includes starting or increasing the dose of statins, antiplatelet agents, β-blockers, or ACE inhibitor the patient is already taking. Moreover, the continuation of the said medicine at the time of hospital discharge reduces the cardiac event-free survival period and should be strongly considered.[6] Medical management as per the laid protocol should be administered for such high-risk patients who develop MI. But one should also see that the benefits outweigh the surgical risks of bleeding. β-blockers and ACE inhibitors are advised for patients who develop MINS and PMI, only in doses that do not cause hemodynamic instability.[6]

Expert cardiovascular consultation should be taken for patients with MINS, and cardiovascular evaluation should be tailored to the patient's condition. Bedside transthoracic echocardiography is one such tool. It could quickly assess parameters such as left ventricular ejection fraction, any preexisting structural abnormalities of the heart, new regional wall motion abnormalities, and chronic or acute valvular lesions. Elevated cTn without an alternative cause warrants further invasive or noninvasive evaluation to identify patients who may benefit from coronary revascularization. Stress testing (exercise or pharmacological), Single-photon emission computed tomography/positron emission tomography-computed tomography (SPECT/PET-CT), stress MPI, and coronary CT angiography are some of the noninvasive cardiac imaging modalities that may be considered. The universal definition of MI is ischemic symptoms, with electrocardiographic changes and or new wall motion abnormalities and raised cTn levels. Patient showing any of these features warrants immediate coronary angiography and further management based on set protocol. However, consideration should be given to associated factors such as clinical scenarios, hemodynamic instability, and risk of bleeding. Routine coronary angiography or stress tests are not advisable but could be considered in high-risk cases depending on the patient condition and resources.

Without extensive and robust clinical trials, no clear guidelines exist on cardiovascular testing in patients suspected or diagnosed with MINS. Serial ECGs/troponins, transthoracic echocardiography, and noninvasive stress testing are recommended. On suspicion of MINS, optimization of modifiable risk factors such as diet and nutrition counseling, blood pressure control, and glycemic control is mandatory. Besides, guideline-directed therapy regarding antiplatelet agents, statins, β-blockers, and ACE inhibitors needs to be followed.

■ FUTURE PERSPECTIVES

Myocardial injury after noncardiac surgery is a relatively novel entity, first described in 2014. The pathophysiology of this entity is still not clearly understood. There are lacunae in many areas, such as understanding the interplay between hypercoagulability, endothelial dysfunction, and platelet membrane in the perioperative setting. Stress-induced inflammatory cascade due to surgical stress and its contribution to the development of MINS requires augmentation in our understanding of the topic. Also, large-scale trials need to be conducted to elucidate the mechanisms, risk stratification, prevention, and management of MINS.

Upcoming clinical trials across the globe are expected to provide more understanding of the subject. The POISE-3 (the PeriOperative ISchemic Evaluation-3) trial is one such trial. It is designed to compare the effect of hypotension versus hypertension prevention management in the perioperative period on all types of cardiovascular events, including MINS. Anti-inflammatory agents like colchicine are being tried to reduce the risk of adverse perioperative cardiovascular events. COPMAN (Colchicine Prevents Myocardial Injury After Non-Cardiac Surgery Pilot Study) and COP-AF (Colchicine for the Prevention of Perioperative Atrial Fibrillation in Patients Undergoing Thoracic Surgery) trial are such trials underway that are hypothesized to test the potential benefits of colchicine in the setting of noncardiac surgery. Perioperative hypothermia induces unnecessary stress and causes excessive afterload on the heart, increasing the risk of bleeding and infections. Perioperative temperature management during surgery is a much-investigated topic; the PROTECT (Perioperative Hypothermia and Myocardial Injury After Non-Cardiac Surgery) trial is one such trial that assesses this aspect of the incidence of MINS. Similarly, other ongoing prospective observational studies aim to understand the mechanisms of MINS. However, more clinical trials are necessary to establish effective and safe prevention and treatment strategies for MINS.

■ CONCLUSION

Myocardial injury after cardiac surgery is preventable. Diligent preoperative evaluation for identifiable risk factors and their early recognition plays a crucial role in managing patients who develop myocardial injury perioperatively. Maintenance of perfusion pressure, the continuation of beta-blockers, and other cardiovascular risk prevention strategies form the cornerstone of its management.

■ REFERENCES

1. Weiser TG, Regenbogen SE, Thompson KD, Haynes AB, Lipsitz SR, Berry WR, et al. An estimation of the global volume of surgery: a modelling strategy based on available data. Lancet. 2008;372:139-44.
2. Thygesen K, Alpert JS, White HD. Universal definition of myocardial infarction. J Am Coll Cardiol. 2007;50:2173-95.
3. Thygesen K, Alpert JS, Jaffe AS, Chaitman BR, Bax JJ, Morrow DA, et al. Fourth universal definition of myocardial infarction. J Am Coll Cardiol. 2018; 72(18):2231-64.
4. Reed-Poysden C, Gupta KJ. Acute coronary syndromes. BJA Educ. 2015;15(6):286-93.
5. Magoon R, Makhija N, Das D. Perioperative myocardial injury and infarction following non-cardiac surgery: a review of the eclipsed epidemic. Saudi J Anaesth. 2020;14:91-9.
6. Ruetzler K, Smilowitz NR, Berger JS, Devereaux PJ, Maron BA, Newby LK, et al. Diagnosis and Management of Patients With Myocardial Injury After Noncardiac Surgery: A Scientific Statement From the American Heart Association. Circulation. 2021;144:e287-305.
7. Botto F, Alonso-Coello P, Chan MTV, Villar JC, Xavier D, Srinathan SK, et al. Myocardial injury after noncardiac surgery: a large, international, prospective cohort study establishing diagnostic criteria, characteristics, predictors, and 30-day outcomes. Anesthesiology. 2014;120(3):564-78.
8. Wijeysundera DN, Pearse RM, Shulman MA, Abbott TEF, Torres E, Ambosta A, et al. Assessment of functional capacity before major non-cardiac surgery: an international, prospective cohort study. Lancet. 2018;391(10140):2631-40.
9. Roshanov PS, Sessler DI, Chow CK, Garg AX, Walsh MW, Lam NN, et al. Predicting myocardial injury and other cardiac complications after elective noncardiac surgery with the revised cardiac risk index: the VISION study. Can J Cardiol. 2021;37(8):1215-24.
10. Chan MTV, Wang CY, Seet E, Tam S, Lai HY, Walker S, et al. Postoperative vascular complications in unrecognised obstructive sleep apnoea (POSA) study protocol: an observational cohort study in moderate-to-high risk patients undergoing non-cardiac surgery. BMJ Open. 2014;4(1):e004097.

11. Rodseth RN, Biccard BM, le Manach Y, Sessler DI, Lurati Buse GA, Thabane L, et al. The prognostic value of pre-operative and post-operative B-type natriuretic peptides in patients undergoing noncardiac surgery: B-type natriuretic peptide and N-terminal fragment of pro-B-type natriuretic peptide: a aystematic review and individual patient data meta-analysis. J Am Coll Cardiol. 2014;63(2):170-80.
12. Duceppe E, Patel A, Chan MTV, Berwanger O, Ackland G, Kavsak PA, et al. Preoperative n-terminal pro-B-type natriuretic peptide and cardiovascular events after noncardiac surgery: a cohort study. Ann Intern Med. 2020;172(2): 96-104.
13. Kristensen SD, Knuuti J, Saraste A, Anker S, Bøtker HE, de Hert S, et al. 2014 ESC/ESA Guidelines on non-cardiac surgery: Cardiovascular assessment and management: the joint task force on non-cardiac surgery: cardiovascular assessment and management of the European Society of Cardiology (ESC) and the European Society of Anaesthesiology (ESA). Eur Heart J. 2014;35(35):2383-431.
14. Khanna AK, Naylor DF, Naylor AJ, Mascha EJ, You J, Reville EM, et al. Early resumption of β blockers is associated with decreased atrial fibrillation after noncardiothoracic and nonvascular surgery a cohort analysis. Anesthesiology. 2018;129(6):1101-10.
15. Garcia S, Rector TS, Zakharova M, Herrmann RR, Adabag S, Bertog S, et al. Cardiac remote ischemic preconditioning prior to elective vascular surgery (CRIPES): a prospective, randomized, sham-controlled phase II clinical trial. J Am Heart Assoc. 2016;5(10):e003916.
16. Saugel B, Sessler DI. Perioperative blood pressure management. Anesthesiology. 2021;134(2):250-61.
17. Salmasi V, Maheshwari K, Yang D, Mascha EJ, Singh A, Sessler DI, et al. Relationship between intraoperative hypotension, defined by either reduction from baseline or absolute thresholds, and acute kidney and myocardial injury after noncardiac surgery. Anesthesiology. 2017;126(1):47-65.
18. de Hert S, Staender S, Fritsch G, Hinkelbein J, Afshari A, Bettelli G, et al. Preoperative evaluation of adults undergoing elective noncardiac surgery: updated guideline from the European Society of Anaesthesiology. Eur J Anaesthesiol. 2018;35(6):407-65.
19. Duceppe E, Parlow J, MacDonald P, Lyons K, McMullen M, Srinathan S, et al. Canadian cardiovascular society guidelines on perioperative cardiac risk assessment and management for patients who undergo noncardiac surgery. Can J Cardiol. 2017;33(1):17-32.
20. Devereaux PJ, Duceppe E, Guyatt G, Tandon V, Rodseth R, Biccard BM, et al. Dabigatran in patients with myocardial injury after non-cardiac surgery (MANAGE): an international, randomised, placebo-controlled trial. Lancet. 2018;391(10137):2325-34.

CHAPTER

9

Anesthesia Management for Carotid Endarterectomy and Stenting

Dheeraj Arora, Jitin Narula

■ ABSTRACT

Atherosclerosis of the carotid vessels is a leading cause of cerebrovascular accidents due to thrombosis or embolization. Stroke is the leading cause of death and long-term disability. It can be prevented by timely intervention in the form of carotid endarterectomy or stenting. Percutaneous carotid artery procedures such as carotid artery angioplasty or carotid artery stenting and percutaneous transcarotid artery revascularization offer a novel, minimally invasive approach to extracranial cerebrovascular occlusive disease. Anesthesia management for these procedures requires thorough preoperative evaluation and intraoperative and postoperative monitoring to prevent cerebral ischemia. Hemodynamic and neurological monitoring is a prerequisite for conducting carotid artery interventions. The choice of anesthesia technique should be based on the patient's profile, surgeon and anesthesiologist skills, and institutional protocol. Although no single anesthetic technique has shown superior results for patients undergoing carotid endarterectomy, it is essential to ensure adequate cerebral perfusion, cardiovascular stability, and patient recovery.

Keywords: Carotid endarterectomy; Carotid artery stenting; Anesthesia; Neurological monitoring.

■ KEY POINTS

- Stroke is the leading cause of death and long-term disability. The most common cause of embolic stroke is atherosclerosis of the carotid vessels. It can be prevented by timely interventions such as carotid endarterectomy or carotid artery stenting.
- Anesthetic management of these procedures is challenging and requires knowledge of cerebral circulation, physiology, and hemodynamic changes during carotid artery manipulation.
- Choice of anesthesia technique, whether general, regional, or combined, may contribute to the outcome of the intervention. The optimal choice for a patient depends on multiple factors.

- Hemodynamic and neurological monitoring during carotid interventions is of utmost importance.
- The role of postoperative care, problems, and management has been explained.

INTRODUCTION

Atherosclerosis of the carotid vessels is a leading cause of cerebrovascular accidents due to thrombosis or embolization. Stroke is the leading cause of death and long-term morbidity. It can be prevented by timely intervention using carotid endarterectomy (CEA) or stenting. Historically, CEA was first published in Lancet in 1954 and has been considered a standard technique since the 1970s.[1,2] Carotid artery stenting was reported in 1980 by Mathias.[3]

There were various trials for the basis of indication of CEA, such as NASCET (North American Symptomatic Carotid Endarterectomy Trial) and ESCET (European Carotid Surgery Trial).[4,5] According to those guidelines, the indication was based on the severity of stenosis, i.e., CEA was indicated in symptomatic and asymptomatic carotid stenosis of >50% and >70%, respectively.

There are recommendations from Cochrane Group[6] also as given here:
- *Highly recommended* in symptomatic patients with carotid artery stenosis of 70-99%
- *Moderately recommended* in patients with *near 100% occlusion*, primarily in men, patients > 75 years and within 2 weeks of the acute event.
- *Some benefits* in patients with 50-69% symptomatic stenosis.
- *Small benefits* in asymptomatic stenosis such as young male patients with bilateral disease.

Since 1994 carotid angioplasty is also considered an alternative treatment modality to CEA. Many studies, like the CAVATAS trial, have shown comparable results between the two treatment modalities.[7]

ANATOMY

The majority of cerebral blood supply (80-90%) is delivered by the two internal carotid arteries and the remainder by the vertebrobasilar system. The Circle of Willis is formed by carotid arteries and basilar arteries. Although this ring protects the brain against the occlusion of one or another vessel, however, it is incomplete in 15% of patients. An atheromatous disease of one of the vessels may lead to cerebrovascular accidents.

CAROTID ENDARTERECTOMY: SURGERY

Regarding CEA surgical steps, firstly surgical incision is given along the anterior border of the sternocleidomastoid muscle (between the mastoid process and sternoclavicular junction) or obliquely starting on the mastoid process, continuing horizontally across the neck to expose the carotid sheath.

Rigorous surgical retraction of the sternocleidomastoid muscle can cause discomfort in an awake patient, which can be alleviated by injecting 5–6 mL of local anesthetic into the muscle sheath. When the carotid sheath has been opened, the vagus nerve can frequently be seen. The common facial vein is then ligated at the crossing point with the internal carotid artery. Ligatures are placed around the common carotid artery and the internal and external carotid arteries. The hypoglossal nerve is frequently retracted where it crosses the artery at the bulb. These may cause nerve damage.

After clamping the external, internal, and common carotid arteries, the carotid bifurcation is isolated from the circulation. Plaque is removed after arteriotomy, and debris from the intimal surface of the artery is also cleaned to prevent postoperative emboli. After that, repair of the artery is done with a patch or venous graft.

ANESTHESIA MANAGEMENT

Main anesthetic considerations for CEA are:
- To provide analgesia during skin incision, insertion of a retromandibular retractor and perivascular preparation.
- To prevent perioperative complications such as cerebrovascular accident and myocardial infarction.

ANESTHESIA TECHNIQUES

- General anesthesia (GA)
- Regional anesthesia—interscalene block, cervical plexus block
- Combination of general and regional anesthesia.

Preoperative Assessment

The prime aim of the preoperative assessment is to sort out high-risk patients as cerebrovascular accidents, and myocardial infarction is the main complications of CEA. The study data from NASCET, ESCT, and Veteran's Administration Trial reported 35 deaths (1.1%) within 30 days of surgery out of 3,248 patients, along with 229 patients having a combined outcome in the form of stroke or death.[8]

Neurological Assessment

- Any history of presenting complaints and any acute event should be assessed and indication for surgery in accordance with recommendations.
- Symptoms and evidence of any existing neurological deficits to decide about anesthesia techniques.

Cardiovascular Assessment

- To identify associated cardiovascular comorbidity, primarily coexisting coronary artery disease. To decide about combining CEA with coronary artery bypass grafting surgery.
- Associated peripheral vascular disease to be assessed.

General Assessment

- Effort tolerance
- Respiratory system assessment and optimization with focus on history of smoking
- Associated comorbidities such as renal, hepatic or coagulopathy, etc., should also be reviewed and optimized.

Medication History

- All medications that reduce cardiovascular and thrombotic complications should be continued such as statins which reduce plaque rupture, and beta blockers. Moreover, statins may be started in a selective group of patients.
- A lower dose of aspirin should also be continued.

Depending upon the findings, the anesthesia plan should be discussed with the operating surgeon and patient. In awake surgery, baseline neurological testing (specific questionnaire) is performed to replicate the same intraoperatively.

Types of Anesthesia: General, Regional or Local

The choice of anesthetic technique should be based on the patient's comorbidities, institutional protocols, the anesthesiologist's expertise, and the surgeon's expertise. Most guidelines state that neither GA nor regional techniques affect the clinical outcome. A randomized trial meta-analysis revealed that the incidence of local hemorrhage was less with a local anesthetic. However, there was no evidence of a reduction in the operative stroke.[9] A meta-analysis of 17 nonrandomized trials also stated a lack of data to draw any conclusion regarding the two techniques.[10,11]

General Anesthesia

A balanced anesthesia technique with opioid, sedative, and volatile agents, along with controlled mechanical ventilation, is used for GA.

Advantages
- The airway is secured with control ventilation
- Ensure comfort and immobility

- Avoids the need for urgent conversion
- Volatile agents may give neuroprotection

Disadvantages
- Clinical neurological monitoring is lacking.
- Perioperative hemodynamic instability (hypo- or hypertension during manipulation)
- Carotid shunt use may increase
- Delayed recovery from GA may mask postop neurological complications.

Regional Anesthesia

Advantages
- *Awake patient:* Clinical neurological monitoring is better
- Coronary and cerebral autoregulation preserved
- Problems associated with GA can be avoided
- Shorter operating times and hospital LOS
- Lower rates of death, stroke, MI.

Disadvantages
- Limited access to the airway
- Supine position with drapes—anxiety/claustrophobia, restlessness
- Access limited to long carotid lesions or high bifurcations
- Anxiety or pain may cause myocardial ischemia in vulnerable patients
- Risk of excess sedation.

Regional Anesthesia for Carotid Endarterectomy
- Superficial cervical plexus block
- Deep cervical plexus block
- Cervical epidural anesthesia.

Superficial cervical plexus block is administered to block (C2-4) the sensation of the superficial neck tissues. The procedure involves injecting 3–5 mL of local anesthetic agent (aiming cephalad then caudal) in the middle of line drawn between the mastoid and C6 transverse process. Other method is to inject at the point where the external jugular vein crosses the sternocleidomastoid muscle at the posterior border.

A deep cervical plexus block is used to anesthetize the cervical plexus (sensory innervation of the deep cervical structures) formed from C2 to C4 anterior rami of the ipsilateral spinal roots. The procedure involves positioning the patient supine with a reverse Trendelenburg position (10–20°) and the head slightly rotated to the contralateral side and extended posteriorly. An imaginary line is drawn for superficial block 1 cm posterior and parallel to the sternocleidomastoid muscle. After identifying C2-C4 transverse processes, 5–6 mL of local anesthetic is injected slowly at C2 and C4 levels.

MONITORING

Neurological Monitoring

The main aim is to avoid cerebral ischemia, especially during arterial cross-clamping. It also aids in determining the placement of the carotid artery shunt. The main drawback of neurological monitoring is a paucity of uniform criteria for ischemia, subjective bias when to intervene, and lack of a gold standard monitor. Various monitors, which are in use, are as follows:

- *Awake testing:*
  - Gold Standard for neurological monitoring
  - Questionnaire (baseline and repeated during carotid clamping)
  - Handgrip strength with a ball or toy to assess motor function
- *Stump pressure:*
  - It is the pressure distal to the carotid clamp to assess contralateral circulation
  - *>50 mm Hg:* High specificity (99%) for good collateral pressure
  - *Drawbacks:* Poor sensitivity (30%) as there is no cutoff for shunt placement
  - It is not a continuous measurement.
- *Transcranial Doppler (TCD):*
  - A probe placed over the petrous temporal bone to measure middle cerebral artery (MCA) flow
  - Measures flow and to detect and quantify emboli
  - 50% reduction in flow has a sensitivity of 100% and specificity of 86% for ischemia.
  - *Drawbacks:* Highly operator dependent and may interfere with the surgical site, and acoustic windows are not found in 10–20% of patients.
- *Near infrared spectroscopy (NIRS):*
  - It measures venous and capillary oxygenation to generate regional cerebral oximetry values by placing sensors over the frontal cortex.
  - It is easy to use and has a high negative predictive value. Trigger for interventions is absolute values rSO_2 <50% or 15–20% decrease from baseline.
  - *Drawbacks:* Poor positive predictive value, small sampling window (frontal cortex) and cannot identify emboli.
- *Jugular venous bulb monitoring ($SjVO_2$):*
  - It measures venous saturation by sampling blood at the ipsilateral internal jugular vein.
  - Jugular venous lactate is a marker of brain ischemia.
  - It is a global, not regional, monitor and has a wide range of normal $SjVO_2$ (55–75%).
  - Not an effective monitor.

- *Somatosensory evoked potentials (SSEPs):*
  - It represents deeper structure activity as EEG is recorded after the stimulus.
  - Highly specific.
  - GA may alter the signal and cannot identify emboli.
- *Electroencephalography (EEG):*
  - Waveforms obtained from scalp electrodes (16) in multichannel sets.
  - Inability to monitor subcortical structures and not a good monitor for intraoperative use.

Cardiovascular Monitoring

Carotid endarterectomy leads to heart rate and blood pressure lability. Moreover, coronary vasospasm, tachycardia, and increased afterload may trigger myocardial ischemia during the intraoperative period.[12] Therefore, close cardiovascular monitoring is required during the perioperative period. CAD is quite commonly associated with carotid disease and warrants combined surgery. Hemodynamic monitoring includes multilead ECG (leads II and V5) with ST segment analysis and invasive arterial and central venous pressure monitoring.[13]

- *Bradycardia:* It may be triggered by the manipulation of the carotid sinus and vagal nerve during surgery. It can be attenuated by injection of 1–2 mL of a local anesthetic before manipulation of vessels and maintaining euvolemia.
- *Tachycardia:* Manipulation of the carotid sinus, stress, pain, or catecholamine release may cause tachycardia. It may lead to adverse outcomes in CAD patients and should be managed with short-acting beta blockers such as esmolol or labetalol.
- *Hypotension:* It may be due to vasodilating and negative inotropic effects of several anesthetics or secondary to hypovolemia and bradycardia. It can happen after carotid unclamping, and cerebral reperfusion secondary to cerebral autoregulatory effect protects the brain from reperfusion injury by reducing the production of renin, vasopressin, and norepinephrine.[14] It can be managed by fluids and small boluses of vasopressors.
- *Hypertension:* Cross clamping of the carotid artery leads to stimulation of baroreceptors in the carotid body. That further causes an intracranial release of renin, vasopressin, and norepinephrine to preserve collateral cerebral perfusion. Persistent hypertension may cause cerebral reperfusion injury, hemorrhage, and wound hematoma. It can be managed by titrated doses of vasodilators.

POSTOPERATIVE MANAGEMENT

- *Slow emergence from anesthesia:* Due to residual anesthetic effects, hypothermia, or hypercarbia.

- *New neurological deficits:* Perioperative stroke may occur 24–48 hours after surgery. Doppler ultrasound is to be done to rule out thrombosis.
- *Hypertension:* It may happen due to baroreceptors or cerebral autoregulation disruption that leads to abnormally increased cerebral blood flow. Postoperative pain can also cause an increase in arterial blood pressure.
- *Cerebral hyperperfusion syndrome:* It may occur 2–7 days postsurgery and manifest as cerebral edema, intracerebral hemorrhage, unilateral headache, or seizures. It can be diagnosed with the TCD showing increased peak MCA velocity.
- *Hypotension:* Sometimes, residual carotid hypersensitivity after plaque excision, MI, or hemorrhage can cause hypotension.
- *Neck hematoma:* It may be due to uncontrolled hypertension, anticoagulation, or inadequate surgical hemostasis. Airway and neck structures may be compromised and sometimes warrant reopening of the wound.
- *Cranial nerve injury and vocal cord paralysis:* Surgical traction and compression of the branches of the facial, hypoglossal, and glossopharyngeal nerve may cause temporary paresis. Vocal cord paralysis may be due to injury to the recurrent laryngeal nerve.

CAROTID ARTERY STENTING

Carotid artery stenting (CAS) has been considered an option in patients with complex surgical anatomy and old age with comorbidities. It was first reported in the 1980s as an alternative to CEA. It was initially done as simple balloon dilatation followed by stent placement in 1994.

In the CAVATAS trial, low-to-moderate risk symptomatic patients underwent either CEA or carotid angioplasty. They found no significant difference concerning ipsilateral stroke or transient ischemic attack.[7] In the International Carotid Stenting Study (ICCS), 1,731 patients who underwent either procedure also found no significant difference concerning fatal stroke CAS (6.4%) and CEA (6.5%) after 5 years in the two groups.[15]

The CREST study also studied 2,502 symptomatic and asymptomatic patients about the composite of stroke, MI, or death during the 30 days after the procedure or any ipsilateral stroke within 4 years. They revealed no significant difference in CAS and CEA (7.2 vs. 6.8%, respectively) regarding 4-year rates of the primary endpoint. However, stroke was more frequent in CAS (4.1 vs. 2.3%, $p = 0.01$), and MI in CEA (2.3 vs. 1.1%, $p = 0.03$). They suggested that CAS may be considered an alternative to CEA in average surgical risk patients.

Carotid artery stenting should ideally be performed with adequate procedural quality levels instead of endarterectomy only in specific conditions:[16,17]

- Clinical situations where endarterectomy is technically challenging to perform, such as patients with a history of radiation therapy in the cervical area, post-CEA or complex cervical anatomy.
- Very high (above the mandible) or low (below the clavicle) lesions
- Contralateral laryngeal nerve palsy
- Patients with carotid artery dissection
- Severe tandem lesions
- Age >80 years
- Conditions such as fibromuscular hyperplasia and Takayasu's arteritis
- Severe vascular, cardiac, or pulmonary comorbidities such as congestive heart failure (New York Heart Association class III/IV) and/or known severe left ventricular dysfunction (ejection fraction <30%); need for open heart surgery within 6 weeks; recent myocardial infarction (>24 hours and <4 weeks); and ongoing unstable angina (Canadian Cardiovascular Society class III/IV); and contralateral carotid occlusion.

Advantages of CAS over CEA

- Less invasive
- Requires light sedation or MAC and GA can be avoided
- Decreased incidence of myocardial infarction, cranial nerve injury, venous thromboembolism, or wound infection
- Less incidence of perioperative hypertension
- Cervical hematoma and airway compromise is less.

Carotid Artery Stenting Procedure

Carotid artery stenting may be performed via transfemoral approach or transcarotid artery approach under local anesthesia (LA) or mild sedation. It involves the intra-arterial placement of a catheter over a guidewire and the deployment of a balloon or a stent. The stent is used to expand the lumen of the carotid artery, with or without an emboli-protection device. Even though the transfemoral technique is believed to provide better maneuverability, it can be limited by aortic arch anatomy and calcifications that can be prevented by the transcarotid artery revascularization (TCAR)[18] approach. The TCAR procedure is a hybrid surgical and endovascular intervention in which the common carotid artery is identified and dissected circumferentially. A vessel loop or umbilical tape is placed around the artery. The common carotid artery is accessed directly using a micropuncture kit, and an angiogram is obtained. This approach reduces the risk of embolization in case of a hostile aortic arch.

Anesthesia Management of Carotid Artery Stenting

Anesthetic considerations for CAS are primarily the same as for CEA. The only difference is that patients have more comorbidities. Thus, the anesthesiologist must tailor an individualized plan to maximize therapeutic benefit and eliminate morbidity. As these procedures are usually performed in a radiology suite, the challenges associated with providing anesthesia in remote locations must always be anticipated. The unique challenges encountered in nonoperating room anesthesia include: a remote location of the suite, difficult airway and intravenous cannula, climate control, hazards associated with the use of radiations and contrast material, etc.[19]

Anesthesia Technique of Carotid Artery Stenting

The transfemoral approach is usually performed under LA with or without sedation to monitor the patient's neurological status. As the transcarotid approach involves direct surgical exposure of the common carotid artery thus, it may require LA with sedation or GA. Access to the airway is usually limited due to the C-arm, and patients with difficult airways may impose unique challenges of patient position and equipment required. Moreover, intravenous access may also be limited due tucking of the limbs by the side of the patient thus, extension lines must be used for administering intravenous fluids and additional drugs. Forced air warmers should be used to keep the patient warm and avoid shivering/hypothermia.

Regardless of the approach, patients should be closely monitored during the procedure, and standard monitoring as per the ASA recommendations mentioned earlier. Invasive hemodynamic monitoring and neurological monitoring, as described earlier, should be considered in cases that are performed under GA.[20] Vascular manipulation around the carotid bulb can cause dramatic changes in the patient's hemodynamics, such as hypotension and/or bradycardia. Administration of prophylactic anticholinergics such as glycopyrrolate can help in mitigating bradycardia associated with carotid sinus manipulation.[21]

Anticoagulation

Carotid artery stenting involves the placement of numerous catheters and guidewires and the manipulation of wires and stents across plaques. Anticoagulation helps prevent thromboembolic complications secondary to these manipulations. A baseline activated clotting time (ACT) must be obtained in all patients, following which a small heparin bolus dose (approximately 100 IU/kg) is administered intravenously to target an ACT of > 250 seconds. Reversal of anticoagulation is usually not required, but protamine should be available to treat any hemorrhage secondary to a prolonged ACT. Dual antiplatelet therapy should be continued in the postoperative period.

Hemodynamic Management

The main aim of hemodynamic management is to prevent cerebral ischemia during the perioperative period. Initially, arterial pressure should be maintained 15-20% above the baseline to ensure adequate cerebral perfusion via the circle of Willis.[22] After the stent deployment and a 3-minute washout period has lapsed, one must consider decreasing or stopping vasopressors as target systolic blood pressure to 110-140 mm Hg to prevent cerebral hyperperfusion. Persistent hypotension is also frequently encountered after stent deployment due to carotid baroreceptor stimulation and may warrant the use of vasopressor support. Prompt management of other physiological parameters such as temperature, glucose, blood rheology, and arterial carbon dioxide tension that can influence cerebral blood flow is also essential.

Postprocedure Care

Cerebral hyperperfusion can happen frequently after CAS for a severely stenosed artery in patients with poor cerebral autoregulation and limited cerebrovascular reserve.[23] It is slow in onset and can occur 2-7 days postprocedure. The patient usually complains of a headache secondary to cerebral edema, which can progress to intracerebral hemorrhage causing focal neurological signs and/or epileptic seizures.[24] Brain imaging, such as contrast angiography or magnetic resonance angiography, can help distinguish hyperperfusion or cerebral vasoconstriction. Admission to an ICU or a high dependency unit for the first 24 hours after the procedure to closely monitor the neurological and hemodynamic status of the patient. Patients with persistent hypotension are also predisposed to cerebral and myocardial hypoperfusion leading to stroke/myocardial ischemia and may require vasopressor support till hemodynamics are completely optimized.[25,26]

Monitoring of distal limb pulsations is an essential aspect of postoperative monitoring as it is frequently overlooked, and nasty vascular complications have been reported. The presence of distal pulses must always be documented after the end of a procedure. Care must be taken when removing large bore sheaths as they may cause complications such as the groin or retroperitoneal hematoma, dissection of major vessels, and/or peripheral thrombosis causing limb ischemia.

■ CONCLUSION

Carotid endarterectomy is an intervention of choice for treating patients with carotid artery stenosis, while the role of carotid angioplasty/stenting is under evaluation in various randomized clinical trials and is gaining acceptance. The primary objective of any of these procedures is to prevent embolic stroke. Perioperative anesthetic management in such situations must be tailored to prevent these by maintaining tight physiological control.

These patients are at high risk of developing adverse perioperative cardiac and neurological sequelae and require close monitoring. Optimizing their cardiovascular status, renal insufficiency, and diabetes mellitus are mandatory during the perioperative period. Carotid clamping during resection and anastomosis predisposes these patients to the risk of cerebral ischemia, which can be minimized by maintaining high perfusion pressure. No single anesthetic technique has shown superior results for patients undergoing CEA. It is essential to ensure that cerebral blood flow is optimized, cardiac stress is minimized, and that anesthetic recovery is rapid. Carotid artery stenting is ideally performed under light sedation with antithrombotic therapy as per guidelines. Tight hemodynamic control and vigilance for bradycardia and hypotension are essential during the procedure and in the immediate postoperative period. Although a CAS is a minimally invasive option still, there is a higher risk of perioperative stroke, and it is primarily reserved for patients with complex neck anatomy and significant systemic comorbidities, making them unsuitable for surgery.

REFERENCES

1. Eastcott HH, Pickering GW, Rob CG. Reconstruction of internal carotid artery in a patient with intermittent attacks of hemiplegia. Lancet. 1954;267(6846):994-6.
2. Radak D, de Waard D, Halliday A, Neskovic M, Tanaskovic S. Carotid endarterectomy has significantly lower risk in the last two decades: should the guidelines now be updated? J Cardiovasc Surg. 2018;59:586-99.
3. Mathias K. Perkutane transluminale Katheterbehandlung supraaortaler Arterienobstruktionen. Angiology. 1981;3:47-50.
4. North American Symptomatic Carotid Endarterectomy Trial Collaborators. Beneficial effect of carotid endarterectomy in symptomatic patients with high-grade carotid stenosis. N Engl J Med. 1991;325(7):445-53.
5. European Carotid Surgery Trialists' Collaborative Group. Randomised trial of endarterectomy for recently symptomatic carotid stenosis: results of the MRC European Carotid Surgery Trial (ECST). Lancet. 1998;351:1379-87.
6. Rerkasem A, Orrapin S, Howard DPJ, Rerkasem K. Carotid endarterectomy for symptomatic carotid stenosis. Cochrane Database Syst Rev. 2020;9: CD001081.
7. Endovascular versus surgical treatment in patients with carotid stenosis in the Carotid and Vertebral Artery Transluminal Angioplasty Study (CAVATAS): a randomised trial. Lancet. 2001;357(9270):1729-37.
8. Rothwell PM, Eliasziw M, Gutnikov SA. Analysis of pooled data from the randomised controlled trials of endarterectomy for symptomatic carotid stenosis. Lancet. 2003;361:107-16.
9. Rerkasem K, Bond R, Rothwell PM. Local versus general anaesthesia for carotid endarterectomy. Cochrane Database Syst Rev. 2004:CD000126.
10. Tangkanakul C, Counsell C, Warlow C. Local-versus general anaesthesia for carotid endarterectomy (Cochrane review). In: The Cochrane Library (Issue 2). Oxford: Update Software; 2003.

11. Harky A, Chan JSK, Kot TKM, Sanli D, Rahimli R, Belamaric Z, et al. General anesthesia versus local anesthesia in carotid endarterectomy: a systematic review and meta-analysis. J Cardiothorac Vasc Anesth. 2020;34:219-34.
12. Choi SS, Lim YJ, Bahk JH, Do SH, Ham BM. Coronary artery spasm induced by carotid sinus stimulation during neck surgery. Br J Anaesth. 2003;90:391-4.
13. Yastrebov K. Intraoperative management: carotid endarterectomies. Anesthesiol Clin N Am. 2004;22:265-87.
14. Gibbs BF. Temporary hypotension following endarterectomy for severe carotid stenosis: should we treat it? J Vasc Endovasc Surg. 2003;37:33-6.
15. Bonati LH, Dobson J, Featherstone RL, International Carotid Stenting Study investigators. Long-term outcomes after stenting versus endarterectomy for treatment of symptomatic carotid stenosis: the International Carotid Stenting Study (ICSS) randomized trial. Lancet. 2015;385(9967):529-38.
16. Brott TG, Hobson RW II, Howard G, Roubin GS, Clark WM, Brooks W, et al; CREST Investigators. Stenting versus endarterectomy for treatment of carotid-artery stenosis. N Engl J Med. 2010;363(1):11-23.
17. Cremonesi A, Setacci C, Bignamini A, Bolognese L, Briganti F, Di Sciascio G, et al. Carotid artery stenting: first consensus document of the ICCS SPREAD Joint Committee. Stroke. 2006;37(9):2400-9.
18. Ankam A, Kinthala S, Madabhushi P. Anesthetic considerations for transcarotid artery revascularization: experience and review of forty cases from a single medical center. Cureus. 2020;12(12):e12250.
19. Goudra B, Alvarez A, Singh PM. Practical considerations in the development of a nonoperating room anesthesia practice. Curr Opin Anaesthesiol. 2016;29(4):526-30.
20. Moritz S, Kasprzak P, Arlt M, Taeger K, Metz C. Accuracy of cerebral monitoring in detecting cerebral ischemia during carotid endarterectomy: a comparison of transcranial Doppler sonography, near-infrared spectroscopy, stump pressure, and somatosensory evoked potentials. Anesthesiology. 2007;107: 563-9.
21. Chung C, Cayne NS, Adelman MA, Riles TS, Lamparello P, Han D, et al. Improved hemodynamic outcomes with glycopyrrolate over atropine in carotid angioplasty and stenting. Perspect Vasc Surg Endovasc Ther. 2010;22:164-70.
22. Vanpeteghem C, Moerman A, De Hert S. Perioperative hemodynamic management of carotid artery surgery. J Cardiothorac Vasc Anesth. 2016;30:491-500.
23. Moulakakis KG, Mylonas SN, Sfyroeras GS, Andrikopoulos V. Hyperperfusion syndrome after carotid revascularization. J Vasc Surg. 2009;49(4):1060-8.
24. Abou-Chebl A, Yadav JS, Reginelli JP, Bajzer C, Bhatt D, Krieger DW. Intracranial hemorrhage and hyperperfusion syndrome following carotid artery stenting: risk factors, prevention, and treatment. J Am Coll Cardiol. 2004;43(9):1596-601.
25. Mylonas SN, Moulakakis KG, Antonopoulos CN, Kakisis JD, Liapis CD. Carotid artery stenting-induced hemodynamic instability. J Endovasc Ther. 2013;20:48-60.
26. Lian X, Lin M, Zhu S, Liu W, Li M, Sun W, et al. Risk factors associated with haemodynamic depression during and after carotid artery stenting. J Clin Neurosci. 2011;18:1325-8.

CHAPTER

Anesthetic Implications in the Intravascular Treatment of Cerebral Aneurysms and Arteriovenous Malformations

Anil Parakh, Joanna S Rodriques

ABSTRACT

Airway protection, adequate monitoring, and cardiovascular and neurological stability are critical in managing patients for intravascular treatment of cerebral aneurysms and arteriovenous malformations. One of the most important considerations for an anesthesiologist should be attempting to achieve hemodynamic stability in the face of potential increased intracranial pressure and subsequent vulnerability of the tissues to ischemic insult.

Keywords: Arteriovenous malformation; Cerebral aneurysm; Anesthesia; Interventional neuroradiology.

KEY POINTS

- The main aim of anesthesia is to provide stable hemodynamics and a rapid emergence for the early assessment of the patient.
- Deliberate hypotension is required during glue injection to prevent embolization of the glue.
- Hyperemic complications may result in cerebral edema and hemorrhage postoperatively.
- For cerebral aneurysms, the popularity of adenosine to provide cardiac standstill is increasing.
- Any change in the transmural gradient should be minimized to prevent rupture of the aneurysm.
- Adequate perfusion pressure is to be maintained with euvolemia or vasopressors.

INTRODUCTION

Arteriovenous malformations (AVMs) are knotted anastomoses of blood vessels of varying levels where arteriovenous shunting occurs in a central nidus. This nidus is defined as the site where multiple feeding arteries converge and where large veins drain.[1] AVMs result due to atypical direct communications between small arteries and veins sans the intervening

capillaries, thereby resulting in low resistance and high-flow shunts. The classical presentation includes:
- Intracranial bleed (30–86% in adults[2] and 75–80% in pediatrics[3])
- Seizure (8–46%)[2]
- Focal neurological deficits (4–23%)[2]
- Hydrocephalus or rarely congestive cardiac failure (CCF).[2]

Cerebral compromise occurs due to:
- "Steal" phenomenon
- Ischemia from the failure of perfusion from CCF
- Hemorrhagic infarction from thrombosis of the aneurysm of the great vein of Galen
- Cerebral atrophy
- Alterations of flow caused by surgery.[4]

Intracranial AVMs are discovered in:
- Supratentorial areas (70-97%)
- Infratentorial areas (3–30%)
- Or in deeper brain structures (5–18%).[2]

Prognostic factors pertaining to higher intra and postoperative complications include:
- The volume of AVM (>20 cm)[5]
- Presence of deep feeding vessels and a deep draining system
- Shunt flow >120 cm/sec[1] and pulsatility index <0.5 as estimated by transcranial Doppler
- Eloquent area of the brain
- History of the previous bleed.

Langer et al. suggested that smaller AVMs are at a higher risk of hemorrhage due to higher perfusion pressure.[6] Treatment of AVMs depends on factors such as the patient's age, neurological condition, and characteristics of AVMs.

The different treatment modalities are:
- Conservative management
- Microsurgical removal with or without endoscopic assistance
- Endovascular embolization
- Stereotactic surgery.

ANESTHETIC CONSIDERATIONS

Anesthesia for Endovascular Embolization

Conscious sedation under monitored anesthesia care (MAC) is usually considered the basic anesthetic approach in cooperative adult patients is conscious sedation.[2,7-8] General anesthesia is required for those patients who are unaccommodating, need controlled ventilation [to minimize movement and improve image quality or if there is a sign of an increase in increased intracranial pressure (ICP)], have comorbid conditions that exempt them from lying supine for long hours (arthritis, chronic cough, and asthma), aiding induced hypotension, augmentation of blood pressure in patients with an occlusive disease, claustrophobic patients or for those having an unstable neurological or cardiovascular status.

1. *Preoperative evaluation:* Barring the regular preanesthetic evaluation, attention to detail must be paid with regards to assessing the neurological status, the physical condition of the patient (CCF), drug history, protamine allergy (including insulin use, fish allergy),[8] histories of prior anticoagulation or coagulation disorders, recent steroid use and contrast reaction. Robust attempts at induced hypotension are dangerous in patients with a history of transient ischemic attacks or cerebrovascular occlusion.[7] The patient's ability to lie supine for many hours is a prerequisite for monitored anesthesia care.

2. *Premedication:* Many centers administer glycopyrrolate and continue the antiepileptic drugs as well as other medication as per the medical comorbidities of the patient.

3. *Room preparation:* An interventional radiology suite should be equipped for anesthetic care exactly as standard operating rooms. All intravenous (IV) lines, including the central venous catheter, should have sufficient slack by attaching long extension tubing to their ports to have free movement of the C-arm of fluoroscopy, and tubing should be prefilled with the desired drugs or saline. Continuous arterial line monitoring should be started before the induction of anesthesia. The patient should be adequately warmed, and care should be taken to administer only warm fluid to avoid excessive cooling. The bladder should also be catheterized to monitor urine output, which helps in fluid management because the contrast medium produces an osmotic load and often leads to vigorous diuresis.[9]

4. *Anesthesia technique:* The agents used for the induction and maintenance of anesthesia should support and result in hemodynamic stability, rapid emergence at the end of the procedure, and the medical and neurological requirements of the patients. Factors favoring the choice of general anesthesia are age (infants or young children), uncooperative patients, potential airway problems (chronic cough, smoking, and snoring), back pain, an anticipated lengthy procedure where complete immobility is needed, and suspected increase in ICP where sedation is contraindicated.[7]

   General anesthesia is administered using propofol, and tracheal intubation is achieved using any muscle relaxant except succinylcholine ventilation goals include moderate hypocapnia, as spontaneous ventilation with the possibility of hypercarbia may be detrimental. A baseline activated clotting time (ACT) is also obtained,[7] and the patient is then anticoagulated with heparin 1 mg/kg IV to keep the ACT 1½ times above its standard value. Heparin should be continued for a further 24 hours.[8] To prevent retrograde thrombosis in the embolized vessels, which transpires due to the thrombogenic effects of endothelial trauma and the inherently thrombogenic materials instilled, 24 hours postprocedure anticoagulation is incorporated.

5. *Deliberate hypotension:* During embolization, the blood pressure should be monitored and controlled, and deliberate hypotension is mandated during glue injection. The idea is to decelerate the flow through the feeding artery and prevent systemic embolization of glue. Sodium nitroprusside (SNP) can be used as an infusion. However, bear in mind that SNP is also a cerebral vasodilator and can cause cerebral steal, but it maintains the best cerebral perfusion among other agents.[10] Cardiac standstills using adenosine are also utilized to decrease the flow through AVM during glue placement.[11]

6. *Deliberate hypertension:* In situations where cerebral ischemia develops, the brain can be protected by an increase in blood pressure, which leads to an increase in the flow in the collateral pathways. This can be achieved using phenylephrine with or without dopamine.

7. *Postprocedure management:* Ideally, the trachea is extubated after the procedure in a straightforward, uncomplicated case. Immediate neurological intervention and consultation are sought in case there is any episode of nausea, vomiting, or headache. Deliberate hypotension or hypertension postembolization is maintained as per the conduct of the case.

Anesthetic Considerations for Surgical Resection

Preoperative or intraoperative embolization, along with surgical resection, is the mainstay of treatment. Intraoperative ultrasonographic examination during the surgical treatment of AVM is picking up steam because of its ability to detect the components of the lesion.[12]

1. *Preoperative evaluation and premedication:* Preoperative evaluation and premedication are similar to the patients scheduled for embolization (as discussed above). However, the development of any new neurological insult during embolization, condition of hydration status, and kidney status keeping in view that a large amount of dye might have been injected during angiography and/or embolization should primarily be evaluated and stabilized. Although preoperative endovascular embolization has been shown to reduce intraoperative blood loss during surgical resection,[13] when it occurs, it can be rapid, massive, and difficult

to control. Hence, appropriate measures should be taken beforehand, including the availability of blood and blood products.
2. *The technique of Anesthesia:* Principle goals are smooth induction and intubation with tight blood pressure control. The anesthesia technique should be directed to suppress the noxious stimuli and evaluate the volume status. The hemodynamic response to laryngoscopy, intubation, and placement of pins for head fixation and skin incision must be anticipated, and the appropriate use of drugs (viz., lidocaine, β-blocker, nitroglycerin, and SNP) at an appropriate time may be beneficial.
3. Monitoring equipment is applied before the induction of anesthesia. After induction but before tracheal intubation, an indwelling arterial catheter should be placed for direct blood pressure measurement. A central venous pressure catheter, pulmonary artery catheter, or transesophageal echocardiography may help monitor fluid replacement therapy, particularly in patients with underlying cardiovascular disease.
4. *Brain protection:* Cerebral protection may be achieved through metabolic suppression with barbiturates, propofol, or etomidate, but at the cost of delayed emergence. Metabolic suppression may be helpful if there is an intraoperative catastrophe. (e.g., uncontrolled bleeding, malignant cerebral swelling). Non-pharmacological methods of cerebral protection include maintenance of stable systemic hemodynamics and cerebral perfusion pressure, cerebral relaxation to decrease retractor pressure [via neutral head position, cerebrospinal fluid (CSF) drainage, diuretics, modest hypocapnia], euglycemia and isotonicity, euvolemia, mild hypothermia, and controlled emergence from anesthesia.
5. *Emergence:* In contemplation of having a swift and trustworthy assessment of the neurological function of the patient, an early emergency is prudent. Adequate blood pressure control is needed to avoid bleeding from the AVM bed.

COMPLICATIONS AND THEIR MANAGEMENT

1. *Management of neurological mishaps during embolization:* Debacles during AVMs can take you by storm, and hence vigilance and careful planning are required. The sole concern is to secure the airway and preserve gas exchange in a sedated patient. Augmentation of blood pressure with or without direct thrombolysis is sought in case of an occlusive issue that increases the distal perfusion. In contrast, if there is a hemorrhage, blood pressure is reduced using SNP, and heparin is reversed using protamine. The rapidity with which heparin is reversed is directly proportional to the excellent outcome from the bleed.[8] Use of a muscle relaxant facilitates trachea intubation as well as prevents a seizure, and helps to maintain ventilation. The contrast medium can cause a variety

of adverse reactions. It may include allergic reaction or osmotic load that further aggravates CCF, especially in neonates, hypovolemia, electrolyte imbalance (osmotic load), and renal impairment, especially in patients with renal compromise.

2. *Complications after surgical resection:* Hyperemic complications may occur due to cerebral edema or hemorrhage. The theories to explain its pathogenesis include "normal perfusion pressure breakthrough" (NPPB) and "occlusive hyperemia", proposed by Spetzler et al.[14] and Al-Rodhan et al.,[15] respectively. Once the shunt is abruptly rectified and removed, the increased cerebral blood flow (CBF) shunts into previously hypoperfused areas leading to cerebral edema and hemorrhage at normal perfusion pressure and hence responsible for all the symptoms and signs.[16]

INTRACRANIAL ANEURYSMS

Cerebral aneurysms are outpouchings of arteries protruding into the subarachnoid space. Hemodynamic stress and turbulent flow lead to vascular bifurcations and aneurysms usually occur at these junctions,[17] aneurysms or AVMs having weakened blood vessels rupture, leading to hemorrhagic strokes. Prevalence is higher in women and patients with polycystic kidney disease or a positive family history of intracranial aneurysms or subarachnoid hemorrhage (SAH).[18] Most cerebral aneurysms (80–85%) are located in the anterior circulation and are more prone to rupture when larger than 7 mm.[19-21] Classically, patients present with:

- The worst headache of their lives (as after aneurysmal rupture, arterial blood flows freely into the subarachnoid space spreading into the cerebrospinal fluid. Intracranial pressure suddenly reaches values equal to arterial pressure).
- Nausea, vomiting, and photophobia
- Altered or lost consciousness
- Seizures
- Meningismus
- And focal neurological deficits.

Many grading scales for SAH have been proposed, but three **(Tables 1 to 3)** are mainly used in clinical practice.[17,22,23]

Non-contrast computed tomography (CT) scans can successfully diagnose an SAH. However, if inconclusive, a lumbar puncture may be inevitable. Angiography is considered the most helpful yardstick to conclude an aneurysm as the etiology of SAH. CT angiography and magnetic resonance imaging (MRI) angiography are noninvasive valuable tools, although less reliable for small aneurysms.[19]

Aneurysmal SAH equates with early and late complications that may inveigle the anesthetic management.

TABLE 1: Hunt and Hess classification after subarachnoid hemorrhage (SAH).

Category	Criteria
Grade I	Asymptomatic, or minimal headache and slight nuchal rigidity
Grade II	Moderate-to-severe headache, nuchal rigidity, no neurological deficit other than cranial nerve palsy
Grade III	Drowsiness, confusion, or mild focal deficit
Grade IV	Stupor, moderate-to-severe hemiparesis, possibly early decerebrate rigidity and vegetative disturbances
Grade V	Deep coma, decerebrate rigidity, and moribund appearance

TABLE 2: World Federation of Neurological Surgeons (WFNS) subarachnoid hemorrhage (SAH) scale.

WFNS grade	Glasgow Coma Scale (GCS) score	Motor deficit
I	15	Absent
II	14–13	Absent
III	14–13	Present
IV	12–7	Present or absent
V	6–3	Present or absent

TABLE 3: Fisher Scale for Grading Subarachnoid Hemorrhage (SAH) on Admission Computed Tomography (CT) Scan.

Grade	CT Scan
I	No blood visualized
II	A diffuse deposition or thin layer with all vertical layers of blood (interhemispheric fissure, insular cistern, ambient cistern) <1 mm thick
III	Localized clots and/or vertical layers of blood 1 mm or greater in thickness
IV	Diffuse or no subarachnoid blood, but with intracerebral or intraventricular clots

Surgical treatment involves obliterating the aneurysm by clipping via the intracranial route or coiling via the endovascular route.

Anesthesia Management for Craniotomy for Aneurysm Clipping

- *Preoperative anesthetic evaluation:*
  - The number, location, and size of the aneurysms should be noted.
  - The patient's baseline vitals, neurological deficits, any complications **(Table 4)**, and treatment received should be documented.

TABLE 4: Complications after subarachnoid hemorrhage (SAH).

Neurological complications	Non-neurological complications
Hydrocephalus	Cardiac dysfunction
Intracranial hypertension	Pulmonary dysfunction (neurogenic or cardiac pulmonary edema, and acute respiratory distress syndrome)
Vasospasm and delayed cerebral ischemia	Electrolyte disturbances (hyponatremia hypomagnesemia, hypocalcemia, hypokalemia)
Rebleeding	Endocrine disturbances (hyperglycemia, hypothalamopituitary dysfunction)
Seizures	Fever

- The anesthetic-related risks, possibilities of cataclysms such as aneurysm rupture or rebleeding, the need for blood transfusions, and postoperative mechanical ventilation should be explained diligently to the patient and the relatives.
- Due to altered mental status and drowsiness in patients with SAH, premedication with benzodiazepines or an opioid should be given gingerly.
- *Monitoring:*
  - Besides standard monitoring, urine catheters and temperature probes are mandatory.
  - Large bore peripheral IV lines should be secured, and an arterial line should be inserted. A central venous line may be deemed necessary in case of poor peripheral access or when large amounts of vasopressors and large blood loss are anticipated.
- *General Goals:*
  - Minimize any change in the aneurysm transmural gradient.
    - The transmural gradient is the difference between the pressure within the aneurysm (mean arterial pressure) and the pressure outside the aneurysm (intracranial pressure).[17] Any sudden increase in this gradient may lead to rupture. Therefore, blood pressure escalations should be avoided and promptly treated with fast-acting agents. Hypertension is frequently encountered during laryngoscopy, pinning, and incision.
  - Maintain adequate cerebral perfusion pressure.
  - Cerebral perfusion pressure is the difference between mean arterial pressure and intracranial pressure. If there is reasonable cerebral perfusion, there is adequate brain oxygenation and no ischemia. This cerebral perfusion pressure is imperative to maintain cerebral autoregulation.[17] Cerebral perfusion pressure should be maintained

with euvolemia and vasopressors such as phenylephrine or norepinephrine.
- *Provide brain relaxation:*
  - Adequate surgical exposure and minimal brain retraction injuries can be facilitated by a relaxed brain. This is usually achieved by unobstructed cerebral venous return, adequate cerebral perfusion pressure and oxygenation, and normal ventilation.
  - Volatile anesthetics above one minimum alveolar concentration produce significant direct cerebral vasodilation resulting in increased cerebral blood volume and brain bulk.
  - Propofol reduces cerebral blood volume and may be preferable over volatile anesthetics if the intracranial pressure is elevated.[17]
  - Mannitol decreases brain water content by generating an osmotic gradient through an intact blood-brain barrier. When used in an injured blood-brain barrier, mannitol may produce rebound edema with secondary intracranial hypertension. Mannitol should not be used if serum osmolality exceeds 330 mOsm/L.
  - Furosemide alone (1 mg/kg) or combined (5–20 mg) with mannitol decreases intracranial pressure and brain bulk.
  - Combined therapy is more effective than either of these drugs alone, but is associated with an even greater loss of free water and electrolytes, possibly leading to hypovolemia and hypotension.[17,24-26] Cerebrospinal fluid drainage via lumbar drain or external ventricular drain may be used to improve the operating condition. It should be used carefully before dural opening to avoid acute elevation of the aneurysm transmural gradient and secondary aneurysm rupture. Transient mild hyperventilation should be avoided as it can cause an excessive reduction in cerebral blood flow. When surgical exposure is adequate, $PaCO_2$ should be kept between 35–38 mm Hg.
- Allow a fast and smooth emergence.
  - Early neurological evaluation is imperative to detect complications that may need intervention. Delayed emergence may be due to iatrogenic drug dosages, intracranial bleeding, stroke, seizures, or tension pneumocephalus. Coughing, bucking, vomiting, and hypertension should all be avoided to minimize brain edema. Patients must be shifted to the intensive care unit for thorough monitoring and evaluation.
- *Neurophysiologic monitoring:*
  - The most frequently incorporated monitoring includes electroencephalography and evoked potentials (somatosensory evoked potentials, motor evoked potentials, and brainstem auditory evoked potentials).[17]

- Anesthesia agents should be carefully administered to elicit a recording while maintaining adequate anesthesia depth and immobility. Volatile anesthetics should remain below 0.5 minimum alveolar concentration when somatosensory evoked potentials and motor evoked potentials are recorded. When motor evoked potentials are monitored, an initial muscle relaxant for intubation may be administered however, after that it should be avoided. Propofol and opioid infusion should be titrated appropriately. Adequate analgesics must be given and bolus drugs must be avoided. Dexmedetomidine is an excellent agent to include in the armamentarium of drugs for this purpose.
- *Temporary arterial occlusion and brain protection:*
  - Temporary occlusion of the proximal artery techniques may be incorporated by surgeons while dealing with giant aneurysms and those likely to rupture intraoperatively. The occlusion time should be limited to 10 minutes as >20 minutes of occlusion is associated with poor outcomes.[27,28] While doing so the blood pressure should be kept at a higher size to maximize the collateral flow.
  - No clear-cut benefits of hypothermia have been proven, nor is there any evidence of its harm.[29,30]
  - Hyperthermia and hyperglycemia should be avoided.
- *Intraoperative rupture:*
  - Any untimely rupture must be communicated to the anesthesiologist by the surgeon, and the target blood pressure must be decided. Temporary-controlled hypotension is associated with poor,[31] although an adenosine-induced transient circulatory arrest has proven beneficial.[32-34]

Anesthetic Considerations for Endovascular Coiling of Cerebral Aneurysms

- The main aim is to prevent vasospasm and elevated intracranial pressure to prevent the aneurysm from rupturing and avoid any disastrous culminations. This can be achieved by reducing systemic pressure. The transmural pressure gradient of the aneurysm should be maintained by preventing increased blood pressure, especially during intubation and pinning.[17,35,36]
- General anesthesia is preferred over sedation as it allows for an immobile patient, thereby minimizing the risk of vessel injury, enabling superior hemodynamic stability and control, ensuring a secure airway, and permitting a comfortable patient to withstand long hours if the procedure is prolonged or if complications arise.[37,38]

- The insertion of an laryngeal mask airways (LMA) bypasses the autonomic nervous system excitation induced by direct laryngoscopy, intubation, and extubation.[36,37] However, some advocate its use for endovascular internal carotid artery (ICA) repair only.
- General anesthesia, when administered with a combination of propofol or sevoflurane, ensures stable hemodynamics, adequate depth, and early recovery.[35,37] However, when sevoflurane is used at an MAC of >2, the cerebral blood flow and CO_2 increase, thus making it unfavorable.[17] Although during angiography and the placement of coil springs in the aneurysm sac, the extent of stimulation is markedly lower than during the induction of anesthesia, it is preferable to secure the airway and intubate the patient to avoid coughing and bucking during the procedure. LMA use is tricky as they may get dislodged during a head turn or 360° turn of the collimator machine. Shifting such a patient postoperatively on the ventilator might not be permissible.
- *Management of intracranial aneurysm rupture:* Any increase in the intracranial pressure may result in aneurysm rupture.[17] If the depth of anesthesia is inadequate, there could be hypertension accompanied by bradycardia. On the contrary, reflex hypotension can cause hypoperfusion, leading to ischemic injuries. Hence standard monitoring, particularly arterial pressure measurements and mean pressure values, must be used.[37,38]

CONCLUSION

Management of intravascular AVMs and aneurysms is challenging but gratifying when positive results are yielded. This can be achieved by providing appropriate anesthesia techniques as the situation demands, incorporating brain protection techniques, and using neuro monitoring to detect potential brain injury and prevent subsequent postoperative complications.

REFERENCES

1. Saleh O, Baluch A, Kaye AJ, Kaye A. Arteriovenous malformation, complications, and perioperative anesthetic management. Middle East J Anaesthesiol. 2008;19(4):737-56.
2. Black S, Sulek CA, Day AL. Cerebral aneurysm and arteriovenous malformation. In: Cucchiara RF, Black S, Michenfelder JD (Eds). Clinical Neuroanaesthesia. 2nd edition. New York: Churchill Livingstone; 2000. pp. 265-318.
3. Di Rocco C, Tamburrini G, Rollo M. Cerebral arteriovenous malformations in children. Acta Neurochir (Wien). 2000;142(2):145-56.
4. Millar C, Bissonnette B, Humphreys RP. Cerebral arteriovenous malformations in children. Can J Anaesth. 1994;41(4):321-31.
5. Hamilton MG, Spetzler RF. The prospective application of a gradient system for arteriovenous malformations. Neurosurgery. 1994;34(1):2-6.

6. Langer DJ, Lasner TM, Hurst RW, Flam ES, Zager EL, King JT Jr. Hypertension small size and deep venous drainage are associated with risk of hemorrhagic presentation of cerebral arteriovenous malformations. Neurosurgery. 1998;42:481-6.
7. O'Mahony BJ, Bolsin SN. Anaesthesia for closed embolisation of cerebral arteriovenous malformations. Anaesth Intens Care. 1998;16(3):318-23.
8. Young WL, Pile-Spellman J. Anesthetic considerations for interventional neuroradiology. Anesthesiology. 1994;80(2):427-56.
9. Jaeger K, Ruschulte H, Herzog T, Heine J, Leuwer M, Piepenbrock S. Anaesthesiological and critical care aspects regarding the treatment of patients with arteriovenous malformations in interventional neuroradiology. Minim Invas Neurosurg. 2000;43:102-5.
10. McDowell GD. Induced hypotension and brain ischaemia. Br J Anaesth. 1985;57:110-9.
11. Pile-Spellman J, Young WL, Joshi S, Duong S, Vang MC, Hartmann A, et al. Adenosine-induced cardiac pause for endovascular embolisation of cerebral arteriovenous malformations: technical case report. Neurosurgery. 1999;44(4):881-6.
12. Cokluk C, Iyigün O, Senel A, Celik F, Rakunt C. The guidance of intraoperative ultrasonography in the surgical treatment of arteriovenous malformation. Minim Invasive Neurosurgery. 2003;46(3):169-72.
13. Viñuela F, Dion JE, Duckwiler G, Martin NA, Lylyk P, Fox A, et al. Combined endovascular embolisation and surgery in the management of cerebral arteriovenous malformations: experience with 101 cases. J Neurosurg. 1991;75(6):856-64.
14. Spetzler RF, Wilson CB, Weinstein P, Mehdorn M, Townsend J, Telles D. Normal perfusion pressure breakthrough. Clin Neurosurg. 1978;25:651-72.
15. Al-Rodhan N, Sundt TM Jr, Piepgras D, Nichols DA, Rüfenacht D, Stevens LN. Occlusive hyperaemia: a theory for hemodynamic complications following resection of intracerebral arteriovenous malformations. J Neurosurg. 1993;78(2):167-75.
16. Macfarlane R, Moskowitz MA, Sakas DE, Tasdemiroglu E, Wei EP, Kontos HA. The role of neuroeffector mechanisms in cerebral hyperperfusion syndromes. J Neurosurg. 1991;75:845-55.
17. Priebe HJ. Aneurysmal subarachnoid haemorrhage and the anaesthetist. Br J Anaesth. 2007;99(1):102-18.
18. Vlak MH, Algra A, Brandenburg R, Rinkel GJ. Prevalence of unruptured intracranial aneurysms, with emphasis on sex, age, comorbidity, country and time period: a systemic review and meta-analysis. Lancet Neurol. 2011;10(7):626-36.
19. Conolly ES Jr, Rabinstein AA, Carhuapoma JR, Derdeyn CP, Dion J, Higashida RT, et al. Guidelines for the management of aneurysmal subarachnoid hemorrhage: a guideline for healthcare professionals from the American Heart Association/American Stroke Association. Stroke. 2012;43(6):1711-37.
20. Wiebers DO, Whisnant JP, Huston J 3rd, Meissner I, Brown RD Jr, Piepgras DG, et al. International study of unruptured intracranial aneurysms investigators.

unruptured intracranial aneurysms: natural history, clinical outcome, and risks of surgical and endovascular treatment. Lancet. 2003;362(9378):103-10.
21. Schievink WI. Intracranial aneurysms. N Engl J Med. 1997;336(1):28-40.
22. Hunt WW, Hess RM. Surgical risk as related to time of intervention in the repair of intracranial aneurysms. J Neurosurg. 1968;28(1):14-20.
23. Rosen DS, Macdonald RL. Subarachnoid hemorrhage grading scales: a systematic review. Neurocrit Care. 2005;2(2):110-8.
24. Drummond JC, Patel PM. Neurosurgical anesthesia. In: Miller RD (Ed). Anesthesia. 7th edition. Philadelphia: Churchill Livingstone Elsevier; 2010. pp. 2045-87.
25. Marsh ML, Marshall LF, Shapiro HM. Neurosurgical intensive care. Anesthesiology. 1977;47:149-63.
26. Stoelting RK, Hillier SC. Diuretics. In: Stoelting RK, Hillier SC (Eds). Pharmacology and Physiology in Anesthesia Practice. 4th edition. Philadelphia: Lippincott Williams and Wilkins; 2006. pp. 490-2.
27. Samson D, Batjer HH, Bowman G, Mootz L, Krippner WJ Jr, Meyer YJ, et al. A clinical study of the parameters and effects of temporary arterial occlusion in the management of intracranial aneurysms. Neurosurgery. 1994;34(1):22-9.
28. Ogilvy CS, Carter BS, Kaplan S, Rich C, Crowell RM. Temporary vessel occlusion for aneurysm surgery: risk factors for stroke in patients protected by induced hypothermia and hypertension and intravenous mannitol administration. J Neurosurg. 1996;84(5):785-91.
29. Todd MM, Hindman B, Clarke WR, Torner JC; Intraoperative Hypothermia for the IHAST Investigators. Mild intraoperative hypothermia during surgery for intracranial aneurysm. N Engl J Med. 2005;352(2):135-45.
30. Li LR, You C, Chaudhary B. Intraoperative mild hypothermia for postoperative neurological deficits in intracranial aneurysm patients. Cochrane Database Syst Rev. 2012;2:CD008445.
31. Giannotta SL, Oppenheimer JH, Levy ML, Zelman V. Management of intraoperative rupture of aneurysm without hypotension. Neurosurgery. 1991;28(4):531-5; discussion 535-6.
32. Bebawy JF, Zeeni C, Sharma S, Kim ES, DeWood MS, Hemmer LB, et al. Adenosine-induced flow arrest to facilitate intracranial aneurysm clip ligation does not worsen neurologic outcome. Anesth Analg. 2013;117(5):1205-10.
33. Luostarinen T, Takala RS, Niemi TT, Katila AJ, Niemelä M, Hernesniemi J, et al. Adenosine-induced cardiac arrest during intraoperative cerebral aneurysm rupture. World Neurosurg. 2010;73(2):79-83; discussion e9.
34. Chowdhury T, Petropolis A, Wilkinson M, Schaller B, Sandu N, Cappellani RB. Controversies in the anesthetic management of intraoperative rupture of intracranial aneurysm. Anesthesiol Res Pract. 2014;2014:595837.
35. Levy DM, Nowicki RWA. Anaesthesia for treatment of cerebral aneurysms. CPD Anaesthesia. 2002:4(3):106-14.
36. Lakhani S, Guhta A, Nahser HC. Anaesthesia for endovascular management of cerebral aneurysms. Eur J Anaesthesiol. 2006;23(11):902-13.
37. Varma MK, Price K, Jayakrishnan V, Manickam B, Kessell G. Anaesthetic consideration for interventional neuroradiology. Br J Anaesth. 2007;99(1):75-85.
38. Lai YC, Manninen PH. Anethesia for cerebral aneurysms: a comparison between interventional neuroradiology and surgery. Can J Anaesth. 2001;48(4):391-5.

CHAPTER 11

Anesthetic Considerations for Functional Neurosurgery

Maria Bustillo

ABSTRACT

Functional neurosurgery is a relatively new branch of neurosurgery that has developed rapidly during the last few years, thanks to advances in the areas of imaging technology. Functional neurosurgery uses structural and functional neuroimaging to localize particular regions of the brain and to perform definite interventions, for example, ablation, neurostimulation, neuromodulation, and neuro-transplantation. These advances have allowed the development of new procedures that use minimally invasive and precise techniques for specific diseases such as Parkinson's disease, essential tremor, epilepsy, and psychiatric disorder like depression. It is fundamental for the anesthesiologist to understand these conditions as well as the goals and the technical difficulties associated with these procedures to be able to provide safe care for these particular groups of patients. In this chapter, we discuss the advances in functional neurosurgery, specifically, the indications for deep brain stimulators, and MR-guided ultrasound. We will review the requirements for the patients undergoing these procedures and evaluate the current recommendations for the anesthesiologist.

Keywords: Neurosurgery; Anesthesiology; Anesthetic techniques; Parkinson's disease (PD); Essential tremor (ET); Dystonia; Deep brain stimulation (DBS); MRI guided Ultrasound (MRgUS).

KEY POINTS

- Parkinson's disease (PD) is a slowly progressive neurodegenerative disease caused by dopamine deficiency in the substantia nigra, locus ceruleus, and other brainstem dopaminergic cell groups. When patients experience wearing-off phenomena or dyskinesias unresponsive to medical management, surgical interventions, such as deep brain stimulation (DBS) and focused ultrasound (FUS) thalamotomy.
- Essential tremor affects approximately 1% of the population worldwide. It is a fine to coarse tremor, usually affecting the hands and head. If not responsive to medical management, DBS and FUS unilateral thalamotomy are safe alternatives for treatment.

- Dystonia is a movement disorder characterized by sustained abnormal postures and disruptions of ongoing movement resulting from alterations in muscle tone. Medical treatment is often unsatisfactory.
- Deep brain stimulation of the thalamic nucleus and the globus pallidus internus has become the preferred stereotactic technique for PD. The globus pallidus internus is the target for dystonia, and the ventral intermediate nucleus of the thalamus is the target for the treatment of essential tremors. Stimulation of the subthalamic nucleus has been shown to cause hyperpolarization and inhibition of neuronal activity. Stimulation of gamma-aminobutyric acidergic neuronal activity results in inhibition of globus pallidus internus (GPi)-target neurons.
- Magnetic resonance imaging (MRI)-guided focused ultrasound (MRgFUS)—the feasibility of noninvasively applying focused ultrasonography through the skull without the necessity of performing craniotomy created a significant transformation that made this technique far more attractive for more general clinical use.
- Magnetic resonance imaging (MRI)-guided focused ultrasound is the treatment for patients with essential tremor refractory to medical treatment. Transcranial MRgFUS is a noninvasive procedure that creates a thalamotomy without the risks of infection or hardware placement.

INTRODUCTION

Functional neurosurgery is a division of neurosurgery that has undergone rapid expansion over the last few years, incited by advances in imaging technology and new treatment modalities. It uses structural and functional neuroimaging to recognize and select specific areas of the brain and to execute specific interventions (ablation, neurostimulation, neuromodulation, and neurotransplantation).

These developments have led to new procedures using minimally invasive and accurate techniques for diseases such as Parkinson's disease (PD), essential tremor, and dystonia. It is fundamental for the anesthesiologist to understand the goals and technical challenges of these procedures to provide safe management of these patients. We center our discussion on the advances in functional neurosurgery, the indications of deep brain stimulators (DBS) and MRI-guided ultrasound (MRgUS), and provide guidelines for the anesthesia care for the patients going through these treatments.

FUNCTIONAL NEUROSURGERY

Functional neurosurgery is a fast-growing and developing area of neurosurgery that is focused on the treatment of neurological disorders that are refractory to medical treatment. These disorders have an alteration of function usually not accompanied by structural or anatomic changes.

Patients with movement disorders (Parkinson's disease, essential tremor, and dystonia), psychiatric diseases (obsessive-compulsive disorder, depression), and chronic pain disorders that are refractory or unresponsive to medical treatment can benefit from functional neurosurgical treatments. The use of frame-based imaging to visualize brain structures and to establish coordinates, electrophysiologic guidance with microelectrode recordings (MERs), and intraoperative clinical testing of awake patients present a challenge to the anesthesiologist as they are demanding, and the patients frequently have complex medical conditions. An organized multidisciplinary team comprised of neurologists, neurosurgeons, neurophysiologists, and anesthesiologists is necessary for good surgical outcomes and patient safety.[1,2]

Parkinson's Disease

Parkinson's disease is a multisystem progressive, a degenerative neurologic disorder that affects 1–2% of persons >60 years of age and is caused by dopamine the lack of adequate levels of dopamine in the substantia nigra. Decreased inhibition of the extrapyramidal motor system produces the characteristic features of the disease, such as resting tremor, bradykinesia, and cogwheel rigidity, as well as shuffling gait, facial immobility, and a monotonous voice. Due to the extensive neurodegeneration, patients also suffer from non-motor characteristics such as seborrhea, orthostatic hypotension, bladder dysfunction, dementia, and depression.[3]

Medical treatment of PD is targeted to increase the action of dopamine relative to acetylcholine in the brain, at the same time minimizing adverse effects of dopamine in the periphery. The most efficacious and widely used drug is levodopa, a dopamine precursor, often mixed with carbidopa, a peripheral decarboxylase inhibitor, to decrease side effects such as nausea, vomiting, and hypotension. Other medical treatment modalities are dopamine-receptor agonists, such as bromocriptine and pramipexole, also selegiline, a type B monoamine oxidase inhibitor (MAOI). Chronic treatment is associated with developing motor complications. The disease is progressive.[4]

When patients present wearing-off phenomena or dyskinesias that do not respond to medical treatment, surgical procedures, such as DBS and MRgFUS thalamotomy, present highly effective and safe options.

Anesthetic concerns for patients with PD are many and are related to the underlying disease, other comorbidities, and medical regimen. The preoperative evaluation must include detailed questions about symptoms and the severity of the disease, particularly bulbar dysfunction, autonomic insufficiency, decreased respiratory reserve, and sleep apnea. PD medications and medications for other comorbidities must be reviewed, including the schedule of the last doses and when the following doses are required, and any side effects associated with therapy.[3]

Essential Tremor

Essential tremor (ET) is one of the most common movement disorders affects approximately 1% of the population worldwide. It is a fine to coarse tremor, usually affecting the hands and head. It can start during childhood, and it tends to increase with age, with no difference in prevalence between men and women.[5] ET is marked by the rhythmic oscillation of agonist and antagonist groups of muscles. It usually affects the head, legs, and voice. The tremor may be unilateral, minimal, or absent at rest. Cognitive dysfunction and gait abnormalities can be also the characteristics of ET, but the disability does not correlate to the severity of the tremor. Although the brain of patients with ET does not appear to have any structural abnormalities, many characteristics indicate an underlying cerebellar or brainstem pathology. Several patients develop exacerbations of ET only with stressful triggers, such as public performances, and as a result, require only intermittent treatment. For others, ET produces persistent disability and, as a result, requires continuous treatment. The initial therapy for essential tremors is medical management; 50% of failure in response to treatment is reported.[6] If ET becomes unresponsive to medical management, DBS and MRgFUS unilateral thalamotomy are the other options. One of the anesthetic considerations for ET is keeping patients still during the procedure under minimal sedation. Other anesthetic concerns are related to the side effects of different treatments.[5]

Dystonia

Dystonia is a movement disorder distinguished by continuous abnormal postures and disruptions of ongoing movement resulting from alterations in muscle tone. Medical treatment is often unsatisfactory. Dystonia can be classified based on clinical presentation or etiology.[7] Generally, dystonia is exacerbated by voluntary movements, whereas rest or sleep can eliminate the symptoms. Frequent locations include the neck (cervical dystonia or torticollis).[7] Symptoms usually begin in childhood. Patients usually do not have other medical conditions but are debilitated by the disease.

There is no cure for dystonia, and the treatment options are primarily symptomatic and usually unsatisfactory. The most promising drug is levodopa but only for the group of patients that are dopa-responsive. Anticholinergic treatments (usually limited by side effects), baclofen, benzodiazepines, muscle relaxants, and anticonvulsant therapy can be helpful. Botulinum toxin injections are considered the primary treatment of cervical dystonia, and they are used with success for spasmodic dysphonia and blepharospasm. The main surgical option for patients that fail medical management is DBS implantation. In some patients, ablation procedures could be a good alternative.[8]

Anesthetic considerations for patients with dystonia include difficulty with positioning and airway challenges. Younger patients with dystonia may require sedation for frame placement and positioning. The anesthetic goal remains to have a patient awake during electrode placement, stimulation, and recording.[9]

DEEP BRAIN STIMULATION

Deep brain stimulation target nuclei differ according to the disease and patient symptoms. The subthalamic nucleus and globus pallidus internus (GPi) are the primary targets for PD. The GPi is the main target for dystonia, and the ventral intermediate nucleus (VIN) of the thalamus is the target for treating ET.[2]

The mechanism of high-frequency stimulation to improve symptoms is not fully known but is likely based on the target nuclei. Stimulation of the subthalamic nucleus has been shown to produce hyperpolarization and inhibition of neuronal activity. Stimulation of gamma-aminobutyric acidergic neuronal activity produces inhibition of GPi-target neurons.[2]

Anesthetic Considerations for Deep Brain Stimulation

The main objective of anesthetic management is to deliver patient comfort and hemodynamic control while facilitating surgical conditions for mapping and implanting the DBS systems. Traditionally, DBS procedures have been done in awake patients with scalp infiltration with local anesthetics. Some patients require mild conscious sedation to help MERs and patient participation during macrostimulation. With advances in intraoperative computed tomography (iCT) and intraoperative MRI that increase target localization precision, some centers report routine use of general anesthesia for DBS placement.[2,3,10]

Preoperative Evaluation

Patients that go through DBS procedures are usually medically complex. In addition to the disease-specific concerns, physicians should evaluate for comorbidities such as hypertension that can increase the risk of intracranial hemorrhage (ICH) during the procedure. The anesthesiologist should consider the approach to the airway and management with the stereotactic frame. The careful evaluation of the airway, ease of mask ventilation with the stereotactic frame on, the Mallampati score, history of difficult intubation, and any other predictors of difficulty with laryngoscopy must be assessed in anticipation of potential obstruction, wheezing, or other potential airway compromises. History of obstructive sleep apnea and obesity can further complicate airway management. Attention must be centered on critical issues for the awake patient undergoing a procedure.[11]

Emphasis on establishing good communication between the patient and the anesthesiologist, as well as the entire team working in the operating room during the case is of the highest importance to make the procedure as safe as possible.[9]

Patients should receive clear instructions on medication management. Anti-PD drugs are usually stopped the evening before surgery to increase the presence of symptoms during the procedure. This will help to demonstrate the accurate placement of the stimulating electrodes as symptoms improve with macrostimulation.

The significance of selecting motivated patients that can cooperate in a different and stressful environment for an extended period is fundamental.[11] Anxiety disorders, low tolerance to pain, and psychiatric diseases could preclude candidacy because there is not much help regarding drugs that can be offered to awake patients with their heads fixed within a stereotactic head holder. Screening of patients should include tests of concentration or personality inventory aimed at discovering problems incompatible with a cooperative patient in the operating room. Claustrophobia may affect cooperation and positioning because, usually, the surgical drapes must hang near the immobilized face may induce a sense of suffocation. Careful placement of the surgical drapes with open access to a patient's face is necessary. Severe uncontrolled movement disorders may cause compromise in the surgical field.

Anesthetic Techniques

Deep brain stimulation implantation may be performed as a two-stage procedure on 1st day or two different days. The initial stage consists of the microelectrode implantation. During this stage, the patient is required to be awake. In the second stage, the implantation of the pulse generator (battery unit) can be done immediately following the initial stage or days later. The second stage is done with the patient under general anesthesia.[11]

For lead implantation, the patient needs to be awake. Standard anesthesia monitors are applied, and oxygen is administered via nasal cannula. Patients are placed in a semi-sitting position. Special attention to positioning is necessary to ensure patient comfort and access to the upper and lower extremities to evaluate the effects on movement during stimulation. Thorough local anesthetic infiltrations, as well as scalp blocks, are critical to achieving patient comfort during the initial stage for lead implantation with the patient awake. Local anesthesia can be supplemented with intravenous sedation, but that will depend on the practice of each institution of lead implantation. Some institutions perform lead placement under general anesthesia.[1-3,10] During awake procedures, sedation should not be administered during microelectrode insertion and recording.

If sedation is required, then effects of sedatives on MER and the respiratory drive should be considered. Medications that can cause respiratory depression should be avoided or used carefully. In addition, plans for emergency airway management should be in place, as access to the airway in patients with stereotactic frames can be extremely difficult. Patients with PD that come for surgery have discontinued their drugs the evening before, making their symptoms very apparent, which in addition to the anxiety associated with the procedure, can induce hypertension even in patients without a previous history. Patients with ET may be taken off their beta-blockers, which can also lead to hypertension. Maintenance of blood pressure within normal parameters is of utmost importance for the anesthesiologist to decrease the risk of intracranial hemorrhage.[1,3]

Surgical Technique for Deep Brain Stimulation Implantation

The first stage is the microelectrode implantation, for this part of the procedure is required for the patient to be awake. Imaging is used to plan a straight path from the parietal surface to the thalamus or structures near-thalamus. This path must avoid vascular structures and the ventricles. Once the stylet electrode lead is in place, the MERs show changes in spontaneous neuronal firing as the electrode goes through the different nuclear or thalamic areas. Recordings of spontaneous neuronal discharges and changes in discharges with patient movement guide the lead placement. Once the lead is in the desired position, macrostimulation begins, and patients are observed for specific symptom amelioration and adverse effects or unpleasant sensations resulting from stimulation. Once the precise location of the microelectrode is achieved and satisfactory feedback observed, the stylet is removed, and the lead is set to be tunneled and connected to the internal pulse generator (IPG).[10,11]

The second stage is the IPG implantation (battery), which may be done immediately after the first stage or days later, and the procedure is done under general anesthesia. During this stage, the leads are tunneled and then connected to the IPG (typically placed in the pectoral region of the chest wall).

Perioperative Complications of Deep Brain Stimulation Procedures

Anesthesiologists need to be attentive to the possible complications associated with DBS placement. It is fundamental to be familiar with the patient's coexisting diseases and to be ready to treat any possible problems associated with the procedure. The incidence of reported problems associated with the procedure varies notably, from 1–25%, accordingly to the center. Reported complications comprise airway obstruction, apnea, aspiration, confusion, agitation, venous air embolism, and uncontrolled hypertension that can lead to cardiac ischemia and intracranial bleeding. Neurologic complications such as seizures and stroke have been reported.[1]

MAGNETIC RESONANCE IMAGING-GUIDED FOCUSED ULTRASOUND

Focused ultrasound for the targeted lesion-based treatment of intracranial abnormalities was first described in the 1950s. Unfortunately, the major limitation of earlier ultrasound-based technology was the significant fading and dissipation of ultrasound waves associated with the intact bony skull, which limited its use.[2] Two significant developments have made possible the use of MRgFUS in clinical practice for neurological diseases. The first development was the ability to marry the ultrasound procedure with magnetic resonance thermometry, permitting visualization of the areas of the brain being heated to different levels of temperature depending on the thresholding of the thermometry output.[12] This is highly important for MRgFUS because it allows identifying the location of the heating concerning the planned target area and the nearby undesired structures. Also, it can reveal the shape of the tissue heated to allow for adjusting parameters that might allow better targeting of the desired tissue.[12] The second development was combining this method with a new helmet technology that allows the focusing of the ultrasound energy on a precise area of the brain.[12] The combination of these two features has permitted for the noninvasive delivery of enough ultrasound energy to allow lesioning of a specific brain target area and, at the same time, monitoring the temperature delivery to guarantee the achievement of lesioning temperatures within a sufficient portion of the target region to be clinically effective and avoid off-target lesioning.[12]

Hemispheric multielement, phased-array transducers defeat the limitations of the intact skull by correcting the phase distortion caused by the variable thickness of the skull and provide specific-targeted cavitation therapy without the need for a craniotomy.[2] Before the final treatment, a pre-procedure computed tomography scan that quantifies the skull thickness and density is fused with an anatomic MRI so that desired targeting and heating are accomplished.[2]

Magnetic Resonance Imaging-guided Focused Ultrasound for Essential Tremor

The most frequent use of MRgFUS in clinical practice during the last several years has been treating ET refractory to medical treatment. Transcranial

MRgFUS for ET uses a noninvasive approach to produce a thalamotomy without exposing the patient to risks of infection or hardware.[2] The VIN of the thalamus is the designated target for controlling the essential ET.[6] Reported side effects related to MRgFUS therapy included transient sensory, cerebellar, motor, and speech abnormalities.[12] Two significant side effects have been observed up to 12 months after treatments, which are gait disturbances and paresthesia/numbness.[2] MRgUS usually is performed only unilaterally because, in some cases, gait, speech, or sensory disorders can persist indefinitely.[12]

Patient Preparation

Magnetic resonance imaging-guided focused ultrasound has several significant advantages over traditional neurosurgical techniques, as it is an incisionless technique that avoids the introduction of hardware and developing infections. Still, there are several limitations to comprehensive embracing. First, a complete and meticulous head shave is a critical step for patient preparation but remains a very unwelcome prerequisite for patients.[6] The entire MRgFUS procedure, from head shaving to completion, could be as long as 3–4 hours for a complex ablation case.[6] This is a more prolonged procedure than a typical unilateral thalamic DBS.[6]

The prolonged procedure time within the MRI scanner may be a problem for patient comfort. Attention to the positioning of the patient in the MRI scanner is critical, all pressure points should be padded, and extremities must be resting comfortably to ensure patients can tolerate the entire procedure in the scanner. Particular attention must be paid to patients with claustrophobia as they can have difficulty in the scanner. Nausea is a frequent side effect during the procedure. Patients should receive antinausea medication before the beginning of the case.[6]

This procedure does not require general anesthesia. Most cases are performed awake without sedation as conscious sedation may obscure clinical signs of treatment, particularly for essential tremor patients. Also, patients need to be tested between cycles to evaluate the effects of the ablations. There are reports of centers where patients may have received sedation to be able to tolerate the procedure.[13] Sedation requirements for MRgUS can vary depending on the institution, the surgeon, and the patient. Blood pressure control during the procedure is necessary to avoid possible intracranial hemorrhage secondary to hypertension, beta-blockers should not be used for blood pressure control for a patient with tremors as beta-blockers can mask clinical signs of treatment. As with DBS procedures, patients undergoing MRgUS have a head frame. The frame can negatively impact airway management during emergencies. Plans to respond to airway emergencies should be in place during these procedures.

ADDITIONAL INDICATIONS FOR FOCUSED ULTRASOUND

Magnetic resonance imaging-guided focused ultrasound lesioning of the VIN of the thalamus has been approved by the Food and Drug Administration (FDA) for the treatment of tremor-dominant PD.[6] Most recently, MRgUS received approval by the FDA for the treatment of dyskinetic PD. Currently, clinical trials are looking at using MRgUS to treat Alzheimer's disease.[6]

CONCLUSION

Deep brain stimulators and MR-guided focus ultrasound are procedures that use minimally invasive techniques. These techniques are being used for the treatment of movement disorders such as Parkinson's disease, essential tremor, and dystonias. Deep brain stimulators have been used successfully to treat Parkinson's disease, essential tremors, dystonias, and some psychiatric diseases like depression. MRI-guided focus ultrasounds have been used for the treatment of essential tremors and the treatment of Parkinson's disease.

Patients undergoing these procedures usually have diseases that have become refractory to medical treatment. The anesthesiologist needs to understand how this can affect the anesthetic plan. Careful airway assessment and managing the airway with the stereotactic frame are critical. History of difficult intubation, as well as any other predictors of possible difficult intubation, must be taken into consideration in case of potential airway compromise because of the stereotactic frame. The selection of motivated patients, as well as establishing good communication between the patient and the anesthesiologist, and the rest of the team in the procedure room, is essential to achieve a successful outcome. Anesthesiologists must familiarize themselves well with these procedures to provide safe patient care.

REFERENCES

1. Venkatraghavan L, Manninen P, Mak P, Lukitto K, Hodaie M, Lozano A. Anesthesia for functional neurosurgery: review of complications. J Neurosurg Anesthesiol. 2006;18(1):64-7.
2. Dunn LK, Durieux ME, Elias WJ, Nemergut EC, Naik BI. Innovations in functional neurosurgery and anesthetic implications. J Neurosurg Anesthesiol. 2018;30(1):18-25.
3. Crawford L, Mueller D, Mathews L. Anesthetic considerations for functional neurosurgery. Anesthesiol Clin. 2021;39(1):227-43.
4. Olanow CW, Stern MB, Sethi K. The scientific and clinical basis for the treatment of Parkinson disease. Neurology. 2009;72(21 Suppl 4):S1-136.
5. Haubenberger D, Hallett M. Essential tremor. N Engl J Med. 2018;378(19):1802-10.
6. Chazen JL, Stavarache M, Kaplitt MG. Cranial MR-guided focused ultrasound: clinical challenges and future directions. World Neurosurg. 2021;145:574-80.

7. Albanese A, Bhatia K, Bressman SB, Delong MR, Fahn S, Fung VS, et al. Phenomenology and classification of dystonia: a consensus update. Mov Disord. 2013;28(7):863-73.
8. Jinnah HA. Medical and surgical treatments for dystonia. Neurol Clin. 2020;38(2):325-48.
9. Osborn IP, Kurtis SD, Alterman RL. Functional neurosurgery: anesthetic considerations. Int Anesthesiol Clin. 2015;53(1):39-52.
10. Venkatraghavan L, Luciano M, Manninen P. Review article: anesthetic management of patients undergoing deep brain stimulator insertion. Anesth Analg. 2010;110(4):1138-45.
11. Erickson KM, Cole DJ. Anesthetic considerations for awake craniotomy for epilepsy and functional neurosurgery. Anesthesiol Clin. 2012;30(2):241-68.
12. Stavarache MA, Chazen JL, Kaplitt MG. Foundations of magnetic resonance-guided focused ultrasonography. World Neurosurg. 2021;145:567-73.
13. Chapman M, Park A, Schwartz M, Tarshis J. Anesthesia considerations of magnetic resonance imaging-guided focused ultrasound thalamotomy for essential tremor: a case series. Can J Anaesth. 2020;67(7):877-84.

CHAPTER

12

Anesthetic Implications in Pediatric Spinal Neurosurgery

Pradeep Sharma, Rahul Yadav

ABSTRACT

Pediatric patients may require neurosurgical procedures in the spinal region for various congenital, traumatic, and neoplastic conditions. These patients represent a complex state and transition of pediatric physiology after birth which gets further compounded by frequent association with other systemic congenital anomalies. Moreover, they have limited physiological reserves and are more prone to adverse cardiorespiratory events (especially in neonates and infants). These patients should be carefully evaluated for a primary neurological condition, associated congenital anomalies or comorbidities, surgical plan, desired intraoperative position, and need for intraoperative neurophysiological monitoring.

Adequate arrangements for airway, fluids, temperature management, and blood products must be undertaken in advance. Most principles of adult neuroanesthesia practice are broadly applicable to pediatric neurosurgery, however, the confines of safety are not well defined due to limited scientific knowledge. The perioperative anesthesia care plan should be tailored based on the primary lesion and risk assessment to improve the functional neurological outcome.

Keywords: Pediatric spinal neurosurgery; Neural tube defects; Anesthesia concerns.

KEY POINTS

- Children may require neurosurgery in the spinal region for various lesions, the most common being neural tube defects. Neonates and infants have immature systemic physiology, thus putting them at elevated risk of perioperative complications.
- The neurological status of the child, congenital lesions, or even syndromic associations should be carefully evaluated during preoperative anesthesia checkups for perioperative risk assessment.
- Preoperative fasting should be kept to a minimum. Recent recommendations allow liberal fluids up to 1 hour before the elective

neurosurgical procedure. Similarly, enteral feeding should be started at the earliest after surgery.
- Sedative premedication should be avoided if the child cannot be kept under supervision. Mass lesions in the spinal region often make conventional airway management impractical and require improvisation such as intubation in a lateral position.
- Patients must be cautiously positioned to prevent position-related injuries. Careful protection of the eyes must be ensured.
- Intravenous or inhalational anesthetics can be used for induction and maintenance of anesthesia. Intraoperative neuromonitoring frequently requires the anesthetic technique to be modified to a great extent.
- Isotonic crystalloid fluids are preferred to maintain normovolemia. Glucose-containing fluid (1–2%) is recommended only in patients susceptible to hypoglycemia. It is desirable to maintain normoglycemia and normothermia. A restrictive transfusion strategy is commonly practiced.
- Patients with anticipated significant blood loss may be started on antifibrinolytic infusion. Multimodal analgesia with acetaminophen, ibuprofen, ketorolac, surgical site local anesthetic infiltration, and parent-controlled analgesia is recommended.

INTRODUCTION

Pediatric age group patients pose a unique challenge to the anesthesiologist as they cannot be simply presumed to be miniature adults. Children often have other systemic congenital anomalies, which may cause adverse neurological outcomes. Congenital neurological deformities, including neural tube defects (NTD) such as spina bifida or tethered cord syndrome (TCS), are amongst the most common spinal neurosurgical procedures in this age group. Other common indications include correction of scoliosis deformity and spinal cord injuries. Spinal cord tumors, arteriovenous malformations (AVM), and intervertebral disk herniations are uncommon. While formulating an anesthesia plan for pediatric spinal neurosurgical procedures, one must consider the pathophysiology of the primary lesion, the effect of age-appropriate systemic physiology, and the influence of other concomitant anomalies. Patient positioning, the feasibility of intraoperative neurophysiological monitoring (IONM), and blood salvage strategies are other critical perioperative factors affecting outcomes.[1] In this chapter, we have delve into common pediatric neurosurgical conditions in the spinal region, followed by neuroanesthesia concerns in conjunction with pediatric considerations.

COMMON NEUROSURGICAL ENTITIES IN THE SPINAL REGION

Neural Tube Defects

Neural tube defect (NTD)/dysraphism (prevalence 1 to 3 per 1,000 live births) is defined as an inadequate midline fusion or closure of a neural tube resulting in defects in nerve roots, spinal cord, or vertebrae. It signifies a defect either during the primary or secondary neurulation process. Primary neurulation consists of the formation of the neural tube, while secondary neurulation involves the hollowing of the neural tube and the formation of the medullary cord and cavities. Neurulation occurs in human embryos between days 17 and 28 after fertilization. NTDs can affect both the cranium and the entire spinal column.[2]

Spinal NTDs can be classified as open (spina bifida aperta) or closed (spina bifida occulta) based upon the presence or absence of exposed neural tissues, respectively. Spina bifida is the most common NTD globally, followed closely by anencephaly or encephalocele. Myelocele and myelomeningocele are the common open spinal NTDs, while spina bifida occulta consists of split cord malformations, lipomyelomeningocele, meningocele, and abnormal filum. Spina bifida occulta have congenital absence of spinous process or lamina, are usually not associated with other anomalies of the central nervous system (CNS), and carry a favorable prognosis.

Myelocele and Meningomyelocele

Varying degrees of the defect in the neural arch result in herniation of meninges or neural tissue, leading to an extensive spectrum of spinal NTDs. If the herniated sac does not contain any neural tissue, it is termed a meningocele. In myelocele, the spinal cord is exposed, so that nerve tissue lies exposed on the surface of the back without even a covering of skin or the meninges. The meningomyelocele has a protruding membranous sac containing cerebrospinal fluid (CSF), meninges, and nerve roots **(Figs. 1 and 2)**. Most often, it affects the lumbosacral region, followed by thoracic and cervical regions with higher levels having complex neurologic deficits and poor prognosis. It is often diagnosed on antenatal ultrasound scans. The child is usually born with a cystic membranous sac on the back. They may have flaccid paralysis, sensory disturbances below the lesion level, and bowel and bladder involvement. Associated neurological conditions include hydrocephalus, Arnold–Chiari malformation (ACM), or a tethered cord. They are likely to have multiple systemic involvements such as tetralogy of Fallot (TOF), atrial septal defect (ASD), renal anomalies, and club feet. Early surgical closure as soon as possible is recommended to prevent CSF leak and meningitis.

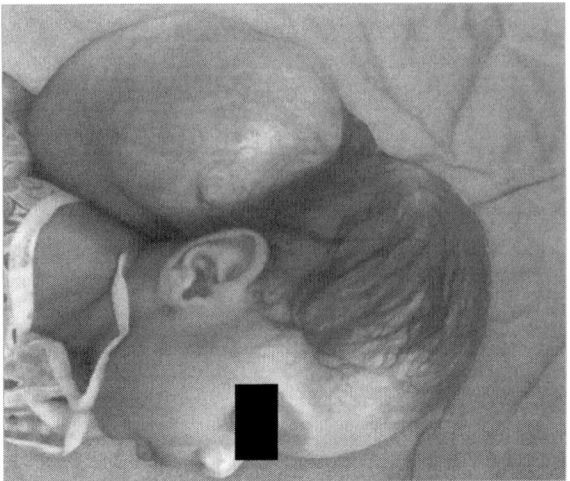

Fig. 1: Cervical meningomyelocele.

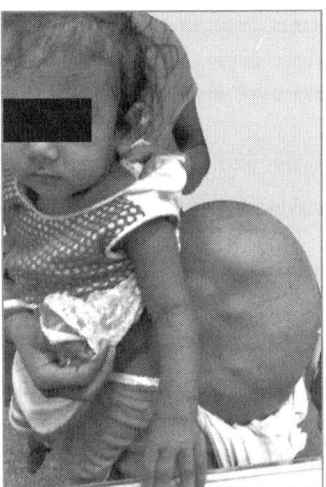

Fig. 2: Lumbar lipomeningomyelocele.

Closed Spinal Neural Tube Defects/Spina Bifida Occulta

They are characterized by the presence of a spinal column bony defect, but the resultant lesion has an intact skin cover which prevents CSF leak. Often, these lesions are accompanied by common cutaneous symptoms such as nevus, hypopigmentation, a tuft of hair, and lipoma.

- *Spinal lipomas* are the most common closed spinal NTD lesions encountered anywhere from the filum, conus, or spinal cord. They are managed by detethering of the cord and removal of lipomatous tissue.
- *Meningoceles*, as the name suggests, have meninges herniated through a defect in the vertebral column. Lumbar and sacral meningoceles are

considered closed NTD, while cervical lesions can be occult or open NTD. Treatment of meningocele entails surgical correction of the defect.[3-5]
- In *split cord malformations (SCM)*, the spinal cord is divided over a portion of its length into two equal or unequal halves. Type I SCM, also known as *diastematomyelia*, has two hemicords. A median bony spur separates them into two separate spinal canals. In type 2 SCM or diplomyelia, two hemicords are housed within a single dural tube separated by a fibrous median septum. Split cord malformations may be asymptomatic or manifest with gait disturbances and sensory-motor or autonomic disturbances. Surgical correction is accomplished with detethering of the spinal cord and removal of the median bony spur or fibrous band.[6]
- *Tethered cord syndrome (TCS)* is a stretch-induced functional disorder of the spinal cord where its caudal portion is anchored by an inelastic structure. Neurological symptoms are caused by restricted spinal cord movement, particularly during flexion and extension of the spine. Typically, children present with leg or back pain, leg weakness, sensory disturbances, and urinary or fecal incontinence. Surgical correction is achieved by detethering of cord and dural repair.[7]
- *Chiari malformation* is a group of congenital malformations involving the hindbrain and spinal cord associated with an array of symptoms due to compression of the medulla, lower cranial nerves, and/ or flow obstruction of cerebrospinal fluid (CSF). The anatomical defect (ACM I to V) ranges from herniation of cerebellar tonsils (type I ACM), cerebellar vermis, lower brainstem, or even occipital lobe through the foramen magnum. It may have other associated neurological conditions such as myelomeningocele, tethered cord, and hydrocephalus. Foramen magnum or posterior fossa decompression surgery, with or without duraplasty, is commonly performed for correction.[8]
- *Primary syringomyelia* is defined as the forming of a fluid-filled cyst within the spinal cord. This cavity may or may not communicate with the CSF pathways. It is frequently seen after spinal injuries, tubercular meningitis, or arachnoiditis due to diagnostic or therapeutic procedures such as lumbar puncture or myelography. It presents with altered temperature sensitivity, pain, paresthesia, and lower motor neuron dysfunction. Surgical correction aims at the restoration of normal CSF flow dynamics.[9]

PRIMARY SPINAL CORD TUMORS

They constitute approximately 10% of the pediatric CNS tumors. They can be classified into intramedullary, intradural/extramedullary, and extradural tumors based on their anatomical location. Extradural spinal tumors account for majority of the lesion while only 25% tumors are intramedullary. The most frequent intramedullary tumors are ependymomas and low-grade astrocytoma.

Extramedullary intradural tumors such as neurofibromas, ganglioneuromas, and meningiomas are mostly benign. Most spinal tumors grow insidiously and commonly present with pain, motor weakness, and gait disturbances. Many of these tumors, particularly extramedullary benign masses, can be completely resected and carry a favorable prognosis.[10,11]

SPINAL CORD INJURY IN PEDIATRIC AGE GROUP

Acute spinal cord injuries are less common in children but are associated with raised morbidity and mortality. Common causes include motor vehicle accidents, sports injuries, falls from height, child abuse, and obstetric injuries. Due to the larger head size compared to the trunk, weak neck musculature, and horizontal orientation of the facets, the higher cervical spine region (65–80%) is more vulnerable to injury. Often these injuries are associated with concomitant traumatic brain injury (25%) and carry a poor prognosis. Immobilization and traction are used for stable spine injuries, while surgical decompression with fixation is recommended for unstable vertebral column injuries.[12]

CRANIOVERTEBRAL JUNCTION ANOMALIES

The craniovertebral junction (CVJ) includes two critical joints, namely "the atlantooccipital and atlantoaxial joints". There exists a complex relationship between the bony, neural, and vascular structures in the vicinity of the cervicomedullary junction. Mobile atlantoaxial dislocation, nonreducible AAD along with different grades of basilar invagination are the most commonly experienced anomalies. These children commonly present with neck pain, limb weakness, and respiratory muscle weakness. Surgical management involves open/microscopic/endoscopic decompression anteriorly or posteriorly with or without fixation.[13]

SPINAL DEFORMITY

A number of congenital or acquired conditions frequently associated with spinal column deformities such as Ehlers–Danlos syndrome, achondroplasia, and neurofibromatosis, require surgical correction of the spinal deformity **(Figs. 3A and B)**. Most elder children present with scoliosis and/or kyphosis. There is a female preponderance among these children. Scoliosis is the abnormal lateral curvature (>10°) and rotation of the thoracolumbar vertebrae as measured by Cobb's angle. Most cases are idiopathic, while the rest may be secondary to neurological conditions or infections. Significant cardiorespiratory involvement occurs once Cobb's angle exceeds 65° leading to elevated morbidity and mortality in the perioperative period.[14,15]

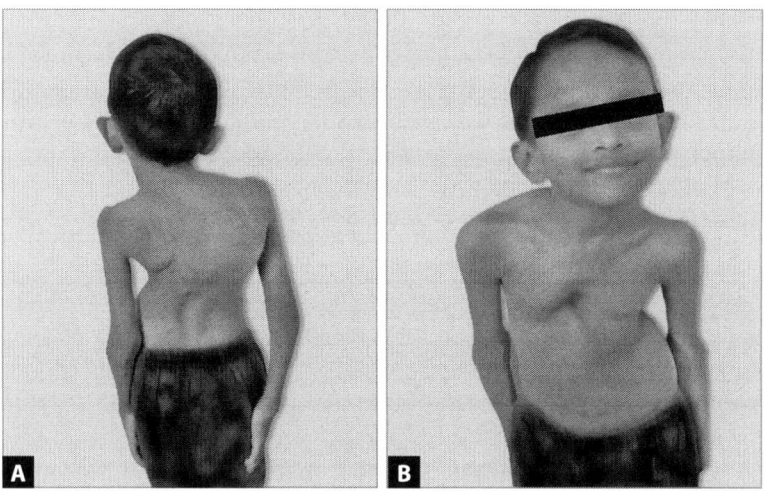

Figs. 3A and B: Severe kyphoscoliosis in Ehlers–Danlos syndrome.

SPINAL CORD VASCULAR MALFORMATIONS

Spinal cord vascular malformations are rare entities and include AVM, cavernous malformations, dural arteriovenous fistulas (AVFs), and capillary telangiectasias. They present with backache, radiculopathy, and bowel or bladder involvement. Vascular malformations can lead to an arterial steal phenomenon diverting blood away from the spinal cord parenchyma. They are generally managed by endovascular embolization.[16]

PREOPERATIVE EVALUATION

Pediatric age group patients range from neonates to adolescents. Moreover, systemic physiology evolves significantly during neonatal and early childhood. Secondly, the immature organ function during this period makes them vulnerable to perioperative stress and requires a neuroanesthesiologist to devise a specific plan. Particular attention should be paid to the systemic, anatomical, and physiological differences, including pediatric airway, with specific consideration for CNS physiology.

Clinical presentation, the evolution of symptoms, current neurological status, ongoing medical management, and proposed surgical plan with desired patient position (mostly prone) should be carefully noted. Often, it may be challenging to complete a neurological examination in children. Features of raised intracranial pressure (ICP) should also be noted if CSF pathway obstruction is suspected. The child should be cautiously assessed for other systemic congenital anomalies, and necessary evaluation, including a cardiologist's opinion, should be sought on a case-to-case basis. Birth history, including the period of gestation, maternal exposure to teratogens such as alcohol and drugs, pregnancy-related complications such as gestational diabetes, and peripartum events such as birth asphyxia and meconium aspiration can have etiopathological implications or perioperative connotations. Airway evaluation in pediatric spinal neurosurgery is critical. Apparent facial anomalies, restricted mouth opening, or neck movement should be ruled out. Particular attention should be paid to children with congenital syndromes associated with airway abnormalities such as Apert's, Crouzon, and Goldenhar syndrome to formulate an airway management plan. Obese children should be evaluated for obstructive sleep apnea (OSA). Neuroradiological imaging should also be reviewed to aid in making plans for anesthesia care.[17,18]

Laboratory testing is a vital component of preoperative evaluation however, the benefits of routine preoperative laboratory testing before elective neurosurgery remain contentious. Abnormal preoperative laboratory values are rare in patients older than two years without any comorbidities undergoing elective neurosurgery. Common predictors of abnormal laboratory parameters include ASA class III–IV, various comorbidities such as diabetes mellitus, hematological, prothrombotic state or cancer, preoperative systemic inflammatory response syndrome (SIRS), and nonelective hospital admission.[19] Preoperative investigations should be ordered based on associated medical conditions and the intended surgical plan. Usually, a complete blood count (CBC) and ABO-Rh blood grouping and typing are all needed since the incidence of critical laboratory values leading to the cancellation of surgery or change in the management plan is minimal. Coagulation profiles, renal or liver function tests, and serum electrolytes are required on a case basis. Spinal neurosurgeries may involve significant blood loss and fluid shifts. Thus, blood products, including packed red blood cells (PRBC), fresh frozen plasma (FFP), platelets, and cryoprecipitate should be ordered in adequate quantity based on the patient's preoperative status and anticipated perioperative blood loss.[18,19]

■ PREOPERATIVE FASTING

The aim of preoperative fasting is to allow adequate gastric emptying and prevent aspiration of gastric contents. However, prolonged fasting times can have harmful effects such as dehydration, hypoglycemia, electrolyte abnormalities, and irritability. Currently, clear fluids such as water with or without sugar and pulp-free juices are encouraged for up to 1 hour (instead of the previous recommendation of 2 hours) before induction of anesthesia for an elective procedure. Similarly, breast milk, formula feed or nonhuman milk, and solid meals are recommended for up to 3 hours, 4 hours, and 6 hours, respectively, before any elective surgery without increasing the risk of pulmonary aspiration. Careful attention should be paid to children with raised ICP, which may lead to poor intake and delayed gastric emptying. If required such patients shall be started on intravenous fluids to ensure adequate hydration and maintain electrolyte balance. Although the current literature suggests liberal fasting regimens in the perioperative period, it needs to be re-emphasized that solid foods should not be given to patients scheduled for emergency neurosurgery.[20]

■ PREMEDICATION

Patients can have their concurrent medications in the preoperative period such as steroids and antiepileptics. Medications that need to be stopped on the day of surgery include insulin, diuretics, and other antihypertensives such as angiotensin-converting enzyme (ACE) inhibitors and angiotensin-receptor blocking agents. Application of the eutectic mixture of 2.5% lignocaine and 2.5% prilocaine local anesthetics (Emla/Prilox cream) 30–60 minutes prior may help in establishing intravenous access with minimal discomfort.

Anxiolysis with sedatives should be considered on a case-to-case basis. Avoid premedication with opioids or benzodiazepines in neonates and infants as it may lead to hypoventilation and raised ICP. However, anxious older children can be sedated with midazolam (oral 0.2–0.5 mg/kg or intravenous 0.1–0.2 mg/kg) provided they are kept under continuous supervision. Other sedative premedications include oral clonidine (4 µg/kg) and transmucosal fentanyl lollipops. Since most spinal neurosurgical procedures are done in the prone position, glycopyrrolate (10 µg/kg) is recommended to reduce the oral secretions.[17,18,21]

■ ANESTHESIA CONCERNS

The pediatric age group includes patients from premature infants to adolescents. Accordingly, the anesthesia-related concerns will vary based on anatomical and physiological variations, type of lesion, the extent of surgery, and associated congenital anomalies or comorbidities.

Most meningoceles and myeloceles are repaired during the initial few days after birth to prevent bacterial contamination due to exposed neural tissue. These neonates who are often premature have significant anesthesia concerns related to maturity of organ systems as summarized in **Table 1**.

Careful attention should be paid to systemic physiology while anesthetizing newborns.[22]

■ PREPARATION OF OPERATING ROOM FOR SURGERY

The operating room (OR) should be prepared meticulously before wheeling in any pediatric patient. The temperature should be maintained at 23–25°C to prevent heat loss. Warm blankets, air mattresses, forced air warmers, and fluid warming devices are used to maintain normothermia. Intravenous (IV)

TABLE 1: Systemic anesthesia concerns in neonates.[22]

Organ system	Neonatal anesthesia concerns
Cardiovascular system	Reversion from adult to fetal type circulation (transitional circulation)
	Tendency toward biventricular failure, poor tolerance to afterload, and sensitivity to volume loading • Heart rate dependent circulation • Myocardium more dependent on extracellular calcium
Respiratory system	Increased resistance to airflow • Respiration is less stimulated by hypercarbia • Hypoxia can lead to sustained respiratory depression
	Elevated postoperative apnea risk till 60 weeks postconceptual age
	Highly compliant airways and chest wall increases risk of atelectasis
	Diaphragm and intercostal muscle fatigue (less type-I muscle fibers)
Hepatic system	• Modify drug dosing intervals and maintenance dosing (immature enzyme system) • Minimal glycogen reserves
Renal system	• Tolerate fluid restriction and fasting poorly • Reduced ability to excrete free water and solutes warrant precise drug dosing
Miscellaneous	Hypothermia

anesthetic drugs should be prepared as per patient weight in low-volume syringes, especially in patients prone to volume overloading. Prewarmed IV fluid should be ready in sufficient volume guided by patient weight. Suitable pediatric airway management equipment is required to be laid out before inducing anesthesia. Patient positioning accessories such as silicone gel pads, bolsters, and headrests should be arranged based on the patient's body habitus. Once the patient is received in the OR, patient identity, diagnosis, surgical plan, premedication, and parental consent must be checked.

■ INDUCTION OF GENERAL ANESTHESIA

All pediatric spinal neurosurgeries are done under general anesthesia with endotracheal intubation and mechanical ventilation. The goal of anesthesia induction is to ensure adequate spinal cord perfusion by maintaining systemic hemodynamics.[1] In patients with secured venous access, IV induction with propofol or thiopentone and appropriate neuromuscular blockade is usually preferred. Children aged below 2 years (2.9 mg/kg) require a higher dose than patients beyond six years of age (2.2 mg/kg).[22] Ketamine can also be used unless contraindicated due to specific comorbidities or raised ICP. Etomidate is recommended in patients with cardiac lesions or compromised hemodynamic parameters.[18] Inhalational anesthesia induction with sevoflurane is necessitated in patients without IV access, and once an IV cannula is secured, supplemental boluses of propofol can be given. Adequate depth of anesthesia should be achieved to blunt the laryngoscopic response and prevent laryngospasm and bronchospasm. Rapid sequence anesthesia induction, if indicated, is done with IV propofol or thiopentone followed by a fast-acting neuromuscular blocker agent (NMBA) such as succinylcholine (1 mg/kg) or rocuronium (1.2 mg/kg). However, succinylcholine should be avoided in spinal cord injuries, denervation syndromes, and/or suspected myopathy. After anesthesia induction, adequate intravenous access should be secured for administering isotonic crystalloid based on anticipated blood loss and fluid shift.[23-25]

■ AIRWAY MANAGEMENT

The difference between adult and pediatric airways may render endotracheal intubation difficult. This difficulty is further exemplified by the primary pathology (spinal cord injuries, CVJ anomaly, kyphoscoliosis, and concomitant hydrocephalus) or airway anatomy distortion in syndromic children (mid-face hypoplasia, restricted mouth opening, and limited neck movement). Thus, it is vital to arrange appropriate size facemasks, oropharyngeal airways, bougie, stylets, and tracheal tube exchangers [8, 11, and 14 Fr size exchangers, which can accommodate sizes 3, 4, and 5 internal diameter (ID) size endotracheal tube (ETT) respectively]. Currently, ETTs with micro-cuff are used against the earlier practice of using uncuffed ETTs. They have a soft polyurethane cuff that symmetrically inflates and is located more distally than standard tubes. This results in more pressure applied to tracheal mucosa and less potential for edema formation in the subglottic region. If the surgical procedure requires considerable neck flexion, then a reinforced ETT should be used.

Conventional laryngoscopy may not be feasible in patients with meningocele or encephalocele. The lesion can be safely secured and positioned inside customized padding or silicone gel pad, and then laryngoscopy is attempted. These patients are often intubated in a lateral position. Lastly, with the help of an assistant, the head of the patient with a cervical meningocele may be allowed to overhang the edge of the OR table. At the same time, it is carefully supported, and after that, a laryngoscopy is done. Movement at the cervical spine should be kept to the bare minimum in children with cervical spine or cord injury and CVJ anomalies by using manual inline stabilization and other airway adjuncts such as videolaryngoscope.[26]

Supraglottic airway devices are not preferred as the definitive airway in neurosurgical procedures, but they have a quintessential role in airway management. They are used as a conduit for endotracheal intubation, rescue airway devices in the "cannot ventilate and cannot intubate" scenario, and accidental extubation. Video laryngoscope (McGrath, Pentax, and C-MAC) can be used during routine and anticipated difficult airway conditions. Finally, fiberoptic bronchoscope-guided intubation is the gold standard for airway management, but general anesthesia has to be induced before bronchoscopy.[27]

■ MAINTENANCE OF ANESTHESIA

Evidence in support of inhalational anesthetic agents or total intravenous anesthesia (TIVA) for neurosurgeries is equivocal.[18] None of the modalities have been proven superior to the other. Most often, amongst volatile anesthetics, sevoflurane or desflurane is used due to their superior recovery profile compared to isoflurane. Careful attention must be paid to the age-related differences in minimum alveolar concentration (MAC) of volatile anesthetics. Preterm neonates have reduced anesthetic requirements than term neonates, while infants require higher MAC values compared to older children or adults **(Table 2)**. Propofol TIVA-based anesthetic management is guided by the state of ICP and the need for intraoperative neuromonitoring (IONM).[22] Nitrous oxide can cause a rise in ICP and cerebral metabolism, interfere with IONM, and is associated with a higher incidence of postoperative nausea and vomiting (PONV), which has led to its decreased utility in pediatric neuroanesthesia. Neuromuscular blocker agents and opioids such as fentanyl or remifentanil are part of any standard anesthetic regime to ensure immobility and pain relief. Use of NMBAs may be precluded if IONM is planned except during initial intubation. One has to be cautious with the accumulation of fentanyl in preterm infants with repeated bolus dosing leading to prolonged sedative effects. Increasingly, dexmedetomidine is used as an adjuvant to reduce overall MAC requirement and propofol dose. Dexmedetomidine is also getting attention due to its minimal effect on IONM.[23-25]

TABLE 2: Age related minimum alveolar concentration (MAC) values in pediatric age group.

Anesthetic agent	MAC-based on age group				
	Neonate	1–6 month	6–12 months	1–3 years	Beyond 5 years
Sevoflurane	3.3%	3.2%	2.5%	2.5%	2.5%
Desflurane	9.2%	9.4%	9.9	8.7%	8%

Monitoring

Routine ASA monitoring should be applied to all spinal neurosurgeries, including electrocardiogram, noninvasive blood pressure (NIBP), pulse oximetry, capnography, and temperature. An arterial line is placed for invasive blood pressure monitoring if there are anticipated hemodynamic changes or significant blood loss. The need for central venous access in the OR should be guided by blood loss/fluid shift/electrolyte imbalance, the risk for venous air embolism (VAE), and the likelihood of prolonged inotropic and ventilatory support. Monitor urine output during prolonged procedures, in cases with anticipated significant blood loss, and when diuretics or osmotic agents are administered. If TIVA is used intraoperatively, it is prudent to employ depth of anesthesia monitoring such as bispectral index (BIS) or entropy.[28]

Advanced IONM such as somatosensory evoked potentials (SSEPs), motor evoked potentials (MEPs), and electromyograms (EMGs), are increasingly used to improve the safety profile in spinal surgeries and prevent postoperative neurologic deficits. However, instituting these monitoring modalities will require appropriate changes in anesthetic technique (avoid NMBA in MEPs and volatile anesthetic agents with SSEPs, institute propofol TIVA during maintenance of anesthesia) to facilitate IONM and draw plausible conclusions.[29-31]

Patient Positioning

Prone positioning (**Fig. 4**) in a small child is a demanding assignment for anesthesiologists since this position entails maximal hemodynamic perturbations. Guiding principles include generous use of padding,

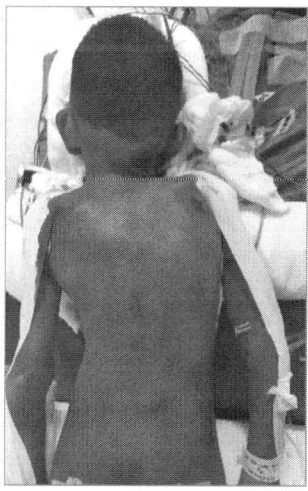

Fig. 4: Prone position with intraoperative neurophysiological monitoring.

preventing pressure on the chest and abdomen to facilitate ventilation, care of eyes with adequate padding, avoidance of head pinning systems in the neonate and small infants, meticulous positioning of the tracheal tube, access to the airway and vascular ports under drapes, and avoidance of extreme head positions with a propensity for brain stem compression and cervical spinal cord ischemia.[32,33]

Fluid Electrolyte Management and Blood Transfusion Strategy

The goal of intraoperative fluid management is to maintain euvolemia. Children can be permitted to have clear fluids till an hour before elective surgery. The fluid requirement in children and infants >4 weeks of age can be calculated using Holliday–Segar's formula **(Table 3)**. For neonates, the fluid requirement is reduced during the initial few weeks of life. Intraoperatively, during the first hour, a fluid bolus of 10 mL/kg can be given for preoperative fluid deficit or 50% of the calculated deficit and the remaining fluid volume over the next two hours. Similarly, maintenance fluid requirement is calculated along with third space losses estimated to be approximately 1–2 mL/kg.[22,34]

Commonly, isotonic crystalloids such as 0.9% saline and Ringer's lactate or balanced crystalloids such as Plasma-Lyte and Isolyte-P are preferred. Glucose-containing solutions (1–2%) are preferred in neonates and small children susceptible to hypoglycemia. Hypotonic saline solutions (including 0.45% NaCl, 0.45% NaCl +5% dextrose) should be avoided as they can worsen cerebral edema. Large volumes of isotonic saline administration can cause hyperchloremic metabolic acidosis. Caution should be exercised while using colloids in infants due to their immature renal system. Fluid therapy should be guided by the child's clinical response such as heart rate, blood pressure, and capillary refill time, and adjustments should be made accordingly. Arterial blood gas (ABG) analysis must be done at regular intervals to assess adequacy of fluid, electrolyte resuscitation, base deficit, serum lactate, and blood transfusion requirement.[35,36]

Both hypoglycemia (serum glucose below 60 mg/dL) as well as hyperglycemia (serum glucose beyond 200 mg/dL) can aggravate

TABLE 3: Holliday–Segar 4-2-1 fluid rule.[34]

Body weight	Fluid requirement
Up to 10 kg	4 mL/kg/h
10 to 20 kg	40 mL/h + 2 mL/kg/h above 10 kg
>20 kg	60 mL/h + 1 mL/kg/h above 20 kg

neurological insult. Careful monitoring of serum glucose should be done to maintain euglycemia (below 180 mg/dL). Similarly, serum electrolytes, particularly potassium, sodium, and calcium should be maintained within the normal range.[37]

Pediatric patients should be closely monitored for blood loss intraoperatively as spinal neurosurgical procedures are prone to excessive blood loss. Careful attention should be paid to the surgical field, suction canisters, surgical sponges, and the blood loss under the surgical drapes, which is often concealed.[18] Hemoglobin (Hb) and hematocrit (Hct) can be reliably followed with regular ABGs during surgery. Some noninvasive Hb monitors are available such as Radical 7 (Masimo Corporation) and Haemospect (MBR Optical Systems). The technology is promising but, in the absence of solid evidence, should be used as supplemental tools only.[38]

The goal of blood transfusion is to increase blood oxygen-carrying capacity. Transfusion requirement is determined by preoperative Hb, Hct, estimated blood volume [Epstein–Barr virus (EBV), determined by age and body weight], ongoing blood loss, and associated comorbidities, as mentioned in **Table 4**. Hematocrit may be allowed to fall by 25% before initiating a blood transfusion. A restrictive transfusion trigger Hb of 7 gm/dL is generally used in children older than 3 years. It is reasonable to maintain higher Hct in patients with cyanotic congenital heart diseases or severe respiratory illness. ABO and Rh group and type-specific PRBC should be used for transfusion. Packed red blood cells (60% Hct) transfusion of 10 mL/kg provides a 2 gm/dL increment of Hb. Patients with anticipated major blood loss may be started on antifibrinolytic agents (tranexamic acid) before incision and continued till surgical closure. In patients with anticipated blood loss of >40% of EBV, the platelets and clotting factors may be transfused to maintain hemostasis. The recommended volume for FFP transfusion is 1 unit/10 kg or 10–15 mL/kg,

TABLE 4: Guide to estimate blood volume and transfusion requirements.[22]

Age group	Estimated blood volume (mL/kg)
Preterm neonate	100–120
Term neonate	90
Infant	70–80
>1 year	70

$$MABL = EBV \times \frac{\text{Starting Hct} - \text{Target Hct}}{\text{Starting Hct}}$$

$$\text{PRBC volume to be transfused} = \frac{(\text{Desired Hct} - \text{Present Hct}) \times EBV}{\text{Hct of PRBCs } (\sim 60\%)}$$

(EBV: estimated blood volume; Hct: hematocrit; MABL: maximum allowable blood loss; PRBCs: packed red blood cells) while the platelet dose for transfusion is 1–2 units/10 kg or 10–15 mL/kg. In patients with major blood loss, component therapy with PRBCs, FFP, and platelets can be initiated in equal ratios or guided by point of care tests (POCT) such as rotational thromboelastogram (ROTEM) and thromboelastography (TEG). One should always look for transfusion complications such as hemolytic transfusion reaction, transfusion-associated circulatory overload (TACO), hypothermia, acid-base disorders, hyperkalemia, and citrate toxicity.[39,40]

Temperature Management

Pediatric patients are vulnerable to hypothermia due to various physiological reasons such as a larger head-to-body surface area, more extensive body surface exposure to a cold environment, inadequate nonshivering thermogenesis, extensive volume resuscitation, and cold blood products. Hyperthermia can aggravate neurological injury, while hypothermia is not of any proven benefit; rather, it is associated with many homeostatic disturbances. The aim is to maintain normothermia using active warming modalities.[41,42]

■ INTRAOPERATIVE COMPLICATIONS

Various surgical complications include hemorrhage, aggravation, or appearance of new neurologic deficit, hydrocephalus, or CSF leak. Anesthesia-related complications include poor hemodynamics, accidental extubation, fluid or electrolyte imbalance, and venous air embolism (VAE).[43] Position-related complications include macroglossia, upper airway edema, pressure point sores, compressive peripheral neuropathy, quadriplegia due to excessive neck flexion, and rare but devastating postoperative vision loss.[32,33]

■ EMERGENCE AND TRACHEAL EXTUBATION

The decision to extubate the trachea depends upon preoperative neurological status, intraoperative course, and anticipated complications. Smooth emergence is vital to good operative outcomes due to its favorable effects on ICP and postoperative bleeding into the closed spinal canals. Adequate nonopioid analgesia with IV paracetamol (10–15 mg/kg) and PONV prophylaxis with 5-HT3 receptor antagonists (ondansetron or palonosetron) is provided for surgical closure. Local anesthetic infiltration at the surgical site is very effective in controlling neuroendocrine stress response. After ensuring the return of spontaneous respiration, adequate neuromuscular blockade reversal must be done. The trachea is extubated once the return of protective airway reflexes is confirmed and the child is fully awake. Various strategies have been tested to blunt the autonomic extubation response, such as fentanyl bolus, IV lignocaine, or combined α and β blockers such as labetalol. Recently, there has been extensive research into dexmedetomidine as an adjuvant during extubation. Patients with prolonged surgery in the prone position, larger fluid shifts, stormy intraoperative course, and not meeting cardiorespiratory criteria for extubation should be shifted to intensive care unit (ICU) for elective mechanical ventilation.[18,22-25]

POSTOPERATIVE MANAGEMENT

All patients should be nursed in a pediatric neurosurgical unit. Inadequate pain relief is associated with poor outcomes. The goal is to have a calm child responsive to verbal stimulation. Acetaminophen is the mainstay of postoperative pain relief. Amongst nonsteroidal anti-inflammatory drugs (NSAIDs), ibuprofen has the least effect on platelet function, and even short-term exposure to ketorolac is not associated with any adverse effects. Nurse-controlled analgesia (NCA) or patient-controlled analgesia (PCA), or nurse and parent-controlled analgesia (N + PCA) with opioids have been used with improved patient satisfaction without fear of increased incidence of respiratory depression. Other adverse effects of opioids include nausea, vomiting, pruritus, and constipation. Postoperative nausea and vomiting prophylaxis should be adequately provided.[44,45] Restrictive fluid management is preferable in the postoperative period. If the child is expected to start oral feeds soon, then the 4-2-1 rule is modified to 2-1-0.5. Patients not started on enteral feeds by 12 hours postoperatively should continue with the 4-2-1 rule of maintenance fluid requirements.[22]

CONCLUSION

Perioperative management of children for spinal neurosurgery is challenging. They may present for surgery any time after birth till adolescence. Careful attention must be paid to age-related physiology to formulate an effective anesthesia care plan. Application of the sound principle of neuroanesthesia such as preoperative assessment, optimization of comorbidities before elective surgery, maintenance of systemic hemodynamics, and preservation of cerebral and spinal cord perfusion, can make a significant difference in the outcome.

REFERENCES

1. Soundararajan N, Cunliffe M. Anaesthesia for spinal surgery in children. Br J Anaesth. 2007;99(1): 86-94.

2. Greene ND, Copp AJ. Neural tube defects. Annu Rev Neurosci. 2014;37:221-42.
3. Avagliano L, Massa V, George TM, Qureshy S, Bulfamante GP, Finnell RH. Overview on neural tube defects: From development to physical characteristics. Birth Defects Res. 2019;111(19):1455-67.
4. McComb JG. A practical clinical classification of spinal neural tube defects. Child Nerv Syst. 2015;31(10):1641-57.
5. Salih MA, Mushid WR, Seidahmed MZ. Classification, clinical features, and genetics of neural tube defects. Saudi Med J. 2014;35(Suppl 1):S5-14.
6. Borkar SA, Mahapatra AK. Split cord malformations: A two years experience at AIIMS. Asian J Neurosurg. 2012;7(2):56-60.
7. Hertzler DA 2nd, DePowell JJ, Stevenson CB, Mangano FT. Tethered cord syndrome: a review of the literature from embryology to adult presentation. Neurosurg Focus. 2010;29(1):E1.
8. Ashfaq ul Hassan, Sabah Yaseen, Mubeen Rashid, Rohul Afza, Manmeet kaur, Moin Javid. Arnold-Chiari malformation: anatomical variations and latest embryological perspective. Review of literature. Int J Contemp Med Res. 2016;3(5):1489-91.
9. Giner J, Pérez López C, Hernández B, Gómez de la Riva Á, Isla A, Roda JM. Siringomielia no secundaria a Chiari. Actualización en fisiopatología y manejo. Neurología. 2019;34(5):318-25.
10. Marrazzo A, Cacchione A, Rossi S, Carboni A, Gandolfo C, Carai A, et al. Intradural pediatric spinal tumors: an overview from imaging to novel molecular findings. Diagnostics. 2021;11(9):1710.
11. Spacca B, Giordano F, Donati P, Genitori L. Spinal tumors in children: long-term retrospective evaluation of a series of 134 cases treated in a single unit of pediatric neurosurgery. Spine J. 2015;15(9):1949-55.
12. Lemley K, Bauer P. Pediatric spinal cord injury: recognition of injury and initial resuscitation, in hospital management, and coordination of care. J Pediatr Intensive Care. 2015;4(1):27-34.
13. Mascarenhas O. Anaesthesia management in craniovertebral junctional anomalies. J Craniovert Jun Spine. 2016;7(4):193-6.
14. Young CD, McLuckie D, Spencer AO. Anaesthetic care for surgical management of adolescent idiopathic scoliosis. BJA Educ. 2019;19(7):232-37.
15. Newton PO, O'Brien MF, Shufflebarger HL, Betz RR, Dickson RA. Anesthesia for scoliosis surgery. In: Newton PO (Ed). Idiopathic scoliosis: The harms study group treatment guide. New York: Thieme; 2011. pp. 123-25.
16. Song D, Garton HJ, Fahim DK, Maher CO. Spinal cord vascular malformations in children. Neurosurg Clin N Am. 2010;21(3):503-10.
17. Moningi S, Padhy N. Preoperative evaluation and preparation of children undergoing neurosurgery. In: Rath GP (Ed). Fundamentals of pediatric neuroanesthesia. Singapore: Springer Nature Singapore Pte Ltd; 2021.
18. Rath GP, Dash HH. Anaesthesia for neurosurgical procedures in paediatric patients. Indian J Anaesth. 2012;56(5):502-10.
19. Dasenbrock HH, Smith TR, Robinson S. Preoperative laboratory testing before pediatric neurosurgery: an NSQIP-Pediatrics analysis. J Neurosurg Pediatr. 2019;24(1):92-103.

20. Frykholm P, Nicola D, Hanna A, Christiane B, Lionel B, Eloise C, et al. Preoperative fasting in children: a guideline from the European Society of Anaesthesiology and Intensive Care. Eur Anaesthesiol. 2022;39(1):4-25.
21. Dave NM. Premedication and induction of anaesthesia in paediatric patients. Indian J Anaesth. 2019;63(9):713-20.
22. Miller R, Eriksson L, Fleisher L, Wiener-Kronish J, Cohen N, Young W. Miller's Anesthesia, 8th edition. Philadelphia: Elsevier; 2015. pp. 2757-98.
23. Soriano SG, McManu ML. Pediatric neuroanesthesia and critical care. In: Cottrell JE, Patel P (Eds). Cottrell and Patel's Neuroanesthesia. Philadelphia: Mosby Elsevier; 2017. pp. 327-42.
24. McClain CD, Soriano SG. Anesthesia for intracranial surgery in infants and children. Curr Opin Anaesthesiol. 2014;27(5):465-9.
25. Kalita N, Goswami A, Goswami P. Making pediatric neuroanesthesia safer. J Pediatr Neurosci. 2017;12(4):305-12.
26. Bhagat H, Bloria S, Kapil S, Kaloria N. Airway considerations in pediatric neurosurgical patients. Indian J Neurosurg. 2020;9(03):179-82.
27. Black AE, Flynn PE, Smith HL, Thomas ML, Wilkinson KA; Association of Pediatric Anaesthetists of Great Britain and Ireland. Development of a guideline for the management of the unanticipated difficult airway in pediatric practice. Paediatr Anaesth. 2015;25(4):346-62.
28. Checketts MR, Alladi R, Ferguson K, Gemmell L, Handy JM, Klein AA, et al. Recommendations for standards of monitoring during anaesthesia and recovery 2015: Association of Anaesthetists of Great Britain and Ireland. Anaesthesia. 2016;71(1):85-93.
29. Levin DN, Strantzas S, Steinberg BE. Intraoperative neuromonitoring in paediatric spinal surgery. BJA Educ. 2019;19(5):165-71.
30. Korn A, Halevi D, Lidar Z, Biron T, Ekstein P, Constantini S. Intraoperative neurophysiological monitoring during resection of intradural extramedullary spinal cord tumors: experience with 100 cases. Acta Neurochir (Wien). 2015; 157(5):819-30.
31. Park JH, Hyun SJ. Intraoperative neurophysiological monitoring in spinal surgery. World J Clin Cases. 2015;3(9):765-73.
32. Rozet I, Vavilala MS. Risks and benefits of patient positioning during neurosurgical care. Anesthesiol Clin. 2007;25(3):631-53,x.
33. DeCuypere M. Special considerations for pediatric positioning for neurosurgical procedures. In: Arthur A, Foley K, Hamm C (Eds). Perioperative considerations and positioning for neurosurgical procedures. Switzerland, Cham: Springer International Publishing AG; 2018.
34. Holliday MA, Segar WE. The maintenance need for water in parenteral fluid therapy. Pediatrics. 1957;19(5):823-32.
35. Karnik HS. Fluid management in infants and children during intracranial surgery. J Neuroanaesthes Crit Care. 2017;4(Suppl_1):S24-9.
36. Ryu T. Fluid management in patients undergoing neurosurgery. Anesth Pain Med (Seoul). 2021;16(3):215-24.
37. Godoy DA, Di Napoli M, Biestro A, Lenhardt R. Perioperative glucose control in neurosurgical patients. Anesthesiol Res Pract. 2012;2012:690362.

38. Lee JH, Park YH, Kim JT. Current use of noninvasive hemoglobin monitoring in anesthesia. Curr Anesthesiol Rep. 2014;4:233-41.
39. New York state council on human blood and transfusion services. (2016). Guidelines for transfusion of pediatric patients. [online] Available from https://www.wadsworth.org/sites/ default/fles/WebDoc/ped_tx_guidelines_2.pdf [Last accessed October, 2022].
40. Steinbicker AU, Wittenmeier E, Goobie SM. Pediatric non-red cell blood product transfusion practices: what's the evidence to guide transfusion of the 'yellow' blood products? Curr Opin Anaesthesiol. 2020;33(2):259-67.
41. Mutchnick I, Thatikunta M, Braun J, Bohn M, Polvika BA, Daniels MW, et al. Protocol-driven prevention of perioperative hypothermia in the pediatric neurosurgical population. J Neurosurg Pediatr. 2020;1-7.
42. Sessler DI. Temperature regulation and monitoring. In: Miller RD (Ed). Miller's anesthesia, 8th edition. Philadelphia: Churchill Livingstone Elsevier; 2015. pp. 1622-46.
43. van Lindert EJ, Arts S, Blok LM, Hendriks MP, Tielens L, van Bilsen M, et al. Intraoperative complications in pediatric neurosurgery: review of 1807 cases. J Neurosurg Pediatr. 2016;18(3):363-71.
44. Vadivelu N, Kai AM, Tran D, Kodumudi G, Legler A, Ayrian E. Options for perioperative pain management in neurosurgery. J Pain Res. 2016;9:37-47.
45. Lee CS, Merchant S, Chidambaran V. Postoperative pain management in pediatric spinal fusion surgery for idiopathic scoliosis. Paediatr Drugs. 2020;22(6):575-601.

CHAPTER

13

Awake Tracheal Intubation

Bindiya Salunke, Jigeeshu V Divatia

ABSTRACT

Awake tracheal intubation (ATI) is the safest option with a high-success rate in anticipated difficult airway situations but is underutilized. The reasons for the underuse of this technique could be attributed to unfamiliarity with the technique or unavailability of instruments, as well as reluctance from anesthesiologists. We summarize various components of ATI, including oxygenation, airway topicalization, sedation, as well as different options of ATI procedures as well as management of complications or unsuccessful ATI. A well-trained anesthesiologist, competent assistants, teamwork, good communication, and adequate preparation are the foundation for successful ATI.

Keywords: Airway topicalization; Awake tracheal intubation; Difficult airway; Retrograde intubation

KEY POINTS

- Awake tracheal intubation (ATI) is the safest option, with a high-success rate in the anticipated difficult airway.
- The components of ATI include sedation, topicalization, oxygenation, and performance.
- It is recommended to use supplemental oxygen during ATI.
- Effective topicalization of the airway with local anesthetics is essential for the successful performance of ATI. The maximum dose of topical lignocaine should never exceed 9 mg/kg lean body weight to avoid local anesthetic toxicity.
- Sedation, if used, should always be used after good airway topicalization is achieved and should not be used as an alternative for incomplete or inadequate topicalization.
- Direct laryngoscopy, video laryngoscopy, fiberoptic intubation, retrograde intubation, blind nasal intubation, and awake front of neck airway are available for ATI in the setting of an anticipated difficult airway.
- Optimization of the situation by stopping or reversing the sedation, clearing airway secretions, optimizing or changing the method of

oxygenation, and topicalizing the airway should be employed to avoid unsuccessful ATI.
- Tracheal extubation should be deferred till the patient is awake and the effect of the local anesthetic used for topicalization wears off.
- Complete informed consent and documentation of oxygenation, topicalization, sedation strategy, device and tracheal tube used, approach (e.g., nasal or oral), number of attempts, and complications, if any, should be maintained.

INTRODUCTION

Airway management is a critical skill for the clinical anesthesiologist and intensivist. Appropriate airway assessment, anticipating a difficult airway, and proper planning should be given utmost importance. During airway evaluation, one should be able to predict or suspect difficulty in facemask ventilation, intubation, use of supraglottic airway device (SAD), and emergency front of neck airway access. Physiological factors such as reduced apnea tolerance, aspiration risk, altered hemodynamics, and technical factors such as expertise and equipment availability should also be considered.

If the airway is not managed appropriately, there is a risk of hypoxia and hemodynamic instability, and even death. In the general population, the approximate incidence of Cormack and Lehane laryngoscopy grades 3 and 4 is 10%, difficult intubation is 1%, and difficult bag-mask ventilation is 0.08–5%.[1,2] The reported incidence of difficult facemask ventilation is 0.66–2.5%,[3-6] difficult SAD placement or ventilation 0.5–4.7%,[7-11] difficult tracheal intubation 1.9–10%,[3,5,12-14] and combined difficulty in both facemask and tracheal intubation 0.3–0.4%.[5] In the United Kingdom (UK), the Fourth National Audit Project (NAP4) estimated the incidence of significant complications of airway management during general anesthesia (GA) in the UK. 133 reports were related to airway management under GA. The incidence of difficult airways is 1 per 22,000 GAs. Anesthesia events led to 16 deaths and three episodes of persistent brain damage with a mortality rate of 1 per 180,000 GAs. Airway management was considered good in 19% of assessable anesthesia cases, and elements of care were judged poor in 75% of cases.[15]

Awake tracheal intubation (ATI) is the safest option when a difficult airway is anticipated. However, it is underutilized. This could be due to unfamiliarity with the technique or unavailability of instruments, but also due to reluctance on the part of anesthesiologists to undertake awake airway management. ATI is the tracheal intubation of a patient who is sufficiently conscious of maintaining a patent airway unassisted, breathing spontaneously to maintain adequate gas exchange and protect the airway against the aspiration of gastric contents or other foreign material. ATI can occur via the nasal or oral route and is facilitated by topical, regional, or local infiltrative airway anesthesia.

ATI could be performed either by direct laryngoscopy, video laryngoscopy, fiberoptic bronchoscopy, blind nasal intubation or retrograde intubation, awake tracheostomy, or cricothyroidotomy.

INDICATIONS

- Clear indications for ATI include conditions where insertion of a direct or video laryngoscope blade into the patient's mouth is impossible. These include anatomical airway deformity or any pathology such as total trismus or minimal mouth opening, or severe flexion deformity of the neck.
- *Suspected difficulty with laryngoscopy and tracheal intubation:* Any of the clinical, anatomical, or radiological features that predict laryngoscopy and intubation
- *Any ventilation method is predicted to be difficult:* If ventilation and maintenance of oxygenation by facemask and SAD utilization are predicted to be difficult, then there is no fallback. Morbid obesity, obstructive sleep apnea, potential bleeding, oral lesion on manipulation, anatomical abnormalities of the face, and previous head–neck surgery or irradiation are a few examples of such situations.
- *In patients with a known physiological compromise where apnea tolerance of the patient is significantly reduced:* For example, a hypoxemic patient with decreased functional residual capacity and increased oxygen consumption, obese pregnant patients, etc.
- Contextual issues such as inexperience of airway manager with the technique needed for planned intubation and unavailability of expert backup help are also an indication for ATI.
- Patients at high risk of aspiration may be candidates for awake intubation.
- A patient with a prior history of difficult or failed intubation or a history of airway mishaps in an unanticipated difficult airway should also be considered as a candidate for ATI.
- Anticipated difficult airway with expected difficulty with emergency invasive airway rescue.
- Patients meeting more than one criterion may be good candidates for awake intubation, e.g., an obese patient (predicted difficult airway, reduced apnea tolerance) who presents for emergency surgery with a full stomach (high risk of aspiration).

CONTRAINDICATIONS

The only absolute contraindication for ATI is patient refusal. Relative contraindications are allergy to local anesthetics, uncooperative patient, or bleeding in the airway (making visualization difficult).

FASTING GUIDELINES

The risk of regurgitation of gastric contents is present in ATI as well. It is advisable to follow standard fasting guidelines in elective cases requiring ATI.

COMPONENTS OF AWAKE TRACHEAL INTUBATION

The components of ATI suggested by Difficult Airway Society (DAS) guideline[16] are sedation, topicalization, oxygenation, and performance *(sTOP)*; here, "s" is written in the small case as sedation is optional.

Oxygenation

Difficult Airway Society recommends supplemental oxygen during ATI with grade B evidence. The incidence of desaturation [oxygen saturation (SpO_2) ≤ 90%] during ATI is 12–16% with low-flow oxygen technique and as low as 0–1.5% with humidified high-flow oxygen technique.[17-21]

Airway Topicalization

A topical nasal vasoconstrictor before nasotracheal intubation is recommended as it reduces the incidence of epistaxis. Antisialogogue use is not mandatory, but decreasing oral secretions may improve visualization. It also helps to increase the efficacy of topical anesthesia. However, it may result in undesirable side effects, including prolonged dry mouth, tachycardia, and arrhythmia. If used, it should be administered 40–60 minutes before the procedure via the intramuscular route.

Effective topicalization of the airway with local anesthetics is essential for the successful performance of ATI. Lignocaine is the most commonly used local anesthetic. Systemic absorption of the drug is variable when administered by different techniques/delivery systems; however, the maximum dose of topical lignocaine should never exceed 9 mg/kg lean body weight to avoid local anesthetic toxicity.

Different Techniques of Airway Topicalization

- 10% lignocaine spray to the base of the tongue and tonsillar pillars. Each spray of 10% lignocaine disperses 0.1 mL of volume, equivalent to 10 mg of lignocaine.
- Lignocaine nebulization
- Transtracheal injection of 4% or 2% lignocaine. It helps to block recurrent laryngeal nerves causing topicalization below the vocal cords. The cricothyroid puncture cannula, used for transtracheal local anesthetic injection, can also provide a rescue airway and serve as a conduit for passage of a guidewire if an emergency tracheostomy is needed.

- *Spray-as-you-go (SAGO):* 4% or 2% lignocaine can be sprayed while advancing the fiberoptic bronchoscopy (FOB) through the patient's airway via a working channel port.
- *Invasive nerve blocks:* The glossopharyngeal nerve and superior laryngeal nerve (SLN) can be blocked invasively. These methods are invasive and are rarely used as there is no evidence that percutaneous nerve blocks are superior to topical airway anesthesia.
  - *Glossopharyngeal nerve block:* The glossopharyngeal nerve provides sensation to the posterior third of the tongue, the anterior surface of the epiglottis, the vallecula, the tonsils, and the pharyngeal walls. This nerve can be blocked by two approaches—intraoral and peristyloid.[22] In the intraoral approach, the local anesthetic agent is injected submucosally at the base of the posterior tonsillar pillars after confirming negative aspiration. In the peristyloid approach, a line is drawn from the angle of the jaw to the mastoid process, and the needle is inserted at the midpoint of this line perpendicular to the skin till it comes in contact with the styloid process. Once the styloid process is reached, the needle is reangled posteriorly, and the local anesthetic agent is deposited there. Another less invasive approach is the application of local anesthetic-soaked pledgets at the tonsillar fossa.
  - *Superior laryngeal block:* The SLN provides sensory innervation to the tongue base, the posterior surface of the epiglottis, the arytenoids, and the aryepiglottic folds. Blocking the SLN anesthetizes the larynx above the vocal cords. The SLN splits into the internal and external branches at the greater cornu of the hyoid bone. The internal branch penetrates the thyrohyoid membrane, continuing submucosally in the piriform recess, and the external branch descends deep into the sternohyoid muscle. The SLN can be blocked by two approaches—internal and external approaches.

In the external approach, the patient is placed supine with neck extension to facilitate identification of the hyoid bone. The hyoid bone is then displaced laterally, and a 25-gauge needle is inserted to reach the greater cornu of the hyoid. Once the needle comes in contact with greater cornu, it is walked off the cartilage caudally, and the local anesthetic agent is deposited here after negative aspiration. Both the internal and external branches are blocked by this approach.

The superior cornu of thyroid cartilage can be used as a landmark if the hyoid bone is difficult to palpate. The superior cornu of thyroid cartilage lies just caudal to the greater cornu of the hyoid bone. The superior cornu is felt as a small round structure by tracing the upper edge of the thyroid notch posteriorly. A 25-gauge needle is inserted to reach the superior cornu of the thyroid cartilage, then walked over its cephalad end, and the local anesthetic agent is deposited.

In the internal approach, local anesthetic-soaked pledgets are deposited in the piriform fossae and left there for around 5–10 minutes for adequate and effective action of the local anesthetic agent.[23] Ultrasound-guided deposition of a local anesthetic around the surface of the greater cornu of the hyoid bone after identification of hyoid bone and SLN showed a >90% success rate.[24]

All blocks mentioned above have to be performed bilaterally. Fowler et al.[25] described a newer approach of a single midline injection for bilateral SLN block. In this approach, the local anesthetic agent (larger volume, around 6 mL) is deposited into the midline of the thyrohyoid membrane, and it results in a bilateral SLN block. The additional advantages of this approach are that it avoids neurovascular injection and identification and manipulation of the hyoid bone. The adequacy of local anesthetic action should be checked in an atraumatic manner (with a suction catheter) before ATI.

Sedation

In patients with a difficult airway, it would be ideal to have the patient fully awake without any sedation. Patient anxiety can be minimized by preoperative counseling and reassurance. However, minimal sedation may be required during ATI as it can decrease anxiety and increase the patient's cooperation. Sedation should not affect spontaneous respiration and the cardiovascular system and should be carefully administered. Excessive sedation in the setting of an anticipated difficult airway can lead to airway obstruction, respiratory depression, and loss of the airway resulting in significant hazards such as respiratory arrest, hypoxia, cardiovascular instability, and even death. It is always advisable to have a second anesthesiologist responsible for administering and monitoring the effects of sedation. Sedation should always be used after good airway topicalization is achieved and should not be used as an alternative for incomplete or inadequate topicalization.

Dexmedetomidine is an excellent agent for sedation for ATI as it causes anterograde amnesia, anxiolysis, and analgesia with minimal effects on respiration. Remifentanil has a rapid onset and offset of action, antitussive action, as well as analgesic properties. Both dexmedetomidine and remifentanil have proven to be most efficient in ATI as they have lower risks of oversedation and airway obstruction.

Propofol is also employed for the same purpose by many anesthesiologists. It is best used as a target-controlled infusion with effect-site concentrations of 0.8–2.0 microgram per mL in combination with remifentanil of 1.5–3.2 ng per mL.[26] The potential for airway obstruction, respiratory depression, apnea, and cardiovascular compromise is higher with propofol than with other agents.

Bolus doses of midazolam and fentanyl, while commonly used, are potentially dangerous and, if used, must be given in small, incremental doses (e.g., 0.25 mg midazolam, 10–20 micrograms of fentanyl) titrated to effect.

Procedure

Direct laryngoscopy, video laryngoscopy, fiberoptic intubation, retrograde intubation, and blind nasal intubation are some of the options available for ATI in the setting of an anticipated difficult airway. A well-trained anesthesiologist, competent assistants, teamwork, good communication, and adequate preparation are the foundations for successful ATI.

Standard monitoring (ECG, noninvasive blood pressure, pulse oximetry, and capnography) should be used during and after the procedure. This will help to recognize any hypoxemia, airway obstruction or hemodynamic instability, arrhythmias, etc., which will point toward oversedation or local anaesthetic (LA) toxicity. Two-point check of tracheal tube placement by capnography and visual confirmation of tracheal tube placement must be done after ATI, before administration of anesthesia to the patient. Endotracheal tube (ETT) fixation after confirming the mark should be done with utmost care to avoid accidental tracheal extubation. Inflation of the cuff could be done before, during, or after induction of GA while taking care patient does not cough causing accidental extubation.

Awake Direct Laryngoscopy

After good topicalization of the airway, one attempt by an experienced anesthesiologist can be made if the mouth opening is adequate to allow passage of the laryngoscope blade. A bougie can be used to guide the intubation.

Awake Video Laryngoscopy

Hyperangulated blades are handy to help visualize the glottis. A shaped stylet or bougie should be used to guide the ETT in the trachea. Video laryngoscopes do require some mouth opening and are associated with a learning curve.

Awake Fiberoptic Bronchoscopy

It is the gold standard in cases of anticipated difficult intubation as it gives direct visualization of the airway to the carina. The fiberscope is either inserted via nose or mouth after good airway topicalization. During FOB, the operator can either stand at the head end or face the patient. The FOB is advanced, slowly visualizing the airway structures, and taking care not to touch the mucosa. The SAYGO method can be used to achieve good topicalization of the airway. The additional working ports of the fiberscope allow the operator to clear any secretion with suction, provide oxygen, and spray local anesthetic agents during the procedure. High-flow oxygen via nasal cannula is also helpful. The carina should be visualized before advancing the ETT over the fiberscope into the trachea, and the tip of the tracheal tube should be placed about 4 cm above the carina (in adults) to avoid both endobronchial intubation and excessively proximal placement of the tracheal tube that could risk accidental extubation. However, the equipment is expensive, needs to be handled with care, requires good maintenance, and is associated with a learning curve to be proficient with fiberoptic intubation.

Combined Fiberoptic-guided Intubation and Video Laryngoscopy

This is often referred to as a hybrid procedure. While fiberoptic intubation is considered the gold standard for ATI as the trachea is visualized by the fiberscope and the tube is seen in the trachea, the passage of the tube over the fiberscope from the oral cavity through the larynx into the trachea is blind. The tube can impinge on the arytenoids or cause trauma during its passage from the nose or mouth into the trachea. A hybrid procedure combining simultaneous video laryngoscopy and fiberoptic intubation ensures that the passage of the fiberscope and tracheal tube is continuously visualized from the oral cavity to the larynx by video laryngoscopy, and the entry of the tracheal tube and its final position in the trachea are visualized by the fiberscope. In case the tracheal tube impinges on any part of the larynx, rotation maneuvers of the tube can be carried out under video laryngoscopic vision to guide the tube through the larynx.

Retrograde Intubation[27]

This procedure is performed chiefly where fiberoptic scopes are unavailable. The cricothyroid membrane is pierced to enter the airway and provide transcricoid local anesthetic infiltration. A guide (mostly epidural catheter) is passed via this cannula to come out via the mouth/nose. The needle is removed, and the ETT is railroaded on this catheter. The advantage of this technique is that it can be successfully utilized in the presence of blood or secretions in the airway and cases with flexed neck deformities. The technique of retrograde intubation is illustrated in **Figure 1**.

Various maneuvers may be required for successful placement ETT:
- Facing the beveled tip of ETT posteriorly.
- Tightening the lower end of the catheter to guide the tube in-between the vocal cords; once the ETT enters the laryngeal inlet, the lower end of the retrograde catheter is loosened.
- Backward pressure on the larynx to facilitate ETT entry into the trachea
- When the ETT cannot be advanced but unobstructed breathing is present, the ETT may be engaged at the laryngeal inlet. Application of steady axial pressure on ETT helps to advance ETT into the trachea.
- Various techniques for inserting the epidural catheter through the ETT lumen or Murphy's eye to harness or guide the ETT into the trachea (**Figs. 2A to E**).

Awake Tracheal Intubation

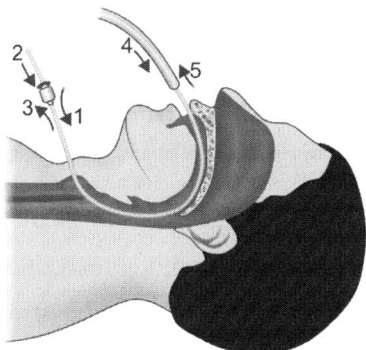

Fig. 1: Steps of retrograde intubation. *Step 1*: Puncture of the cricothyroid membrane to enter the laryngeal cavity. *Step 2*: Insertion of a guide (either epidural catheter or any adequate length (around 70 cm in adult) venous access guidewire inserted through the above needle. *Step 3*: Puncture needle is removed once the guidewire is retrieved from the nasal cavity or the mouth. *Step 4*: The endotracheal tube is railroaded over this guidewire. *Step 5*: Once the confirmation of the endotracheal tube is confirmed by capnography and auscultation, the guidewire is pulled out, and the patient is induced with general anesthesia.

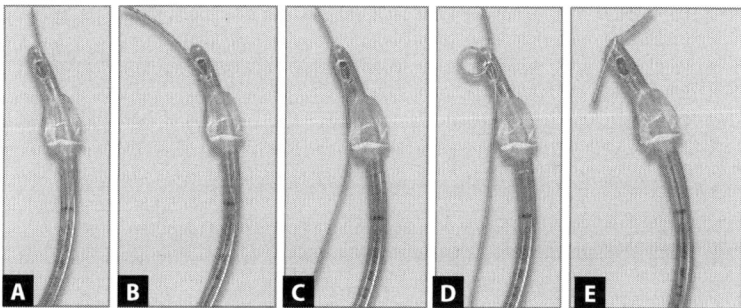

Figs. 2A to E: The various techniques of guiding endotracheal tube (ETT) over the retrograde guide. (A) The ETT is railroaded straight over the retrograde guide inserted through the central lumen of the ETT; (B) The retrograde catheter is guided from Murphy's eye to enter the ETT lumen directed toward the machine end of ETT; (C) The retrograde catheter is passed through the end of the tracheal tube and out from the Murphy eye; (D) The guide is looped through the Murphy's eye; (E) A stitch is taken at the tip of ETT. In A, B, and C, the ETT is guided over the retrograde guide, whereas in D and E, the retrograde catheter is pulled down from the pharynx into the larynx along with the catheter.[27]

Anterograde Guided Retrograde Intubation

The disparity in the thickness of the epidural catheter to the lumen of the ETT makes it difficult at times to railroad the ETT over the epidural catheter into the larynx and trachea. In anterograde-guided retrograde intubation, a hollow anterograde guide such as a ventilating bougie, Aintree catheter, or guidewire sheath is threaded over the retrograde catheter. The end-tidal carbon dioxide monitor is used to confirm its entry into the trachea. Once the anterograde guide is confirmed to enter the trachea, the ETT is passed over it. Decreasing the disparity between the external diameter of the anterograde guide and the internal diameter of the ETT, lumen makes it easier for the ETT to follow the guide into the trachea.

Tracheal Intubation Facilitated by a Retrograde Guide

In challenging situations such as blood and secretions in the airway or abnormal airway anatomy, the retrograde guide can be used to guide FOB-guided intubation. In such situations, the retrograde guide is passed through the suction channel of FOB, which is guided over it. Once the trachea or anatomically identifiable/visible dry field is identified, the retrograde guide is removed under vision, and tracheal intubation is accomplished over the fiberoptic guide.

Blind Nasal Intubation

This method does not require any particular instrument, but does require a skilled operator. Like retrograde intubation, even blind nasal can be successfully utilized in the presence of blood or secretion in the airway. The average reported success rate was 58.0–72.2%.[28-30] During blind nasal intubation, the patient is placed in the sniffing position, and a well-lubricated ETT is passed along the floor of the nose beneath the inferior turbinate while listening to breath sounds to guide the passage of the tube through the glottis into the trachea. If it fails, the patient's head can be repositioned, external laryngeal manipulation could be applied, or tracheal tube cuff is inflated to elevate the tube for easy passage of the ETT.[31] However, this is an entirely blind procedure, and not generally recommended.

■ FAILED AWAKE INTUBATION RESCUE

A failure rate of ATI has been reported as 1–2%.[21,32,33] As mentioned by the DAS guideline, if 3 + 1 attempts of ATI have failed, it is referred to as an unsuccessful ATI. There could be several reasons for failed ATI such as an uncooperative patient, inadequate topical anesthesia, oversedation, adverse anatomy, or an inexperienced/unskilled operator. The options available in this situation are to either postpone the procedure or to secure the airway awake surgically. Optimization of the situation by stopping or reversing the sedation, clearing airway secretion, optimizing or changing the method of oxygenation, and topicalization of the airway should be considered simultaneously. Awake tracheostomy or cricothyrotomy is unavoidable if either airway patency or ventilation is compromised or neurologically the patient has worsened, or surgery is required to be performed urgently, or expected clinical deterioration in the patient.

MANAGING COMPLICATIONS

The reported overall complication rate in patients undergoing either flexible bronchoscopic or video laryngoscopic ATI is about 18%.[21,32-36] Any unplanned removal of the flexible bronchoscope, video laryngoscope, or tracheal tube from the airway is defined as an unsuccessful attempt at ATI. The inadequate or improper implication of sTOP could be considered an essential factor of failure. The likely complications such as airway trauma, airway obstruction, bleeding, and unsuccessful ATI are more likely seen with ATI,[15,37-39] and this risk increases with increased attempts. Reassessing the adequacy of sTOP and reconsidering expert help should be done after each failed attempt. This will assure more success rate, lesser complications, and better patient cooperation.

TRACHEAL EXTUBATION

Extubation should also be done when the patient is fully awake and can maintain the patency of his airway and clear oral secretions. Extubation should be planned well with good preparation as per standard guidelines.[40]

Extubation should be deferred till the patient is awake and the effect of the local anesthetic used for topicalization wears off. Usually, the action of topical lignocaine lasts for about 40 minutes,[41,42] but the terminal elimination half-life of lignocaine is up to 2 hours.[43] Hence, it is advisable to wait till 2 hours after topicalization to extubate these patients. It is also advisable to extubate patients over an airway exchange catheter (AEC) in such situations. AEC acts as a guide and facilitates reintubation and also provides a conduit for oxygenation in an immediate postextubation period. This AEC can be left in situ till the need for reintubation is unlikely.

DOCUMENTATION

Informed written consent must be taken after explaining the risks associated with ATI and alternatives in case of failed ATI. A detailed record of oxygenation, topicalization, sedation strategy, device and tracheal tube used, approach (e.g., nasal or oral), number of attempts, and complications, if any, should be maintained as well as explained in detail to the patient. This will provide ease in deciding strategies if the patient has to undergo any sort of anesthesia in the future.

CONCLUSION

Awake tracheal intubation is underutilized by many anesthesiologists, perhaps due to the unavailability of expertise or instruments. Conducting ATI needs a lot of patience and patient cooperation, as well as surgeons' cooperation. Adequate training to make anesthesiologists familiar with the technique by manikins and simulation workshops followed by conducting FOB-guided/VL-guided intubation on an asleep patient with normal airway can help to reduce this gap by boosting confidence in anesthesiologists who are novices in awake intubation.

In uncooperative patients or situations with altered sensorium patients, pediatric patients, or critically ill patients warranting immediate airway security, we can proceed with induction of GA and tracheal intubation while keeping everything ready for emergency front of neck access.

REFERENCES

1. Cheney FW, Posner KL, Lee LA, Caplan RA, Domino KB. Trends in anesthesia-related death and brain damage: a closed claims analysis. Anesthesiology. 2006;105:1081-6.
2. Apfelbaum JL, Hagberg CA, Caplan RA, Blitt CD, Connis RT, Nickinovich DG, et al. Practice guidelines for management of the difficult airway: an updated report by the American Society of Anesthesiologists Task Force on Management of the Difficult Airway. Anesthesiology. 2013;118:251-70.
3. Norskov AK, Rosenstock CV, Wetterslev J, Astrup G, Afshari A, Lundstrøm LH. Diagnostic accuracy of anaesthesiologists' prediction of difficult airway management in daily clinical practice: a cohort study of 188,064 patients registered in the Danish Anaesthesia Database. Anaesthesia. 2015;70:272-81.
4. Norskov AK, Wetterslev J, Rosenstock CV, Afshari A, Astrup G, Jakobsen JC, et al. Prediction of difficult mask ventilation using a systematic assessment of risk factors vs. existing practice: a cluster randomised clinical trial in 94,006 patients. Anaesthesia. 2017;72:296-308.
5. Kheterpal S, Healy D, Aziz MF, Shanks AM, Freundlich RE, Linton F, et al. Incidence, predictors, and outcome of difficult mask ventilation combined with difficult laryngoscopy: a report from the multicenter perioperative outcomes group. Anesthesiology. 2013;119:1360-9.
6. Kheterpal S, Martin L, Shanks AM, Tremper KK. Prediction and outcomes of impossible mask ventilation: a review of 50,000 anesthetics. Anesthesiology. 2009;110:891-7.
7. Verghese C, Brimacombe JR. Survey of laryngeal mask airway usage in 11,910 patients: safety and efficacy for conventional and non-conventional usage. Anesth Analg. 1996;82:129-33.
8. Saito T, Liu W, Chew STH, Ti LK. Incidence of and risk factors for difficult ventilation via a supraglottic airway device in a population of 14,480 patients from South-East Asia. Anaesthesia. 2015;70:1079-83.
9. Francksen H, Renner J, Hanss R, Scholz J, Doerges V, Bein B. A comparison of the i-gel with the LMA-Unique in non-paralysed anaesthetised adult patients. Anaesthesia. 2009;64:1118-24.
10. Rose DK, Cohen MM. The airway: problems and predictions in 18,500 patients. Can J Anesth. 1994;41:372-83.
11. Cook TM, Trumpelmann P, Beringer R, Stedeford J. A randomised comparison of the Portex Soft seal TM laryngeal mask airway with the LMA-Unique TM during anaesthesia. Anaesthesia. 2005;60:1218-25.

12. Shiga T, Wajima Z, Inoue T, Sakamoto A. Predicting difficult intubation in apparently normal patients: a meta-analysis of bedside screening test performance. Anesthesiology. 2005;103:429-37.
13. Lundstrøm LH, Møller AM, Rosenstock C, Astrup G, Gatke MR, Wetterslev J. A documented previous difficult tracheal intubation as a prognostic test for a subsequent difficult tracheal intubation in adults. Anaesthesia. 2009;64:1081-8.
14. Detsky ME, Jivraj N, Adhikari NK, Friedrich JO, Pinto R, Simel DL, et al. Will this patient be difficult to intubate? The rational clinical examination systematic review. JAMA. 2019;321:493-503.
15. Cook TM, Woodall N, Frerk C; Fourth National Audit Project. Major complications of airway management in the UK: results of the Fourth National Audit Project of the Royal College of Anaesthetists and the Difficult Airway Society. Part 1: anaesthesia. Br J Anaesth. 2011;106(5):617-31.
16. Ahmad I, El-Boghdadly K, Bhagrath R, Hodzovic I, McNarry AF, Mir F, et al. Difficult Airway Society guidelines for awake tracheal intubation (ATI) in adults. Anaesthesia. 2020;75(4):509-28.
17. Rosenstock CV, Thogersen B, Afshari A, Christensen AL, Eriksen C, Gatke MR. Awake fiberoptic or awake video laryngoscopic tracheal intubation in patients with anticipated difficult airway management: a randomized clinical trial. Anesthesiology. 2012;116:1210-6.
18. Sidhu VS, Whitehead EM, Ainsworth QP, Smith M, Calder I. A technique of awake fibreoptic intubation. Experience in patients with cervical spine disease. Anaesthesia. 1993;48:910-3.
19. Fuchs G, Schwarz G, Baumgartner A, Kaltenbock F, Voit-Augustin H, Planinz W. Fiberoptic intubation in 327 neurosurgical patients with lesions of the cervical spine. J Neurosurg Anesthesiol. 1999;11:11-6.
20. Badiger S, John M, Fearnley RA, Ahmad I, Asai T. Optimizing oxygenation and intubation conditions during awake fibreoptic intubation using a high-flow nasal oxygen-delivery system. Br J Anaesth. 2015;115:629-32.
21. El-Boghdadly K, Onwochei DN, Cuddihy J, Ahmad I. A prospective cohort study of awake fibreoptic intubation practice at a tertiary centre. Anaesthesia. 2017;72:694-703.
22. Simmons ST, Schleich AR. Airway regional anesthesia for awake fiberoptic intubation. Reg Anesth Pain Med. 2002;27:180-92.
23. Kostyk P, Francois K, Salik I. Airway anesthesia for awake tracheal intubation: a review of the literature. Cureus. 2021;13(7):e16315.
24. Manikandan S, Neema PK, Rathod RC. Ultrasound-guided bilateral superior laryngeal nerve block to aid awake endotracheal intubation in a patient with cervical spine disease for emergency surgery. Anaesth Intensive Care. 2010;38:946-8.
25. Fowler JG, VanEenenaam DP Jr, Johnson KN, Courtemanche CD, Strathman AJ, Reynolds JE. Single midline injection for bilateral superior laryngeal nerve block. J Clin Anesth. 2020;66:109922.
26. Johnston KD, Rai MR. Conscious sedation for awake fibreoptic intubation: a review of the literature. Can J Anaesth. 2013;60:584-99.
27. Dhara SS. Retrograde tracheal intubation. Anaesthesia. 2009;64:1094-104.
28. O'Brien DJ, Danzl DF, Hooker EA, Daniel LM, Dolan MC. Prehospital blind nasotracheal intubation by paramedics. Ann Emerg Med. 1989;18:612-7.

29. Dronen SC, Merigian KS, Hedges JR, Hoekstra JW, Borron SW. A comparison of blind nasotracheal and succinylcholine assisted intubation in the poisoned patient. Ann Emerg Med. 1987;16:650-2.
30. O'Connor RE, Megargel RE, Schnyder ME, Madden JF, Bitner M, Ross R. Paramedic success rate for blind nasotracheal intubation is improved with the use of an endotracheal tube with directional tip control. Ann Emerg Med. 2000;36:328-32.
31. Gorback MS. Inflation of the endotracheal tube cuff as an aid to blind nasal endotracheal intubation. Anesth Analg. 1987;66:916-7.
32. Law JA, Morris IR, Brousseau PA, de la Ronde S, Milne AD. The incidence, success rate, and complications of awake tracheal intubation in 1,554 patients over 12 years: an historical cohort study. Can J Anesthesia. 2015;62:736-44.
33. Joseph TT, Gal JS, DeMaria SJ, Lin HM, Levine AI, Hyman JB. A retrospective study of success, failure, and time needed to perform awake intubation. Anesthesiology. 2016;125:105-14.
34. Merry AF, Mitchell SJ. Complications of anaesthesia. Anaesthesia. 2018;73:7-11.
35. Wahba SS, Tammam TF, Saeed AM. Comparative study of awake endotracheal intubation with Glidescope video laryngoscope versus flexible fiberoptic bronchoscope in patients with traumatic cervical spine injury. Egy J Anaesth. 2012;28:257-60.
36. Kramer A, Müller D, Pförtner R, Mohr C, Groeben H. Fibreoptic vs. videolaryngoscopic (C-MAC_ D-BLADE) nasal awake intubation under local anaesthesia. Anaesthesia. 2015;70:400-6.
37. Heidegger T, Gerig HJ, Ulrich B, Schnider TW. Structure and process quality illustrated by fibreoptic intubation: analysis of 1612 cases. Anaesthesia. 2003;58:734-9.
38. Ho AM, Chung DC, To EW, Karmakar MK. Total airway obstruction during local anesthesia in a non-sedated patient with a compromised airway. Can J Anesth. 2004;51:838-41.
39. Ovassapian A, Yelich SJ, Dykes MH, Brunner EE. Fiberoptic nasotracheal intubation–incidence and causes of failure. Anesth Analg. 1983;62:692-5.
40. Kundra P, Garg R, Patwa A, Ahmed SM, Ramkumar V, Shah A, et al. All India Difficult Airway Association 2016 guidelines for the management of anticipated difficult extubation. Indian J Anaesth. 2016;60(12):915-21.
41. Kirkpatrick MB, Sanders RV, Bass JB. Physiologic effects and serum lidocaine concentrations after inhalation of lidocaine from a compressed gas-powered jet nebulizer. Am Rev Resp Dis. 1987;136:447-9.
42. Schonemann NK, van der Burght M, Arendt-Nielsen L, Bjerring P. Onset and duration of hypoalgesia of lidocaine spray applied to oral mucosa – a dose response study. Acta Anaesthesiol Scand. 1992;36:733-5.
43. Roberts MH, Gildersleve CD. Lignocaine topicalization of the pediatric airway. Ped Anesth. 2016;26:337-44.

CHAPTER 14

Anesthesia for Tracheal Reconstruction Surgeries

Raj Sahajanandan, Rahul Pillai, Amit Mathew

ABSTRACT

Anesthesia for tracheal resection and carinal surgeries can be challenging as it involves sharing the airway with the surgeons and maintaining oxygenation and ventilation. Perioperative care of these patients involves multidisciplinary planning and tailoring care for the individual patient based on the pathology and the proposed surgery. A good understanding of surgical steps and familiarity with nonintubated techniques, cross-field ventilation, and anesthesia for interventional pulmonology, as well as extracorporeal membrane oxygenation techniques, are essential skills for anesthesiologists. A combination of meticulous preoperative assessment to pick up red flags and combining with investigation helps the team to plan a successful perioperative course. Extubation is equally important and has to be guided by an algorithm to avoid postoperative respiratory events, which can lead to morbidity. Meticulous preparation and close communication with the team are the keys to successfully managing these cases.

Keywords: Cross-field ventilation; Trachea; Resection; Stenosis; Jet ventilation.

KEY POINTS

- Individualized preoperative assessment and investigations to do a risk assessment
- The location, severity of stenosis, comorbidities, and the proposed surgical resection will determine the safest anesthetic approach for the individual patient.
- Understanding surgical plans and communication is crucial for managing shared airway and cross-ventilation strategies.
- Be familiar with techniques such as tubeless airway, jet ventilation, and extracorporeal membrane oxygenation (ECMO).
- Extubation and emergence can be challenging.

INTRODUCTION

Anesthesia for tracheal resection and carinal surgeries is challenging as it involves sharing of the airway with the surgeon as well as maintaining oxygenation and ventilatory function. Often, the patient will have a compromised airway which adds to the difficulty. Multidisciplinary planning, teamwork, and close communication are needed for the successful perioperative management of these cases. Anesthesia challenges involve induction and airway management in the presence of airway pathology, coordination with the surgeons, perfusionists, and theater staff, as well as concerns during tracheal extubation and emergence.

The location, stenosis severity, comorbidities, and the proposed surgical resection will determine the safest anesthetic approach for the individual patient. The conventional anesthetic approach is to secure the airway awake or after induction of anesthesia and then use cross-field ventilation or jet ventilation once the airway is opened. Interventional pulmonology and less invasive techniques are currently in vogue, and regional anesthesia and nonintubated techniques are used to manage these cases.[1]

APPLIED ANATOMY

The trachea in adults is approximately 10–11-cm long. It extends from the larynx (C6) to the carina (T5) and divides into right and left main bronchi. One-third of the trachea is extrathoracic, and the remaining is intrathoracic. Tracheal length varies with neck position, with approximately a 2-cm increase from neck flexion to extension in healthy adults.[2] Proximity of the trachea to the aorta on the left side limits the dissection of the left main bronchus during carinoplasty. Maintaining the blood supply to the trachea by avoiding circumferential dissection is a cardinal principle of tracheal resection and reconstruction (TRR) operations. Bronchial arteries vary in number, usually two on the left and one on the right, which makes the right main bronchus more susceptible to ischemia. The recurrent laryngeal nerves are subject to permanent or temporary injury in tracheal pathology and surgical manipulation. Left recurrent laryngeal nerve arises near ligament arteriosum and courses behind and ascends in the tracheopharyngeal groove, which makes it more susceptible to injury.[3]

PREOPERATIVE EVALUATION

Shortness of breath is a cardinal symptom to seek during preoperative evaluation. Worsening of symptoms during exertion is a sign of a dynamic component. Exertional dyspnea occurs when the tracheal diameter decreases below 50% (usually <8 mm in an adult). When the patient has dyspnea at rest, the tracheal diameter is expected to be between 5 and 6 mm.[4] However, even patients with severe tracheal stenosis may present without stridor or dyspnea during quiet breathing.

Another ominous sign is a *stridor*. The pattern of stridor (inspiratory/expiratory/biphasic) helps in determining whether the pathology is intrathoracic/extrathoracic and whether the lesion is a fixed obstruction or a dynamic obstruction. Inspiratory stridor is associated with fixed obstruction of the larynx and upper trachea. In contrast, expiratory stridor is more commonly seen with the dynamic collapse of the lower trachea (tracheomalacia) and lower airway tumors.[5]

History of coughing and expectoration/*hemoptysis* should be sought. *Cough* on lying down or worsening breathlessness on lying down flat is a sign of airway obstruction and may predict loss of airway with induction of general anesthesia (GA). The position in which the patient is most comfortable (*rescue position*) has to be determined preoperatively and should be communicated with the team.

A *change in voice* may indicate recurrent laryngeal nerve involvement. If there is unilateral partial injury, that side's vocal cord (VC) may be in adducted position with the other side compensating. Induction of anesthesia or topicalization can take away this compensation and result in airway obstruction.

A review of the recent computed tomography (CT) scan or bronchoscopy is mandatory. Radiological imaging (CT/MRI) helps in determining the type (benign-fibrous stenosis vs. malignancy, which can be intraluminal or extraluminal), location (intrathoracic vs. extrathoracic, as well as the distance from the VC and carina), friability, degree and extent of airway narrowing, and involvement of other mediastinal structures. 3D reconstruction and 3D printing can add to the anesthetist's and the surgical teams' plan, especially during the initial airway management.[3]

Anesthetists should remember that these lesions can *progress fast*. Tracheal obstruction, either caused by inflammation (as in benign postintubation stenosis) or tumors, can worsen quickly, over weeks or even days, so the information obtained in the previous surgical notes or earlier imaging may not be actual at the time of presentation for the current surgery.

Attention to *age, comorbidities, and functional status* has an important bearing on anesthesia techniques. The plan for intraoperative jet ventilation may result in hypercapnia and right ventricular (RV) strain. Hence, a baseline arterial blood gas and transthoracic echocardiogram (TTE) to assess RV function may be worthwhile. Avoiding hypercapnia by monitoring arterial CO_2 levels is crucial in patients with pulmonary hypertension and coronary artery disease, especially during tubeless ventilation or high-flow nasal oxygenation techniques. It is prudent to check the arterial partial pressure of carbon dioxide (pCO_2) every 30 minutes during THRIVE or manual jet ventilation.

Baseline pulmonary function tests (PFTs) can offer important information about the patient's respiratory reserve but has questionable value as the ability to tolerate these tests is often suboptimal, and the test itself can induce respiratory crisis.[1] Diffusion capacity of carbon monoxide (DLCO) is a useful indicator of the success of techniques that rely on diffusion of gases such as apneic oxygenation/THRIVE/jet ventilation.[6]

Role of Flow–Volume Loops

The typical graphs of variable intrathoracic/extrathoracic obstructions and fixed obstructions are diagnostic, but it does not add significantly to the information we have from imaging.[7]

Preoperative Bronchoscopy

It has a significant role as it gives real-time information about the anatomy, extent, and the degree of narrowing, distance from the VC to the lesion, and helps in answering questions such as:
1. Will you be able to park a cuffed endotracheal tube (ETT) below the VC and above the lesion?
2. Distance from the carina (Is there a landing zone—can we negotiate an ETT beyond the tumor and keep the tip above the carina? The outer diameter of the bronchoscope, which can be negotiated beyond the lesion, helps the anesthetists decide on the initial ID of the ETT)
3. Is there a dynamic component to the airway obstruction? (If the airway diameter changes from supine to sitting, there is a dynamic component to the obstruction).

Classification and Grading

The earlier classifications were Cotton and Myers (diameter),[8] and McCaffrey (diameter and length)[9] predominantly looked at upper trachea and subglottis **(Figs. 1 and 2)**.

Nowadays, as we are dealing with more and more low tracheal lesions, it is important to have a classification for the teams to speak a common language. Freitag proposed a classification for central airway stenosis **(Figs. 3A to H)**, which classifies the central airway stenosis as schematic representations of the basic types of stenosis and the transition or abruptness of change between the normal lumen and the most narrowed part. (a) Intraluminal tumor or granulation; (b) distortion or buckling; (c) extrinsic compression; (d) scar stricture; (e) scabbard trachea; (f) floppy membrane; (g) abrupt transition (web stenosis); (h) tapered transition (hourglass stenosis).[10]

Red Flags in the Preoperative Assessment

Hypercapnia strongly predicts the potential failure of both spontaneous and mechanical ventilation during GA. Critical fixed narrowing through which anesthetized patients can spontaneously breathe without increasing pCO_2

Anesthesia for Tracheal Reconstruction Surgeries

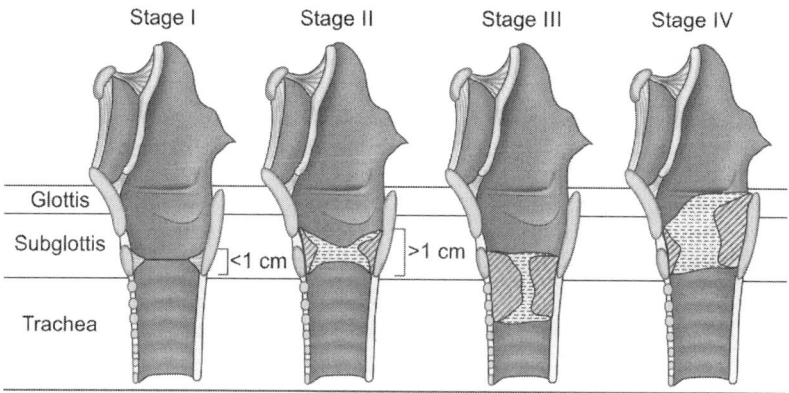

Fig. 1: Cotton and Myers classification (diameter).

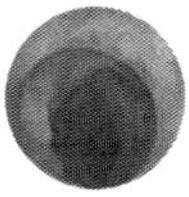

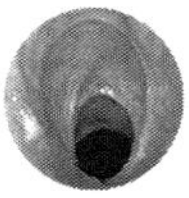

Fig. 2: McCaffrey classification (diameter and length).

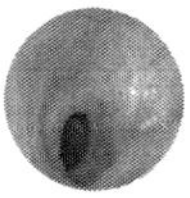

is 4–4.5-mm ID. Critical stenosis for mechanical ventilation in anesthetized patients is not apparent. *Documented VC palsy, hemoptysis, inability to lie flat/cough, or syncope on lying flat suggests significant compression on the trachea and the heart.*

■ OPTIMIZATION

Prehabilitation can be achieved by a combination of strategies such as smoking cessation, improving effort tolerance, and chest physiotherapy, which has to be individualized depending on the pathology, acuity of symptoms, and the premorbid functional status of the patient. The team can consider *tracheal dilatation* as a bridge to achieve this goal. This is normally

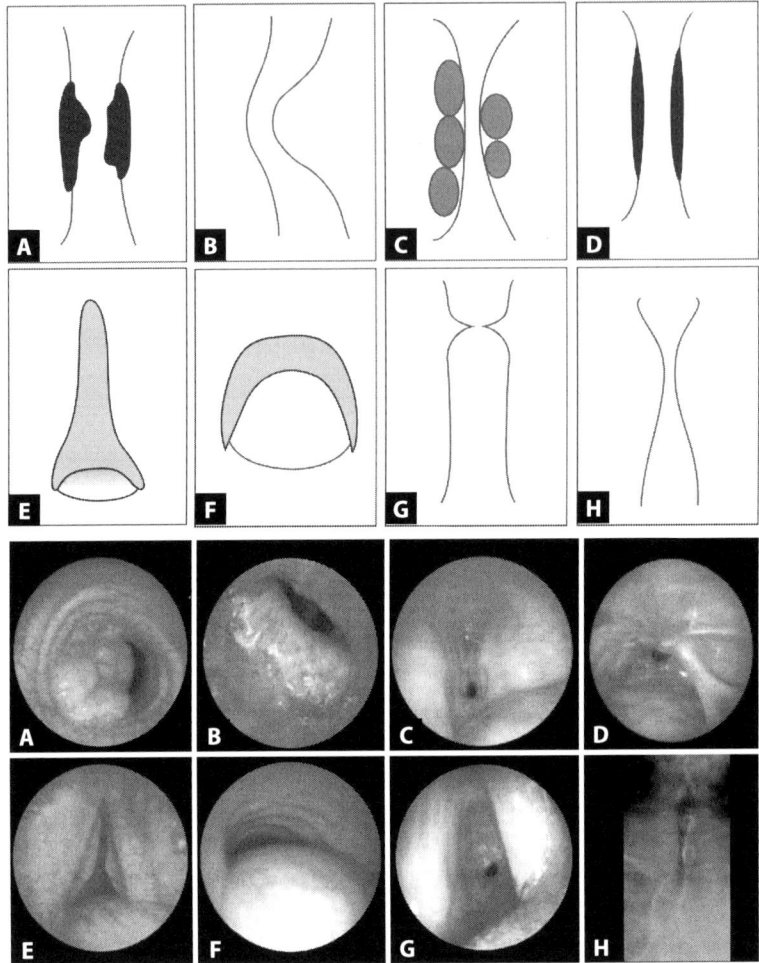

Figs. 3A to H: Freitag classification.

done via supraglottic airway (SGA) over a wire to dilate with a balloon or via a rigid bronchoscope. We should ensure a period of apnea during dilatation to avoid negative pressure pulmonary edema.

Airway management strategy will depend on the complexity and extent of the lesion, proposed surgery, comorbidities, and patient's preference. Factors such as the nature of the lesion, location of the lesion, growth pattern, degree of narrowing, distance from VCs, and distance from carina will also influence airway management.

■ MULTIDISCIPLINARY DISCUSSION

Planning for TRR surgeries requires meticulous discussion between surgeons' anesthetists and intensive care unit (ICU) teams to discuss primary airway plans, surgical steps including fire safety (cautery), strategy for oxygenation and ventilation during shared airway, backup plans including cardiac surgical/perfusionists inputs if cardiopulmonary bypass (CPB)/ extracorporeal membrane oxygenation (ECMO) is planned.

Theater Preparation

Apart from the usual check of the anesthesia machines and monitoring, a Difficult-Airway cart should be in the operation room. Flexible bronchoscopes size 3 and 4, equipment for one-lung ventilation (OLV), equipment for cross-field ventilation (sterile circuits and tubes, swivel connection), equipment for jet ventilation [ideally high-frequency jet ventilation (HFJV) and Hunsaker tubes] appropriate for the patient should be kept ready. If the airway is a critically narrow airway with dynamic/fixed intrathoracic obstruction, it is imperative to arrange a rigid bronchoscope as guided by imaging and personnel capable of using it. Also, a plan for ECMO should be discussed, and appropriate arrangements should be made.

Monitoring

The American Society of Anesthesiologists (ASA) standard monitoring, including capnography, is a must. An arterial line should preferably be inserted on the left arm or femoral if a right thoracotomy is planned to prevent arterial trace dampening if the right innominate is compressed or retracted. It is preferable to put a pulse oximeter on the right arm to alert about innominate compression. Depth of anesthesia monitor is desirable (NICE guideline) if using total intravenous anesthesia (TIVA) with neuromuscular blocking agents (NMBA). Transcutaneous CO_2, if available, is useful in jet ventilation.

Anesthesia for Tracheal Resection Surgeries

The anesthesia for tracheal resection surgeries (TRS) is divided into five phases. The first phase, induction and intubation, is a critical period. The second phase, or the dissection phase, is a relative calm period during which a lesion is defined. The third phase is the open airway, a crucial period of the shared airway in which anastomosis is constructed. The fourth phase is closure and emergence, and the final or fifth phase is extubation. The emergence and tracheal extubation are also extremely crucial.[11]

■ AIRWAY MANAGEMENT STRATEGY

The location, extent, and internal diameter of the section to be removed are the pivotal determinants of airway management strategy.

The airway management includes intubation with the tip of the ETT placed above the lesion, negotiating the tube through the lesion, laryngeal mask airway (LMA), and Jet ventilation through a narrow lumen catheter or a rigid bronchoscope **(Figs. 4A and B)**.

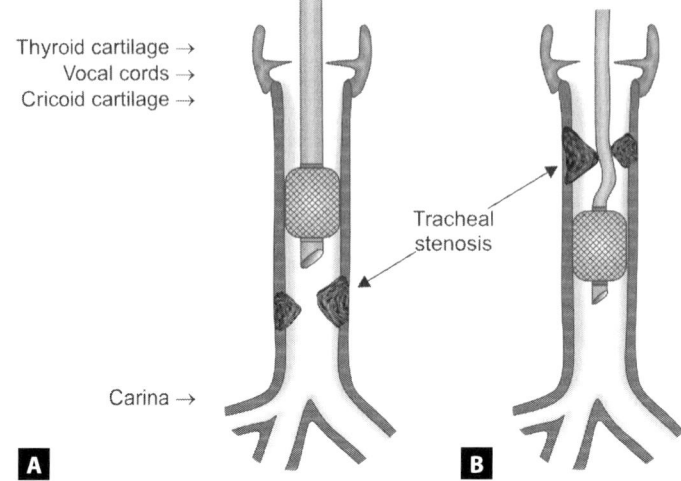

Figs. 4A and B: Location of the lesion and suggested airway management.

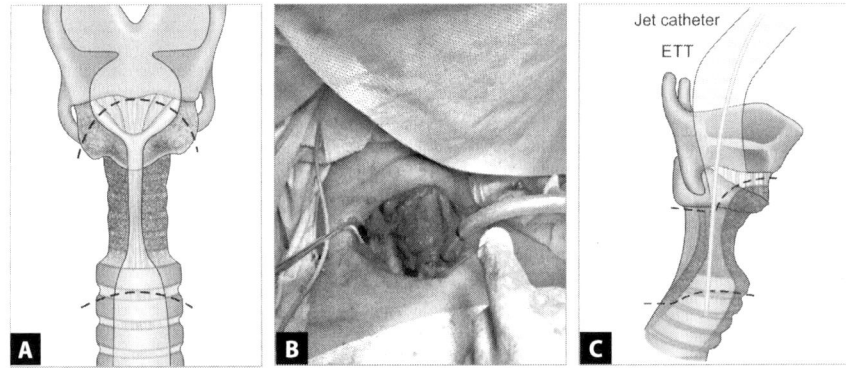

Figs. 5A to C: An airway exchange catheter with a jet ventilation connector passed through the endotracheal tube beyond the stenosis.

Cricotracheal and Upper Tracheal Resections

When dealing with cricotracheal and upper tracheal resections, we need to address a few salient questions:
1. What is the grade of stricture?
2. Is cricoid resection planned?
3. What is the largest ETT (external diameter) that can be passed through?
4. Is there an adequate landing zone above stricture? (4–5 cm between the VC and the lesion to allow the cuff beyond the VC)

If not, a 4–5-mm ID MLS tube can be placed above the larynx to guide the jet catheter **(Figs. 5A to C)**.

Clinical Pearls

Enough landing zone means that the ETT can be stabilized in that position. The smallest ETT size preferred in adults will be a 5.0-mm ID MLS tube.

A Cooks airway exchange catheter (AEC) with a jet ventilation connector can be used for trans-stenotic ventilation before opening the trachea and can be continued during tumor excision. It also acts as a support to help stabilize the ETT above the stenosis and for railroading the ETT distal to the anastomosis after the closure of the trachea **(Figs. 5A to C)**.

High lesions (subglottic stenosis and tumors near or involving the larynx) are easier to manage during cross-field ventilation but can make the initial airway management challenging. Ideally, 30–40 mm of space between the VCs and the lesion is required for the "landing zone" of a standard ETT, which allows the cuff to be inflated below the VCs.

Historically, common approaches included using supraglottic or transtracheal jet ventilation, subglottic HFJV with 2–3-mm Hunsaker catheters, or intubation with 4–5-mm ID microlaryngeal surgery tubes (MLS tube). For the former, an ETT can be placed in the larynx as a guide for the jet catheter and later advanced past after the anastomosis. The latter option is elegant if the stenosis allows, as the MLT can be used for the entire case if ventilation is satisfactory.

Surgical Steps

Cervical approach with transverse low-collar incision: If a stoma is present, the skin around the stoma is excised **(Fig. 6A)**. Pre-excision fiberoptic bronchoscopy (FOB) may be required to confirm the extent of resection.

Release procedures are done when the surgeon deems tension at the anastomotic site may be high.

Incision over the trachea **(Fig. 6B)**: The thyroid isthmus is divided. Circumferential dissection is done at the level of the lesion and up to a centimeter above and below **(Fig. 7A)**. Traction sutures are taken **(Fig. 7B)** and a combination of release procedures—suprahyoid, infrahyoid, and inferior constrictor release is done depending on the length of the trachea resected.

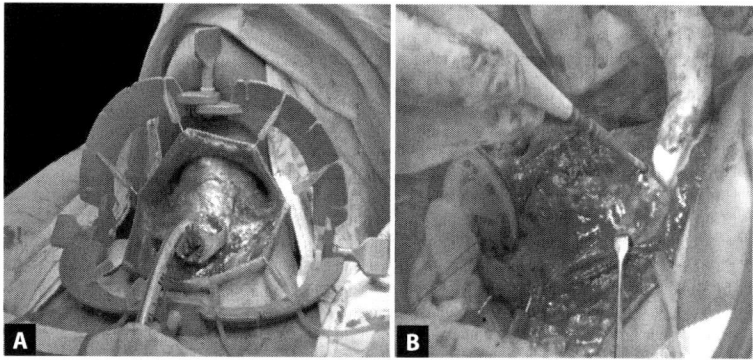

Figs. 6A and B: (A) Lower cervical incision with excision of skin around the stoma; (B) Incision over thyroid cartilage with the division of isthmus.

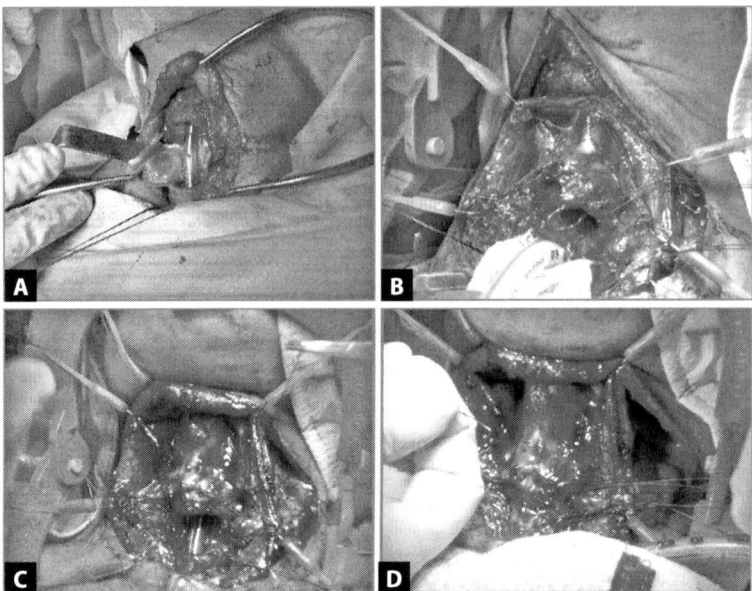

Figs. 7A to D: (A) Excision of tumor with adequate margins; (B) Cross-field ventilation; (C) Endotracheal tube (ETT) introduced to lower trachea after posterior anastomosis; (D) Closure of anterior anastomosis.

Cross-field ventilation is initiated after the opening of the trachea **(Fig. 7B)**. After resection of the tumor, posterior tracheal suturing is done first with intermittent cross-field ventilation or cross-field ventilation with a catheter from the upper airway. The oral/nasal ETT is then advanced into the lower trachea with a cuff beyond the anastomotic site after the removal of cross-field ventilation **(Fig. 7C)**. This may be achieved over an AEC or retrograde over a red rubber catheter. This is followed by the closure of anterior sutures **(Fig. 7D)**.

Tracheal Resection Surgeries via Supraglottic Airway

An emerging method in the management of TRS is the use of a SGA for airway management and ventilation. This avoids the challenges with the correct placement of an ETT. The SGA is a good conduit for flexible bronchoscopy to confirm the extent of the lesion before the start of the surgery. It can then function as a conduit for a jet ventilation cannula or can be used for conventional ventilation till distal tracheal/bronchial intubation is achieved **(Fig. 8)**. The SGA can be left inside during the procedure, which helps to isolate the airway from oral secretions. The anterior tracheal anastomosis can be achieved with a brief period of apneic oxygenation or an MLS tube passed through the SGA. During extubation, return to spontaneous ventilation and emergence can be done with SGA, avoiding risks of trauma and loss of the airway during ETT removal. In addition, SGA can be used as a conduit to

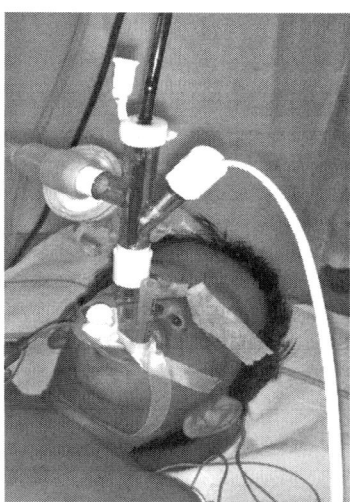

Fig. 8: TRS in a child using supraglottic airway. An Arndt multiport adapter being used for airtight seal for FOB, ventilation, as well as a jet ventilation/oxygenation catheter. (FOB: fiberoptic bronchoscopy; TRS: tracheal resection surgery)

assess VC function. It is advisable to use a second-generation SGA with good sealing capabilities, which is designed for intubation.

Mid-tracheal Lesions

A mid-tracheal lesion will allow intubation after induction of GA, with the ETT cuff above the segment for resection and normal positive pressure ventilation **(Fig. 9A)**. Once the initial dissection and mobilization of the trachea have been performed, the trachea is opened and divided. A sterile ETT is passed to the distal segment by the surgeons, followed by inflation of the cuff **(Fig. 9B)**. A sterile circuit is connected to this ETT, allowing cross-field ventilation. If a sterile circuit is not available, a laparoscopy camera cover can be used as a sterile cover for the circuit connected to a sterile swivel mount. Ideally, a hook-/hockey-stick-shaped reinforced tube (Montando tube) with a short distal tip is used, but any reinforced ETT is suitable. The diseased section is resected, and then the posterior wall of the trachea (or graft) is anastomosed **(Fig. 9C)**. After that, the cross-field ETT is removed, and the original (or a new) reinforced oral ETT is advanced beyond the anastomosis **(Fig. 9D)**. Before each manipulation of the ETTs, the patient should be adequately preoxygenated. A flexible bronchoscope should be used to clear any secretions and careful confirmation of tube position.[12]

Low Tracheal/Carinal Resection

When it comes to low tracheal and carinal resections, it is better to perform it in a large-volume center that does these cases regularly. Before starting

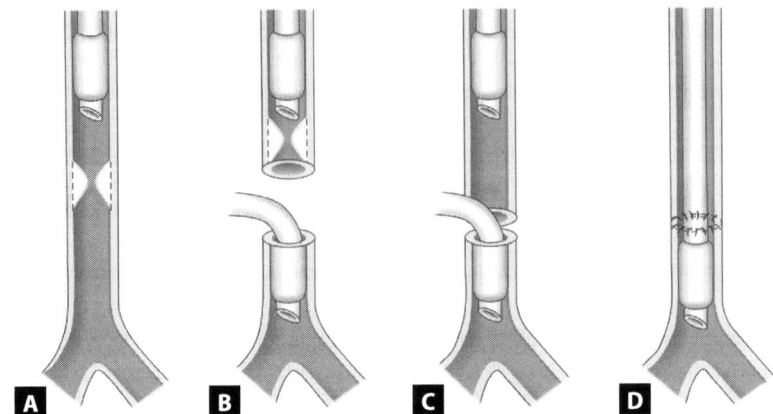

Figs. 9A to D: Mid-tracheal lesions (ETT kept above the lesion during initial intubation followed by cross-field ventilation after tracheotomy). (ETT: endotracheal tube)

the case, it is important to have a multidisciplinary meeting to discuss the challenges and solutions.

As the lesion is lower tracheal/carinal, the initial ventilatory attempt is most likely suprastenotic. We must understand that *the conventional backup plans (Plans B, C, and D) described in the difficult airway algorithms (SGA/FONA) may not help in these situations.* It is crucial to establish backup plans or use them as the primary plan (e.g., doing the case after establishing ECMO). This, however, is a team decision weighing the risks of loss of airway, bleeding, options of cross-field ventilation, costs, as well as the age of the patient.

The airway management plans should include an assessment of images to determine the risks of inadequate ventilation due to auto-positive end-expiratory pressure (PEEP) and carinal flow alterations, which may need selective one-lung ventilation.

Additional questions, which should be discussed, are: (1) the surgical plans for lobar resection or pneumonectomy? (2) Does the surgeon require lung isolation? (3) Will the patient tolerate one lung ventilation? (4) What are the options for dual/split lung ventilation?

It is important to use *lung-protective strategies* during ventilation and take all measures to reduce ALI (acute lung injury). Radiology assessment should look for associated vascular and esophageal involvement. This might help to predict cardiovascular collapse and in planning vascular access.

The other questions, which should be discussed in the team meeting, are: (1) Whether there is space for dissection and suturing? (2) Will mediastinoscopy be performed to assess resectability?

Since most patients with the significant cardiopulmonary disease are not candidates for carinal resection, adequate oxygenation can be achieved in most cases. In patients with complex anatomical repairs or where the

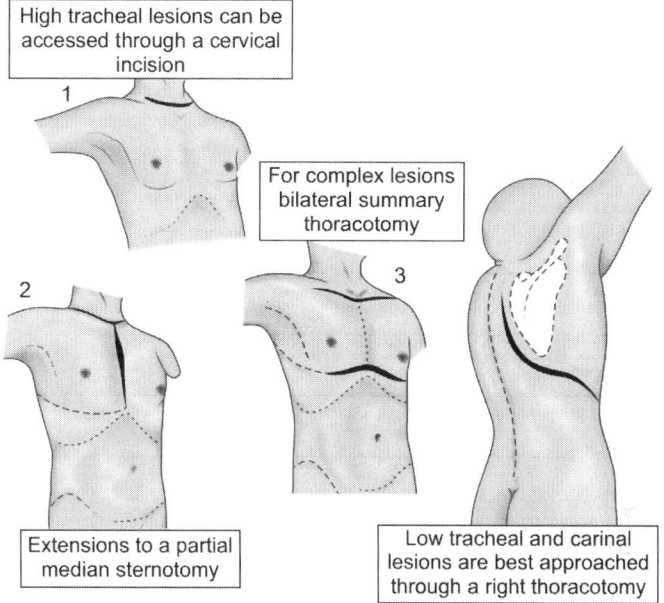

Fig. 10: Surgical approach.

presence of ventilating tubes interferes with surgery, a venovenous ECMO is a good option. However, the team must weigh the risks of bleeding due to heparinization versus the benefits.

Surgical Approach

Lower tracheal lesions can be approached through cervical incisions with the neck extended or by extending this incision to a partial medial sternotomy. Lower tracheal and carinal lesions are best approached by a right posterolateral thoracotomy. While bilateral submammary transsternal thoracotomy may be used for complex lower tracheal lesions **(Fig. 10)**. Sleeve pneumonectomy is usually done for right-sided tumors mainly as the left main bronchus is longer. Isolated carinal resection is for low-grade midline tumors. Median sternotomy and clamshell incision are required for carinal resection/left sleeve pneumonectomy. Isolated carinal resection is possible through right thoracotomy also. However, this may need extensive release procedures such as inferior pulmonary ligament division, hilar release with pericardial opening.

■ ANESTHETIC MANAGEMENT

Anesthesiologists should be able to always control the airway, ensuring maximal free access with unobstructed airways and, in some cases, without an ETT. Anesthesiologists must be able to provide ventilation and oxygenation and have backup plans during all stages of airway management.

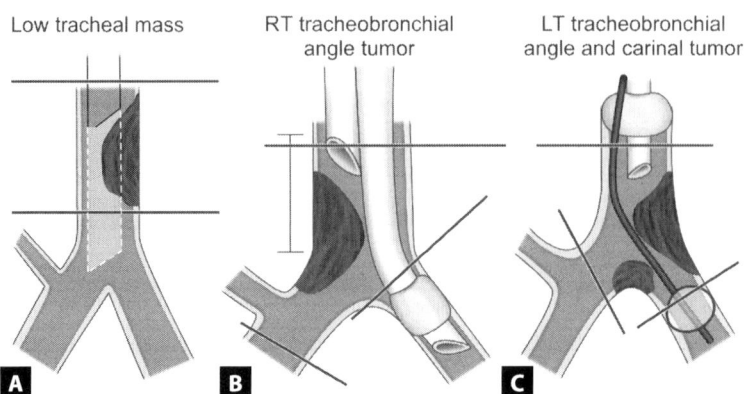

Figs. 11A to C: The lines represent the resection margins. (LT: left; RT: right)

- Initial precarious narrowing
- During trans-section of the airway with plans for cross-field ventilation
- Postoperative precarious airway edema, guardian stitch flexion sedated patient
- Surgical approaches.

Airway Approaches for Various Lower Tracheal and Carinal Lesions

Lower tracheal lesions, unless the lesion is critically narrow or is at risk of airway collapse, may be easy to manage initially by placing the single lumen tube above the lesion, but cross-field ventilation can be difficult. Resection of the carina, especially with right pneumonectomy, can be challenging. The initial airway approach should be individualized and can be a long single-lumen tube (MLS tube) above the lesion with increased airway resistance or a left endobronchial tube. Cross-field ventilation is easier in the left main bronchus **(Fig. 12A)**. The V/Q matching is not good in the supine position, and the other lung may need oxygen insufflation/jet ventilation via a catheter/blocker with the cuff deflated so that the surgical access is not compromised **(Fig. 12B)**.

■ SPECIAL CONSIDERATIONS

During VATS resection and anastomosis, an ETT/jet catheter is introduced through a separate port. Cross-field jet ventilation through a blocker (cuff deflated) or ventilating catheter is preferable in VATS.

Jet ventilation techniques are preferred in pediatric carinal resection or when ETT interferes with suturing or the patient does not tolerate apneic periods. The jet catheter can be introduced through the ETT from above or by a surgeon like in conventional cross-field ventilation. If the surgeon needs to remove distal ETT for periods of difficult suturing, oxygen can be insufflated

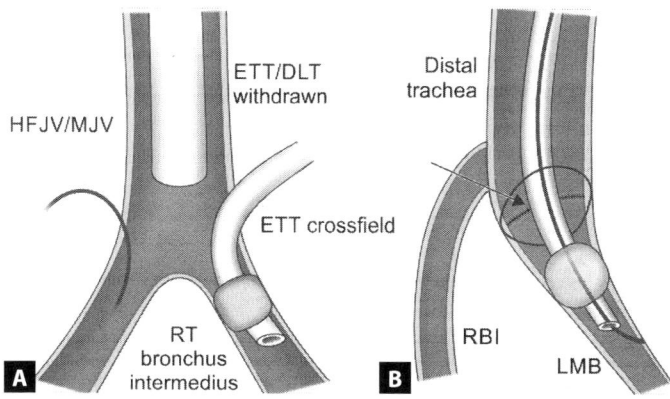

Figs. 12A and B: Intubation of the bronchus with a long single-lumen tube for lower tracheal and carinal lesions (ETT: endotracheal tube; HFJV: high-frequency jet ventilation; MJV: manual jet ventilation; LMB: left main bronchus)

instead of during apneic periods, using a narrow catheter when a jet facility is unavailable. Resection is followed by anastomosis in a similar clock face pattern. Air leak checked while ventilation is carried out by the ETT.

EVOLVING TECHNIQUES

Tubeless Airway Techniques

High-flow nasal oxygen (HFNO) or THRIVE or a combination of TIVA and THRIVE while the patient is on spontaneous ventilation (STRIVE–Hi) is being used, especially in upper tracheal lesions. High-flow oxygenation techniques have been shown to prolong the apneic time during airway surgeries. Once the airway is open, high-flow oxygen through the ETT above the anastomosis is insufflated at 35–40 L/min. These techniques have given apnea time of 20 minutes without desaturation and are the usual anastomotic time. However, this can lead to significant metabolic acidosis and hypercapnia, detrimental in patients with pulmonary hypertension and coronary artery disease. The advantage of these techniques is a tubeless surgical field that is completely spacious and provides the optimal conditions for anastomosis. The incidence of complications of arrhythmia, pneumothorax, hemothorax, and pulmonary barotrauma is minimal.[13] The same techniques can be used to bridge the apneic period during carinal and lower tracheal resections, provided the upper airway is patent.[14]

CASE SCENARIOS

Case 1: Left main bronchus tumor extending to the carina where the surgeon planned a left pneumonectomy with tracheal resection and anastomosis **(Figs. 13A and B)**. The airway can be managed with rigid bronchoscopy and coring followed by a right-sided double lumen tube.

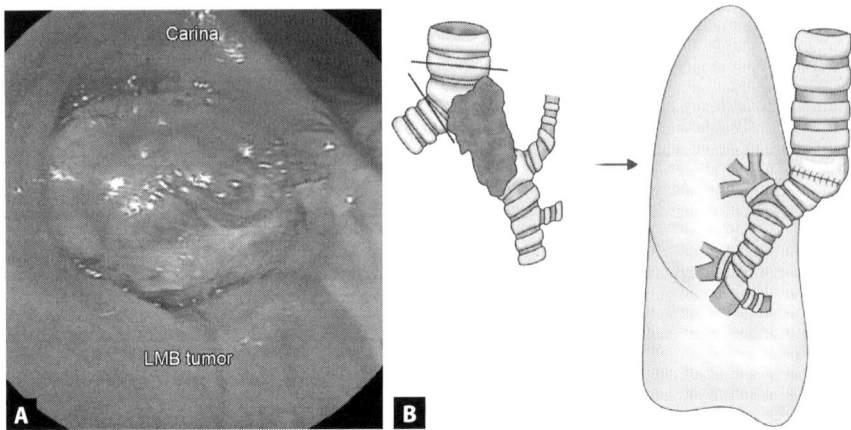

Figs. 13A and B: Left main bronchus tumor extending to the carina—a left pneumonectomy with tracheal resection and anastomosis done.

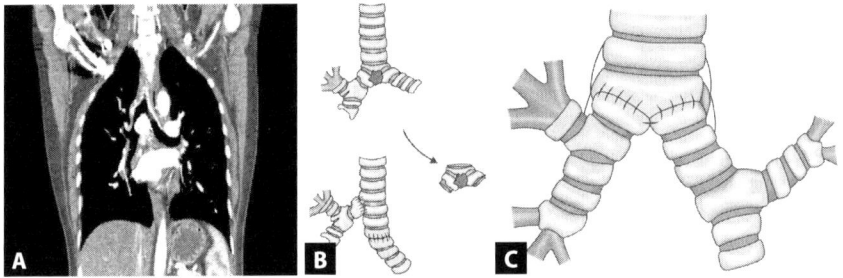

Figs. 14A to C: Isolated carinal resections in smaller midline tumors.

Case 2: Smaller midline tumor—Isolated carinal resections are usually done for smaller midline tumors **(Figs. 14A to C)**.

Case 3: Lower tracheal tumor managed with single lumen tube, and AEC/blocker advanced over the guidewire **(Figs. 15A to C)**.

Extreme Lesions (Figs. 16A and B)

In extreme cases like this, where there is an option to do the STRIVE-Hi, the risk of loss of airway is high. As the backup plans may not prevent morbidity due to hypoxia, it may be worthwhile considering multidisciplinary planning along with pulmonologists and surgeons to discuss the options of rigid bronchoscopy and coring or a venovenous ECMO.

ROLE OF ECMO

Venovenous ECMO under local anesthesia may be established before anesthetizing the patient. Femoral access is established with a 21-F cannula in the inferior vena cava (IVC), which will be the outflow, and a 17-F cannula in the internal jugular vein (IJV) into the RA will be the inflow. Heparin-coated

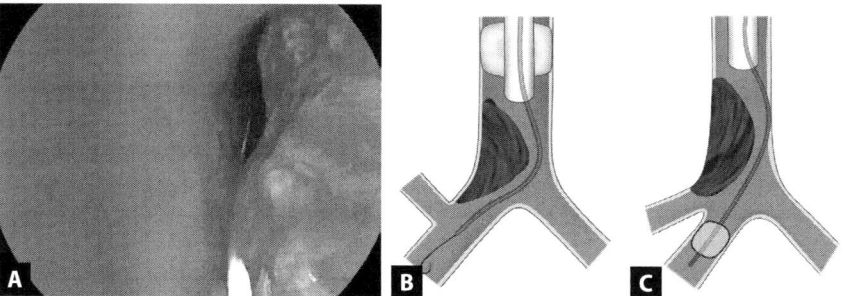

Figs. 15A to C: Lower tracheal tumor managed with single lumen tube, and AEC/blocker advanced over the guidewire.

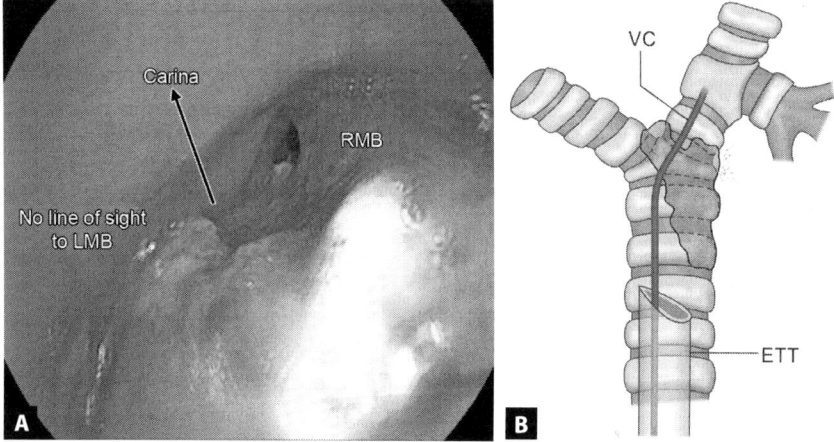

Figs. 16A and B: Extreme tracheal lesion with involvement of lower trachea and carina. (ETT: endotracheal tube; VC: vocal cord)

circuits are used. Before the initiation of cannulation and ECMO, 2,000U heparin is given intravenously to achieve a target ACT of 250 seconds. Establish 3–4 L/min flow with 100% O_2. TIVA with propofol, fentanyl, and atracurium is administered to a target Bi-spectral Index (BIS) of 40–60. No ventilation till tracheal reconstruction is completed.

Once the reconstruction is complete, FOB is done to check the adequacy of the lumen and to ensure tracheobronchial toileting. Oral/nasotracheal intubation is performed. Ensure that cuff is not compressing the anastomotic site under FOB visualization. Pressure-controlled ventilation (PCV) is used to deliver a tidal volume (VT) of 5–6 mL/kg while maintaining a Paw <30 cmH_2O. Once the patient develops adequate respiratory efforts, the patient may be weaned off from the ECMO. Leave the deflated tube as a stent or extubate the patient.

■ EMERGENCE

Complications occur in 5–20% of cases. Anastomotic dehiscence and breakdown led to poor outcomes. Bleeding, infections, tracheomalacia, and restenosis are known complications of TRS. Long-segment tracheal resections, extensive disease, malignancy, poor functional status, postoperative ventilation, infection, and use of steroids are risk factors for developing complications.[12]

■ EXTUBATION

Tracheal extubation is an essential goal at the end of surgery as postoperative mechanical ventilation is implicated in anastomotic dehiscence.[13] Premature extubation may result in the patient becoming apneic and unresponsive necessitating neck extension to maintain the airway or reintubation. Delayed extubation may result in uncontrolled neck extension and coughing, which can compromise the anastomosis. Also, inappropriate use of opiates may lead to loss of airway, necessitating airway manipulation in challenging situations or emergency tracheostomy.[5]

Follow the basic extubation guidelines of Difficult Airway Society (DAS) or All India Difficult Airway Association (AIDAA) for high-risk extubation.

Pre-extubation Assessment

(1) Was the airway difficult [intubation/SGA/difficult mask ventilation (DMV)]? (2) Was there a nerve injury/glottic function either prior or iatrogenic? (3) Are there any concerns with anastomosis? (Luminal narrowing/anastomosis under tension—needs to assess with FOB) (4) Is there airway edema and whether antiedema measures been taken? (5) Number of segments resected: Is there a Guardian stitch **(Fig. 17)**? It is crucial to maintain the neck in flexion and assess tracheal bleeding/obstruction/laryngeal swelling as well as VC dysfunction.[5,15]

If there is an anticipated difficulty 4Ds (difficult intubation, DMV, difficulty due to pre-existent diseases, or delayed recovery) or 3Ss (suspected airway edema, suspected airway collapse, or a surgical cause of airway compromise) plan for high-risk extubation should be done.[16] Leak test is done to rule out airway edema.[13]

Option 1: To use a SGA by modified Bailey's maneuver.[17] Allow the patient to wake up with an LMA and extubate. If there are concerns about anastomosis—lumen/edema/VC function. FOB may be performed through LMA. If the patient develops postoperative stridor, try adrenaline nebulizations/antiedema measures followed by reintubation. AEC can be used for at-risk extubations.

Option 2—awake extubation: The patient may be started on dexmedetomidine or remifentanil infusion to ensure a calm airway. Withdraw the nasal tube over a FOB/AEC if there are concerns.

Immediately after extubation, the VC function needs to be assessed with either a fiberscope or ultrasound to rule out recurrent laryngeal injury.

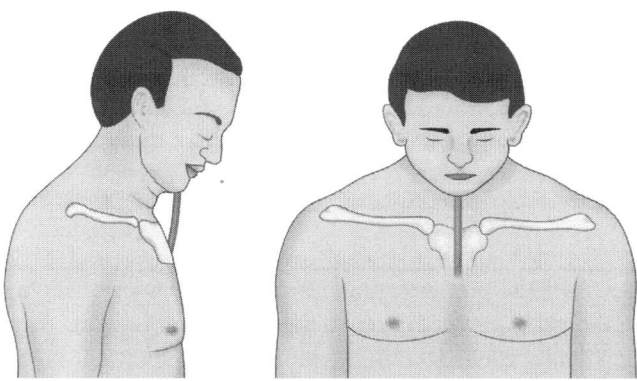

Fig. 17: Gaurdian Stitch

The patient is nursed head up, and mild stridor can easily be managed with nebulized adrenaline.

Precautions with AEC

When using AEC (Cooks AECs), ensure that the marking at the lips is not >25 cm, and the tip should be in the trachea (not into either bronchus). If you are doing jet ventilation and oxygen insufflation via the AEC, it should be done only under anesthetists' supervision.

Carinal resections may require excellent analgesia with a thoracic epidural. These patients often require 12–24 hours of ventilation as their ability to cough and clear secretion is impaired. Postoperative pulmonary edema or ALI is a risk, and ventilatory precautions to reduce ALI and restricting fluids to <1 liter during the case or using dynamic indices to optimize fluid management are recommended.[5]

Postextubation Respiratory Failure

Postextubation respiratory failure is a dreaded complication, which may occur secondary to early tracheal extubation, inadequate neuromuscular reversal, or airway obstruction. For the first two situations, maintenance of the upper airway with nasopharyngeal/oropharyngeal airway or LMA is done while correcting the primary cause with either naloxone or a further dose of reversal or Sugammadex if rocuronium was used. Airway obstruction due to VC edema or dysfunction or anastomotic narrowing (blood clot/mucosal flap) needs a bronchoscopy to confirm the diagnosis. This can be achieved via a second-generation LMA such as AMBU AuraGain or i-gel designed for reintubation. Reintubation with guardian stitch and airway edema/blood can be a daunting task. Bronchoscopic approach/combined video laryngoscopy D blade (no need to align the oral–pharyngeal–laryngeal access) + FOB offers some advantages. LMA-facilitated intubation is a useful technique as it helps in identifying the pathology, which resulted in airway obstruction. Regardless of the technique, use a smaller size tube, preferably 5- or 6-mm ETT, preferably uncuffed, or leave the cuff deflated. The tube should be positioned either above or well below the anastomosis. If the anesthetist cannot establish the airway, the surgeon will need to do a tracheostomy below the level of anastomosis.[5]

CONCLUSION

There is no best choice anesthesia or airway plan. Anesthesia management must be a tailored approach based on the symptoms, imaging bronchoscopy, and surgical needs. Close communication with surgeons and the other team members is paramount. Extubation is equally or rather more important.

REFERENCES

1. Schieren M, Wappler F, Defosse J. Anesthesia for tracheal and carinal resection and reconstruction. Curr Opin Anesthesiol. 2022;35(1):75-81.
2. Wong DT, Weng H, Lam E, Song HB, Liu J. Lengthening of the trachea during neck extension: which part of the trachea is stretched? Anesth Analg. 2008;107(3):989-93.
3. Smeltz AM, Bhatia M, Arora H, Long J, Kumar PA. Anesthesia for resection and reconstruction of the trachea and carina. J Cardiothorac Vasc Anesth. 2020;34(7):1902-13.
4. Sherani K, Vakil A, Dodhia C, Fein A. Malignant tracheal tumors: a review of current diagnostic and management strategies. Curr Opin Pulm Med. 2015;21(4):322-6.
5. Hobai IA, Chhangani SV, Alfille PH. Anesthesia for tracheal resection and reconstruction. Anesthesiol Clin. 2012;30(4):709-30.
6. Jagannathan N, Burjek N. Transnasal humidified rapid-insufflation ventilatory exchange (THRIVE) in children: a step forward in apnoeic oxygenation, paradigm-shift in ventilation, or both? Br J Anaesth. 2017;118(2):150-2.
7. Slinger P. Management of the patient with a central airway obstruction. Saudi J Anaesth. 2011;5(3):241.
8. Myer CM, O'Connor DM, Cotton RT. Proposed grading system for subglottic stenosis based on endotracheal tube sizes. Ann Otol Rhinol Laryngol. 1994;103 (4 Pt 1):319-23.
9. McCaffrey TV. Classification of laryngotracheal stenosis. Laryngoscope. 1992;102(12 Pt 1):1335-40.
10. Freitag L, Ernst A, Unger M, Kovitz K, Marquette CH. A proposed classification system of central airway stenosis. Eur Respir J. 2007;30(1):7-12.
11. Pinsonneault C, Fortier J, Donati F. Tracheal resection and reconstruction. Can J Anesth. 1999;46(5):439-55.
12. OpenAirway. (2019). TRR: Tracheal Resection and Reconstruction. [online] Available from https://openairway.org/wp-content/uploads/2019/01/Hofmeyr-Tracheal-Resection-and-Reconstruction-v2019_0118.pdf. [Last accessed October, 2022].

13. Ly NM, Van Dinh N, Trang DTT, Hai NV, Hung TX. Apnoeic oxygenation with high-flow oxygen for tracheal resection and reconstruction surgery. BMC Anesthesiol. 2022;22(1):73.
14. Garg R, Pandey K. Anesthesia for tracheal resection and anastomosis: What is new! J Anaesthesiol Clin Pharmacol. 2022;38(1):58-60.
15. Membership of the Difficult Airway Society Extubation Guidelines Group; Popat M, Mitchell V, Dravid R, Patel A, Swampillai C, Higgs A. Difficult Airway Society Guidelines for the management of tracheal extubation. Anaesthesia. 2012;67:318-40.
16. Kundra P, Garg R, Patwa A, Ahmed SM, Ramkumar V, Shah A, et al. All India Difficult Airway Association 2016 guidelines for the management of anticipated difficult extubation. Indian J Anaesth. 2016;60(12):915-21.
17. Sorbello M, Cortese G, Gaçonnet C, Skinner M. A modified Bailey's manoeuvre for supraglottic airway continuum using LMA Protector™. Indian J Anaesth. 2019;63(1):78-80.

CHAPTER

15

Anesthesia for Pancreas and Islet Cell Transplantation

Cody Tidwell, Vinh Huu Nguyen, Serjey Ghercuic, Kumar Belani

ABSTRACT

Pancreas transplantation is an effective therapeutic means to treat patients with diabetes mellitus and is often performed as a simultaneous pancreas and kidney transplant procedure. Clinicians are constantly faced with specific underlying comorbidities related to poor glycemic control. This review will touch upon perioperative management from an anesthesiologist's perspective. Attention to preoperative evaluation and patient-specific selection is essential for a good outcome. A discussion of intraoperative management during vascular reperfusion and strict glycemic control requires vigilant monitoring. Postoperative pain control tailored toward multimodal analgesia—including regional anesthesia—is paramount to successful transplantation of the pancreas, kidney, and islet cells.

Keywords: Anesthesia; Diabetes mellitus; Pancreas transplant alone (PTA); Simultaneous pancreas kidney transplant (SPK); Total pancreatectomy with islet autotransplantation (TPIAT)

KEY POINTS

- Pancreas transplant can involve the entire solid organ from a deceased donor, a partial organ from a living donor, or the isolated beta islet cells from an autologous or one or more donor sources.
- Pancreatic tissue transplantation is most performed in patients with diabetes mellitus, and simultaneous pancreas kidney transplant (SPK) is the most frequent transplantation procedure involving the pancreas.
- Diabetes mellitus is a complex disease that affects every organ system of the body. Pancreas transplantation may decrease or cure the disease depending on etiology and severity.
- Organ transplantations are complex surgeries requiring extensive patient screening and optimization preoperatively. Intraoperative management may be complicated by numerous comorbidities involving the need for invasive monitoring equipment.
- Postoperative pain management can be difficult as patients often present on chronic opioid therapy. Multimodal analgesia, including nonopioid, opioid, and regional anesthetic techniques, is required to offer satisfactory analgesia.

INTRODUCTION

Transplantation of the pancreas in humans was first described by Kelly et al. in 1966 after a patient underwent the first simultaneous pancreas and kidney (SPK) procedure to treat diabetic nephropathy. Shortly after, Najarian et al. reported a successful transplant of an isolated islet of Langerhans cells in 1974. The International Pancreas Transplant Registry (IPTR), formed in 1980, estimates nearly 30,000 transplants have been performed in the United States and over 48,000 internationally. Of these transplants, the most common procedure was SPK (~77%) followed by pancreas after kidney (PAK) (~14%) and pancreas transplant alone (PTA) (~9%). 5-year survival rates for SPK, PAK, and PTA were 87, 83, and 91%, respectively.[1,2] The most common indication for pancreas transplantation is type 1 diabetes mellitus (T1DM) with an increasing number of patients with type 2 diabetes mellitus (T2DM) undergoing transplantation.[3]

DIABETES MELLITUS

Diabetes mellitus (DM) is a complex metabolic disorder with various classifications related to type and etiology. The prolonged disruption of glycemic homeostasis and macro- and microangiopathies appears to be the predominant driving factors, among many, that facilitate the physiologic consequences manifested in long-standing DM **(Table 1)**.

Type 1 DM is characterized by autoimmune, T-cell mediated destruction of β-islet cells. Onset is often sudden (especially in children), presenting with symptoms of diabetic ketoacidosis secondary to severe or complete deficiencies in insulin and C-peptide with concurrent hyperglycemia. A number of autoantibodies are implicated in this process: anti-glutamic acid decarboxylase 65 (GAD65), anti-islet cell antibodies (ICAs), anti-zinc transporter isoform 8 (ZnT8), and insulin autoantibodies (IAAs). GAD65 is the most common to be present at the time of diagnosis (80%) followed by ICAs (70–90%) and IA-2α (<75%). Patients with T1DM are, therefore, dependent on exogenous insulin administration to prevent life-threatening hyperglycemia.

Type 2 DM is characterized by a combination of prolonged insulin resistance and subsequent pancreatic β-islet cell dysfunction. Development of T2DM is often later in life compared to T1DM, frequently with a more subtle onset, and is not necessarily an exogenous insulin-dependent process (this entity is referred to as noninsulin-dependent diabetes mellitus or NIDDM). Several risk factors exist for the development of this disease including obesity, family history, insulin resistance, presence of polycystic ovarian syndrome, and sedentary lifestyle. Treatment is multifactorial, beginning with behavior modifications including diet and increased aerobic exercise, oral or injectable antihyperglycemics, insulin injection, and pancreas transplant.

TABLE 1: Consequences of suboptimally controlled diabetes mellitus by organ system.[4-11]

Organ system	Pathologic manifestations
Neurologic	• Sensory neuropathy—often causing burning paresthesias of the hands and feet • Autonomic neuropathy—gustatory sweating, impotence, bladder and stomach hypotonia • Increased risk of CVA/TIA
Ophthalmologic	• Retinopathy—most common ocular complication of diabetes and most common cause of blindness in the United States • Neovascular glaucoma • Cataract formation—risk increased two- to fivefold • Dry-eye syndrome—increased risk of abrasive keratopathy
Cardiovascular	• Hypertension • Dyslipidemia • Diabetic cardiomyopathy • Accelerated arterial (including coronary) atherosclerosis • Peripheral vascular disease—claudication, vasodilation, and edema • Altered autoregulation and vascular tone response—orthostasis
Gastrointestinal	• Esophageal dysmotility • Gastroesophageal reflux disease (GERD) • Gastroparesis • Enteropathy—diarrhea, constipation, or fecal incontinence • Nonalcoholic fatty liver disease (NAFLD) • Glycogenic hepatopathy
Genitourinary	• Nephropathy—leads to hypertension and renal failure • Cystopathy—hypotonia leading to micturition hesitance and urine retention • Impotence
Musculoskeletal	• Osteoporosis and impaired healing of fractures • *Soft-tissue fibroproliferative disorders*: Dupuytren's contracture, carpal tunnel syndrome, adhesive capsulitis, and flexor tenosynovitis • *Arthropathies*: Rheumatoid arthritis, osteoarthritis, and Charcot joint • *Skeletal myopathies*—diabetic amyotrophy and infarction
Immune	• Increased risk of infection—impaired phagocytosis, suppressed cytokine production • Hyperglycemic environment favors infectious organism growth

(CVA: cerebrovascular accident; TIA: transient ischemic attack)

Other types of DM, such as maturity-onset diabetes of the young (MODY), gestational diabetes mellitus (GDM), and secondary diabetes, are listed for completion but are out of the scope of discussion of this review. A summary of the different types and characteristics can be found in **Table 2**.[4]

TABLE 2: Classifications of the most common types of diabetes mellitus and their common attributes.[1,4]

Classification of diabetes mellitus	Characteristics
Type 1	- Second most common type of diabetes (5–10%) - Autoimmune etiology involving the β-islet cells or insulin polypeptide - More often develops in children and adolescents with acute onset - Exogenous insulin dependence due to near- or total insulin deficiency - Latent autoimmune diabetes in adults (LADA) subtype is the most common adult form autoimmune diabetes
Type 2	- Most common type of diabetes (90–95%) - Etiology involves cellular resistance to insulin and β-islet cell dysfunction - Strong genetic predisposition often with insidious onset
Gestational	- New-onset insulin tolerance during pregnancy (1–14% of pregnancies) - Increases lifetime risk of development of T2DM
Maturity-onset diabetes of the young (MODY)	- Rare disorder, often confused for T1DM or T2DM, in which there are genetic abnormalities in β-islet cell glucose detection or insulin release - End-organ insulin sensitivity is unaltered - At least 13 known variants with MODY2 and MODY3 types comprising >80% of MODY cases
Secondary	- Other etiologies that cause β-islet cell dysfunction or decreased insulin sensitivity including infectious, drug-related, traumatic, or syndromic associations

(T1DM: type 1 diabetes mellitus; T2DM: type 2 diabetes mellitus)

■ PANCREAS ANATOMY AND PHYSIOLOGY

The pancreas is an unencapsulated retroperitoneal organ found lying transversely between the duodenum and spleen and anterior to the first and second lumbar vertebrae. The pancreas is segmented into four separate parts from right to left—head, neck, body, and tail. The pancreatic head lies anterior to the inferior vena cava and right renal vein and posterior to the second and third portion, or "C loop", of the duodenum. The neck traverses over the abdominal aorta. The body is the largest portion of the pancreas and overlies the superior mesenteric artery, left kidney, left adrenal gland, and left renal vasculature. Finally, the tail of the pancreas is found extending up to the splenic hilum into the peritoneum.[12,13]

The physiology of the pancreas can be separated into two categories—exocrine and endocrine functions. The exocrine functions are carried out by the acinar cells and their ducts which make up ~80% of the pancreas' tissue.[14] Acinar cells store digestive enzymes in secretory vesicles, the Golgi complexes, which are released by exocytosis when stimulated either by vagal or hormonal input during feeding. Of most clinical importance is the release of enzymes such as amylase, lipase, and inactive proteolytic enzymes such as trypsinogen, chymotrypsinogen, and procarboxypeptidase.[15,16]

The endocrine functions of the pancreas are governed by various types of islet of Langerhans cells designated by Greek letters: α-cells (produce glucagon), β-cells (insulin), γ-cells (pancreatic polypeptide), δ-cells (somatostatin), and ε-cells (ghrelin). In humans, β-cells are most predominant (~60%) followed by α-cells (~30%). The goal of pancreas transplantation, either solid organ or isolated islet cells, is the successful integration of insulin and glucagon producing β- and α-cells to liberate a patient from supplemental insulin and effectively cure their diabetes.[17]

PATIENT SELECTION

There are numerous factors considered when matching a donor and recipient beyond ABO and human leukocyte antigen (HLA) compatibility. Both parties must not be significantly overweight [institutional, but most data support body mass index (BMI) <32 kg/m^2] and no active drug use, systemic infections, or malignancies. Donor exclusion factors may also include previous upper gastrointestinal (GI) surgery, history of alcoholism, or signs of acute pancreatic pathology (histologically seen as glandular edema, hematoma, fatty infiltration, or necrosis). Exclusion criteria are similar for the recipient; a summary of recipient contraindications can be seen in **Table 3**. A number of

TABLE 3: Absolute and relative contraindications to receive donor pancreatic tissue.[16]

Absolute contraindications	Relative contraindications

• Age >65
• *Significant cardiovascular risk:*
  – Myocardial infarction within 6 months
  – Uncorrectable CAD
  – LVEF <30%
  – PA systolic pressure >50 mm Hg
• Incurable malignancy (excluding localized skin)
• Active sepsis
• Peptic ulcer disease
• Inability to maintain medication adherence
	• CVA with significant chronic deficits
	• Active HBV or HCV infections
	• BMI >30 kg/m^2
	• Insulin requirements >1.5 units/kg/day
	• *Extensive vascular disease:*
	  – Aorta
	  – Iliac
	  – Significant peripheral
	• Active drug abuse, including alcohol, and tobacco

(BMI: body mass index; CAD: coronary artery disease; CVA: cerebrovascular accident; HBV: hepatitis B virus; HCV: hepatitis C virus; LVEF: left ventricular ejection fraction)

objective scoring systems have been developed to assist the multidisciplinary transplant team in appropriate patient matching: pre-procurement pancreas allocation suitability score (P-PASS) and pancreas donor risk index (pDRI) are two commonly used in Europe.[18]

IMMUNOSUPPRESSION AND PROPHYLAXIS

Immunosuppression regimens vary by surgical team and facility but follow principles common to most solid organ transplants: induction and maintenance of antilymphocyte activity. Induction often involves the administration of thymoglobulin, basiliximab, or alemtuzumab. Maintenance is frequently achieved with a combination of tacrolimus, mycophenolate, and steroids. Infection prophylaxis is individualized to the patient's community and medical facility policies as well as the donor's serology. Commonly, antivirals for cytomegalovirus (CMV), antifungals, and broad-spectrum antibacterials are administered for a duration of months to lifetime.[3,16]

OVERVIEW OF SURGICAL TECHNIQUE

The surgical technique selected to perform pancreas transplantation varies depending on the patient and their comorbidities **(Table 4)**.[1,4] Solid organ transplantation involves total cadaveric organ or partial living-donor tissue taken from the tail of the living donor's pancreas. When only the islet of Langerhans cells is transplanted, a patient may undergo total pancreatectomy with islet autotransplantation (TPIAT) or allograft islet cells from one or more donors.

TABLE 4: The various types of single- or multiorgan transplantation with expected selection criteria and outcomes.[13]

Type of transplantation	Indications and organ longevity
Simultaneous pancreas and kidney (SPK)	• For insulin-dependent diabetics with renal failure • ~10–15 years of organ function
Pancreas transplant alone (PTA)	• For insulin-dependent diabetics with normal renal function • ~5–7 years of organ function
Pancreas after kidney (PAK)	• ~5–7 years of organ function
Simultaneous islet and kidney (SIK)	• For insulin-dependent diabetics with renal failure • ~5–7 years of organ function
Islet after kidney	• ~5–7 years of tissue function
Islet transplant (TPIAT versus allograft)	• ~5–7 years of tissue function

In most cases of abdominal solid organ transplantation, the native organ is left in place. Except for TPIAT or individual patient anatomic situations, this is also true for pancreas transplant recipients. The venous, arterial, and exocrine duct drainage anastomoses are important surgical considerations. The arterial supply for the new pancreas is produced via a Y-shaped graft of donor superior mesenteric and splenic arteries anastomosed to the patient's iliac artery. Venous drainage is achieved via the portal venous system or systemically via the iliac vein or inferior vena cava. The pancreatic duct was traditionally drained to the bladder, but due to significant complications (urethritis, pancreatitis, dehydration, and electrolyte abnormalities), it is now often drained enterically. As of today, over 80% of pancreatic transplants are currently performed using this technique with success. The donor pancreas may include a segment of donor duodenum allowing the surgical team to form a side-to-side duodenojejunal anastomosis and thereby reduce the likelihood of stricture or leak **(Fig. 1)**. In general, an SPK takes ~6–8 hours to complete while a PTA takes ~3–4 hours.[1,3,16]

For patients undergoing islet cell transplantation, either allograft or as part of TPIAT, the islets must first be isolated from the predominating pancreatic parenchyma (acini). This is a lengthy process, established by Ricordi et al. in 1987, involving dissection of the nonpancreatic tissue (fat, lymph nodes, and vessels), multiple stages of duct perfusion and immersed agitation with specific dissolving agents under strict temperature conditions, washing of debris, and storage of separated islets in cold preservation solution. Once the islets are isolated, they are thoroughly

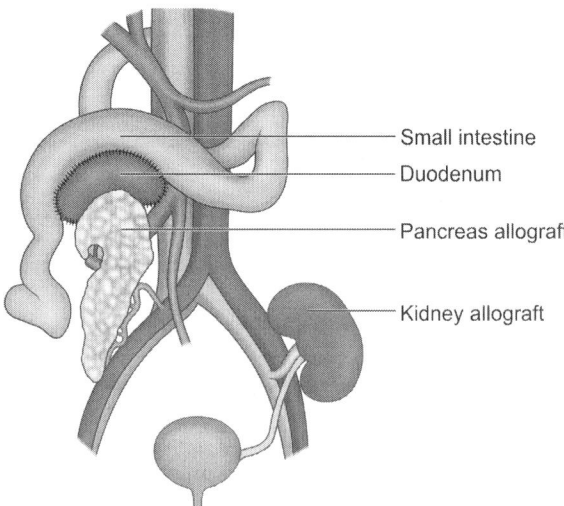

Fig. 1: Surgical vascularization of the pancreas and renal allografts during a simultaneous pancreas and kidney transplantation procedure. The pancreas graft is shown draining enterically with its original duodenal drainage.

tested for sterility, cell count, purity, potency, stability, viability, and total tissue volume; the target is >5,000 islet equivalents with a total volume of ~5 mL. The isolated cells are viable for up to 72 hours. The islets are then introduced percutaneously into the hepatic vein or surgically into the mesenteric artery for delivery to the hepatic parenchyma. Once venous cannulation is confirmed, the cells are transfused by gravity over 30–60 minutes. During this time, portal venous pressures are measured to avoid acute portal hypertension (portal vein pressure >22 mm Hg).[3,19,20]

▇ PREOPERATIVE EVALUATION

Preoperative evaluation of transplant recipients is paramount for safe provision of anesthesia. Mortality after pancreas transplant is most often linked to coronary artery disease necessitating a thorough history and physical examination, with particular attention to the cardiovascular system, before formulating an anesthetic plan. Coronary revascularization was found to reduce the risk of adverse cardiac events in this patient population.[3] In patients undergoing SPK, the renal function should also be extensively investigated.[21] Common comorbidities such as DM, hypertension, anemia, autonomic dysfunction, and electrolyte abnormalities should be medically optimized prior to proceeding with transplantation. In those with long-standing DM, the anesthesiologist may encounter difficult laryngoscopy, if the patient has positive palm print or prayer signs.[22]

▇ ANESTHETIC CONSIDERATIONS

Pancreas transplant patients should undergo general anesthesia tailored to their individual medical needs. Intraoperative management involves patient-appropriate induction with consideration of rapid sequence intubation (RSI) for patients with comorbid gastroparesis. Skeletal muscle paralysis with cisatracurium that undergoes nonenzymatic Hoffman elimination[23] may be used when there is concern for renal or hepatic clearance of more commonly used paralytic agents such as rocuronium. When renal function is adequate, rocuronium-sugammadex reversal was found to have significantly lower incidence of severe hypoxemia, shorter postanesthesia care unit (PACU) stay, and reduced intensive care unit (ICU) admission compared to cisatracurium-neostigmine reversal in patients undergoing kidney transplantation.[24]

Significant hemodynamic shifts can occur in patients with cardiac disease, thus invasive blood pressure monitoring, transesophageal echocardiography (TEE), and pulmonary artery (PA) catheter utilization should be considered. Placement of a central venous catheter for the administration of potent vasopressors and immunosuppressants is required. At least one large-bore IV catheter is recommended to provide rapid transfusion in the event of hemorrhage. Standard hemodynamic, temperature, and metabolic goals should be followed.

Vigilance during vascular unclamping and organ reperfusion is important to maintain graft health and stable systemic perfusion; at this time, the patient may require fluids, vasopressors, and/or blood products to prevent hemodynamic collapse.[3] In preparation for reperfusion, potent inhaled anesthetic should be decreased to minimize systemic vascular resistance (SVR) reduction. Metabolic derangements including electrolyte abnormalities and acid-base imbalance should be corrected. Calcium replacement may be required to help optimize cardiac output and protect from hyperkalemia-induced arrhythmia. Optimal fluid goal for noncardiac patients is achieved with central venous pressure in the range of 12–14 mm Hg and systolic pressure at least 140 mm Hg.[25] Alternatively, in patients with cardiac disease, optimization of intravascular fluid status should be based on PA catheter or TEE. Crystalloids are the mainstay for volume resuscitation, but colloids such as albumin can be an alternative.

Strict glycemic control and monitoring is required with a goal glucose range of 100–150 mg/dL. The importance is twofold: islet cell dysfunction has been seen in hyperglycemic animal studies and trending post-transplantation serum glucose may help to determine new islet cell function (transplanted β-islet cells will be glucose responsive within 5 minutes of reperfusion).[3] Furthermore, hyperglycemia has been shown to decrease immune function, further exacerbating the risk of infection in a patient receiving immunosuppression.[11]

Satisfactory pain management can be difficult to establish in this patient population due to frequent dependence on multiple analgesics at presentation. A multimodal analgesic regimen should be implemented in all patients undergoing pancreatic transplantation. The World Health Organization (WHO) analgesic ladder provides a foundational approach for incremental pain control: begin with nonopioid medications, such as acetaminophen, with escalation to include adjuvant medications (including nonsteroidal anti-inflammatory drugs, tricyclic antidepressants, gabapentinoids, serotonin–norepinephrine reuptake inhibitors, and skeletal muscle relaxants), opioids, and invasive procedures.[26] Ketamine may be particularly efficacious in patients with high-opioid requirements.[27]

Regional anesthesia is often utilized in abdominal cases, and several techniques have been positively described in patients undergoing pancreas transplant. Thoracic epidural analgesia (TEA) is considered the standard of care, but peripheral nerve-blocking procedures such as rectus sheath block (RSB) and transversus abdominis plane (TAP) blocks are beneficial in patients that cannot tolerate or have contraindications to epidural placement. In a study of 29 patients, RSB showed similar postoperative intravenous (IV) morphine equivalent (MEQ) use compared to TEA.[27] The TAP block, either with plain bupivacaine via catheters or liposomal bupivacaine via single-shot technique, was also found to decrease postoperative opioid use.

When compared to IV analgesic administration alone, TAP block showed faster time to intestinal function return, but overall inferior pain control likely due to lack of visceral antinociception.[28,29]

POSTOPERATIVE COMPLICATIONS

Pancreas transplantation carries a particularly high risk of complications compared to other solid organ transplant procedures. Most significant are hemorrhage, infection (intra-abdominal, systemic, or mycotic aneurysm formation), thrombosis, anastomotic leak, pancreatitis, pancreatic-enteric fistula, and rejection. Overall rejection rates range from 5 to 25%. Technical failure, defined by graft loss within the first 3 months, is most often due to thrombosis (50%), pancreatitis (20%), or infection (18%). With respect to islet transplantation, portal vein thrombosis is the most common complication, and it is estimated that 30% of islet cell recipients will require a repeat operation even in the absence of complications from the original procedure.[3,16]

CONCLUSION

Pancreas transplantation is most performed in T1DM patients in order to relieve their exogenous insulin dependence. These patients often have comorbidities significant to anesthetic management including hypertension, coronary artery disease, neuropathies, and chronic kidney disease. The SPK procedure is the most common form of transplantation involving the pancreas and is indicated in patients with concurrent pancreas and kidney disease. Patients are extensively screened for medical and psychosocial issues before being medically optimized as an eligible organ recipient. Individualized anesthetic management should focus on the patient's health with particular attention to cardiovascular disease. Additional invasive monitoring is often necessary to safely complete surgery especially during the significant hemodynamic and metabolic abnormalities associated with organ reperfusion. Pain control may be difficult and should include multimodal analgesic technique with narcotics, adjuncts, and regional anesthesia.

REFERENCES

1. Giorgakis E, Mathur AK, Chakkera HA, Reddy KS, Moss AA, Singer AL. Solid pancreas transplant: Pushing forward. World J Transplant. 2018;8(7):237-51.
2. El-Hennawy H, Stratta RJ, Smith F. Exocrine drainage in vascularized pancreas transplantation in the new millennium. World J Transplant. 2016;6(2):255-71.
3. Longnecker DE, Newman MF, Mackey S, Sandberg WS, Zapol WM, Remskar Konia M, et al. Chapter 59: Anesthesia for Kidney, Pancreas, or Other Organ Transplantation. Anesthesiology. New Delhi: McGraw-Hill Education; 2012. pp. 1094-104.

4. Banday MZ, Sameer AS, Nissar S. Pathophysiology of diabetes: an overview. Avicenna J Med. 2020;10(4):174-88.
5. Watkins PJ, Thomas PK. Diabetes mellitus and the nervous system. J Neurol Neurosurg Psychiatr. 1998;65:620-32.
6. Sayin N, Kara N, Pekel G. Ocular complications of diabetes mellitus. World J Diabetes. 2015;6(1):92-108.
7. Leon BM, Maddox TM. Diabetes and cardiovascular disease: Epidemiology, biological mechanisms, treatment recommendations and future research. World J Diabetes. 2015;6(13):1246-58.
8. Krishnan B, Babu S, Walker J, Walker AB, Pappachan JM. Gastrointestinal complications of diabetes mellitus. World J Diabetes. 2013;4(3):51-63.
9. Min TZ, Stephens MW, Kumar P, Chudleigh RA. Renal complications of diabetes. Brit Med Bull. 104(1):113-27.
10. Sözen T, Başaran NÇ, Tınazlı M, Özışık L. Musculoskeletal problems in diabetes mellitus. Eur J Rheumatol. 2018;5(4):258-65.
11. Berbudi A, Rahmadika N, Tjahjadi AI, Ruslami R. Type 2 diabetes and its impact on the immune system. Curr Diabetes Rev. 2020;16(5):442-9.
12. National Health Service. Types of pancreas transplant. NHS choices. [online] Available from https://www.nhsbt.nhs.uk/organ-transplantation/pancreas/is-a-pancreas-transplant-right-for-you/types-of-pancreas-transplant/. [Last accessed October, 2022].
13. Pandol SJ. The Exocrine Pancreas. San Rafael (CA): Morgan & Claypool Life Sciences; 2010. Anatomy. [online] Available from https://www.ncbi.nlm.nih.gov/books/NBK54134/. [Last accessed October, 2022].
14. A-Kader HH, Ghishan FK. The Pancreas. Textbook of Clinical Pediatrics, 2nd edition. New York City: Springer; 2012. pp. 1925-36.
15. Talathi SS, Zimmerman R, Young M, StatPearls [Internet]. Anatomy, Abdomen and Pelvis, Pancreas. [Updated 2021 Jul 26]. Treasure Island (FL): StatPearls Publishing; 2022.
16. Bahar SG, Devulapally P, StatPearls [Internet]. Pancreas transplantation. Treasure Island (FL): StatPearls Publishing; 2022.
17. Da Silva Xavier G. The cells of the islets of langerhans. J Clin Med. 2018;7(3):54.
18. Piemonti L. Islet Transplantation. In: Feingold KR, Anawalt B, Boyce A, et al. (Eds). Endotext [Internet]. South Dartmouth (MA): MDText.com, Inc.; 2000. [online] Available from https://www.ncbi.nlm.nih.gov/books/NBK278966/. [Last accessed October, 2022].
19. Bellin MD, Gelrud A, Arreaza-Rubin G, Dunn TB, Humar A, Morgan KA, et al. Total pancreatectomy with islet autotransplantation: summary of a National Institute of Diabetes and Digestive and Kidney diseases workshop. Pancreas. 2014;43(8):1163-71.
20. Spence KT, Ladie DE. Islets Transplantation. In: StatPearls [Internet]. Treasure Island (FL): StatPearls Publishing; 2022. [online] Available from https://www.ncbi.nlm.nih.gov/books/NBK562272/. [Last accessed October, 2022].
21. Kumar L, Surendran S, Kesavan R, Menon RN. Simultaneous pancreas-kidney transplant for type I diabetes with renal failure: Anaesthetic considerations. Indian J Anaesth. 2016;60(2):131-4.
22. Carron M, Andreatta G, Pesenti E, De Cassai A, Feltracco P, Linassi F, et al. Impact on grafted kidney function of rocuronium-sugammadex vs.

cisatracurium-neostigmine strategy for neuromuscular block management. An Italian single-center, 2014-2017 retrospective cohort case-control study. Perioper Med (Lond). 2022;11(1):3.
23. Kisor DF, Schmith VD. Clinical pharmacokinetics of cisatracurium besilate. Clin Pharmacokinet. 1999;36(1):27-40.
24. Hashim K, Thomas M. Sensitivity of palm print sign in prediction of difficult laryngoscopy in diabetes: a comparison with other airway indices. Indian J Anaesth. 2014;58(3):298-302.
25. Koehntop DE, Beebe DS, Belani KG. Perioperative anesthetic management of the kidney-pancreas transplant recipient. Curr Opin Anaesthesiol. 2000;13(3):341-7.
26. Shah I, Sheth SG, Kothari DJ. Pain management in chronic pancreatitis incorporating safe opioid practices: Challenge accepted. World J Gastroenterol. 2021;27(23):3142-7.
27. Schwenk ES, Viscusi ER, Buvanendran A, Hurley RW, Wasan AD, Narouze S, et al. Consensus guidelines on the use of intravenous ketamine infusions for acute pain management from the American Society of Regional Anesthesia and Pain Medicine, the American Academy of Pain Medicine, and the American Society of Anesthesiologists. Reg Anesth Pain Med. 2018;43(5):456-66.
28. Hausken J, Rydenfelt K, Horneland R, Ullensvang K, Kjøsen G, Tønnessen TI, et al. First experience with rectus sheath block for postoperative analgesia after pancreas transplant: a retrospective observational study. Transplant Proc. 2019;51(2):479-84.
29. Yeap YL, Fridell JA, Wu D, Mangus RS, Kroepfl E, Wolfe J, et al. Comparison of methods of providing analgesia after pancreas transplant: IV opioid analgesia versus transversus abdominis plane block with liposomal bupivacaine or continuous catheter infusion. Clin Transplant. 2019;33(6):e13581.

CHAPTER

16

Anesthetic Implications in Gastroenterological Interventions Outside the Operating Room

Venkatesan Thiruvenkatarajan, Roelof MAW van Wijk

ABSTRACT

Gastroenterological interventions are often performed outside the operating room in suites that may not be as adequately resourced as standard operating room suites. The demand for such interventions to be performed with the participation of anesthesiologists is steadily growing. The comorbidity burden in this patient population is increasing, and more complex interventions of longer duration are currently being performed. Hence, it offers unique challenges to anesthesiologists. Often, these interventions are undertaken on a semi-urgent basis with variable time for pre-procedure optimization in a rapid turnaround setting. Newer modes of oxygen supplementation and airway management are now available. Preparation and organizational logistics of these areas must be standardized and constantly monitored with collaboration between various stakeholders. A comprehensive understanding of the patients' risk factors, and procedure requirements, along with an improved appreciation of the oxygenation and airway management strategies coupled with the application of optimum pharmacological principles of sedation, will improve the outcome.

Keywords: Airway; Anesthesia; Colonoscopy; Endoscopy; Outside the operating room.

KEY POINTS

- The volume of gastroenterological (GE) interventions performed outside the operating room with the involvement of anesthesiologists is growing progressively.
- The environment is different from a traditional operating room setting.
- Evidence supports that significant cardiorespiratory events are frequent in patients undergoing gastrointestinal endoscopy.
- Advanced therapeutic interventions of longer duration are frequently performed in patients with significant underlying comorbidities.
- Often, presentations are semiurgent in nature with less time for preprocedure optimization.
- Advanced oxygenation and airway management strategies to assist procedural sedation are now available.

- Preprocedure risk stratification should identify those at higher risk and manage appropriately.
- Outside operating room GE intervention suites should be equipped at par with that of the established operating room suites.
- A thorough understanding of the strengths and limitations of the oxygenation strategies and pharmacological agents of sedation at the anesthesiologists' disposal is vital.

INTRODUCTION

The demand for diagnostic and therapeutic gastroenterological (GE) interventions has been steadily increasing recently around the globe.[1] Medicare statistics from the United States indicate that the rates of anesthesiologists-assisted propofol sedation for outpatient endoscopic procedures have grown four times from 14 to 48% between 2003 and 2013.[2] Real-world data suggest that in 2016, roughly 50 million GE interventions were performed in the United States.[3] Anecdotally, it appears that the utilization of this service has witnessed rapid growth in the Indian subcontinent within the last couple of decades. GE interventions present unique challenges in contemporary anesthesia practice. This is due to the extended indications and increased complexity of the interventions performed on patients with significant comorbidity burden.[1] Often, these procedures are performed outside the operating room (OR) in dedicated endoscopy and radiology suites where facilities may not be at par with a standard OR environment.[4] This chapter will discuss the anesthesia implications for GE interventions performed outside the OR, focusing on those that are elective or semiurgent in nature and performed without the requirement of tracheal intubation.

PREPROCEDURAL RISK ASSESSMENT AND OPTIMIZATION

Patients presenting for gastrointestinal endoscopy under anesthesiologist-managed sedation have a high-risk profile. The incidence of significant unplanned intraoperative events such as hypoxemia and hypotension is surprisingly high.[5] The list of routinely performed upper gastroenterological interventions (UGEs) includes esophagogastroduodenoscopy (EGD), endoscopic ultrasound, and endoscopic retrograde cholangiopancreatography (ERCP), enteroscopy, percutaneous endoscopic gastrostomy (PEG), and radiologically inserted gastrostomy tube (RIG). ERCP and enteroscopy facilitate advanced and prolonged interventions within the biliary tract and small bowel. Colonoscopy facilitates interventions of the rectum, large bowel, and a portion of the small bowel. At the same time, flexible sigmoidoscopy involves examination and interventions of the rectum and a portion of the large intestine. Preprocedural assessment should be based on standard guidelines such as the American Society of Anesthesiologists (ASA). Evaluation should focus on identifying risk factors to avoid periprocedural complications.[6] An individualized risk assessment centered on underlying comorbidities and those linked to the procedure should be performed to avoid a wide range of investigations. Routine blood tests are unnecessary for uncomplicated presentations.

Standard fasting guidelines would suffice for UGE procedures, whereas colonoscopy requires bowel preparation with a cathartic to attain optimal conditions. Although bowel preparation regimens differ internationally,[7] they generally include four phases: phase one, a low-fiber diet for 2-3 days; phase two, clear fluids the day before colonoscopy; phase three, commencing bowel emptying with a cathartic the evening before; phase four, fasting for clear fluids 2-10 hours depending on whether the procedure is planned in the morning or afternoon. The diet regimen on the day before a colonoscopy is largely directed by local guidelines, with some sources advocating a low-residue diet for outpatient procedures.[7] In patients at risk of dehydration and electrolyte depletion, such as the elderly who may be on large doses of diuretics, it may be worth reassessing the fluid and electrolyte status after bowel preparation. Further evaluations should focus on the manifestation of other adverse effects of bowel preparation that can potentially impact sedation management, such as ongoing severe nausea and vomiting.

Perioperative medication management, especially for antiplatelets, anticoagulants, and glucose-lowering agents, should be based on guidelines developed and implemented locally as per international recommendations.[8,9] These guidelines should be regulated by practicing interventionalists and clinical pharmacists, with regular reviews and updates.

Preoperative optimization is often not feasible in cases that are semiurgent in nature; for instance, an ERCP for a biliary stent. However, a careful assessment to identify imminent correctable or modifiable risk factors should be attempted. Cases that are unsuitable to be performed outside the OR should be judged.

MONITORING

Standard monitoring according to governing body recommendations should be routinely employed, with more invasive monitoring instituted as needed. The British Society of Gastroenterology and the American Society for Gastrointestinal Endoscopy recommend pulse oximetry, continuous assessment of ventilation, consciousness, heart rate, and blood pressures, with electrocardiogram reserved for high-risk cardiac patients.[1] The role of capnography is discussed separately in the following sections. Appropriate postprocedure monitoring should also be routinely used in the postanesthesia care area.

■ PHARMACOLOGICAL PRINCIPLES OF SEDATION

Sedation is a continuum, and clinicians must limit this parameter between minimal and moderate and avoid the progression to deep sedation.[1] While sedation trajectory is expected to progress in a dose-response continuum, in practice, it is not easy to predict individual patient responses to a given dose.[10] Whenever there is an increasing need for further sedation and/or analgesia, the anesthesiologist should be vigilant about the possibility of an evolving state of general anesthesia (GA), as there is a fine line between deep sedation and GA.[1] A trivial change in the plane of sedation can lead to airway instability and profound unconsciousness.[1] Hence, adequate monitoring of the cardiorespiratory functions should be in place to alert the clinician of an impending respiratory compromise or airway obstruction.[11] Importantly, practitioners should be well equipped and prepared to rescue when the level of sedation becomes deeper than intended.[10] The various levels of central nervous system depression and body functions across a spectrum of sedation to GA as outlined by the American Society of Anesthesiologists may be used as guide **(Table 1)**.[6]

A thorough understanding of the basic pharmacokinetic and pharmacodynamic principles of commonly used sedation agents is vital for their safe administration. As the desired effects of these agents can range across several levels of sedation to GA, factors influencing the onset, duration, recovery profile, and cardiorespiratory stability of the agents administered

TABLE 1: Trajectory of sedation across various levels till general anesthesia.

	Minimal sedation (anxiolysis)	Moderate sedation (conscious sedation)	Deep sedation	General anesthesia
Responsiveness	Normal response to verbal stimulation	Purposeful response to verbal or tactile stimulation	Purposeful response after repeated or painful stimulation	Unarousable even with painful stimulus
Airway	Unaffected	No intervention required	Intervention may be required	Intervention often required
Spontaneous ventilation	Unaffected	Adequate	May be inadequate	Frequently inadequate
Cardiovascular function	Unaffected	Usually maintained	Usually maintained	May be impaired

Source: Adapted from Leslie K, Allen M, Hessian E, Peyton PJ, Kasza J, Courtney A, et al. Safety of sedation for gastrointestinal endoscopy in a group of university-affiliated hospitals: a prospective cohort study. Br J Anaesth. 2017;118:90-9.

either alone or in combination should be thoroughly appreciated.[11] Clinicians should appreciate the potential cardiorespiratory adverse effects of sedative agents and their impact on airway patency, as well as the potential synergistic effect of coadministered drugs.

A detailed description of the pharmacology of the many agents and combinations used for procedural sedation is beyond the scope of this chapter. The salient features of the commonly used medications[10,12-17] are listed in **Table 2**. Common practices include using a sole agent or a combination of agents. Continuous infusion regimens, especially target-controlled infusions (TCIs), can potentially avoid oscillations in the desired serum concentration as encountered with intermittent bolus techniques.[16] Adoption of infusion techniques necessitates a comprehensive understanding of pharmacokinetic principles.[16]

On a practical note, navigating the gastroscope behind the laryngeal inlet may stimulate a cough or laryngospasm; hence, it is imperative to establish an adequate plane of sedation/analgesia before this endeavor. Once the instrument has surpassed the cricopharyngeal muscle, the stimulation is less intense except during maneuvers such as dilatation, balloon use, or cutting.[17] If the gastroscope insertion provokes movement or cough, aggressive attempts to deepen the plane of sedation should be avoided as it may precipitate a respiratory adverse event.[17] To reduce this stimulus, some practitioners may topicalize the oropharynx with a commercial preparation of lidocaine 5 mg and phenylephrine hydrochloride 500 µg. Whenever oropharyngeal topicalization is used, a delayed return of protective airway reflexes should be anticipated and communicated to the personnel involved in postprocedure care.

ORGANIZATIONAL LOGISTICS OF GASTROENTEROLOGICAL PROCEDURES IN SUITES OUTSIDE OPERATING ROOM

The intervention suite should be equipped identical to general ORs. It should include advanced airway and hemodynamic equipment[1] and ready access to pharmacological antagonists such as naloxone and flumazenil.[11] There should be ongoing education and simulation-based training for the teams involved in these areas. Help should be readily available through a medical emergency response team or similar system. The social issues of patient care, such as accompanying escorts and assistance for the next 24 hours, should be adequately scrutinized on admission. Postprocedure recovery monitoring and discharge pathways should be protocolized based on local needs.[1] A backup clinician should be available to assess patients in the recovery suite, if the situation merits a review, and adequate pathways for hospital admissions should be established.[1]

TABLE 2: Commonly used medications for GI sedation.

Medication (group)	Dose regime	Onset of action	Duration of effect	Remarks
Propofol (GABA agonist)	*Bolus:* 0.30–0.5 mg/kg, titrate as necessary *Infusion:* Continuous—50–150 µg/kg/min (3–6 mg/kg/h) TCI: e.g., Marsh model Plasma target 1.5–3.0 µg/mL	30–45 seconds	4–8 minutes (bolus)	• Hypotension and respiratory depression • Pain during injection • Decreased doses in elderly
Midazolam (Benzodiazepine)	0.02–0.03 mg/kg *Bolus:* 0.5–2 mg titrated to effect *Repeat:* Every 2–5 minutes Cumulative dose 5 mg Limit in elderly	2–5 minutes	30–60 minutes	• Dose-dependent respiratory depression especially when given with other agents • Prolonged sedation in elderly, obese, renal, or hepatic impairment
Dexmedetomidine (α_2 agonist)	*Loading:* 0.5–1 µg/kg over 10–20 minutes *Maintenance:* 0.2–0.7 µg/kg/h	Less than 5 minutes Peak effect at 15 minutes		• Context-sensitive half-life is duration of infusion dependent • 4 minutes after a 10-minute infusion • 250 minutes after an 8-hour infusion • Caution with bradycardia and hypotension
Ketamine (NMDA agonist)	0.3–0.5 mg/kg IV	1–2 minutes	20–50 minutes	• Dissociative anesthesia • Emergence delirium is a concern • Benzodiazepines can minimize delirium
Alfentanil (opioid)	*Bolus:* Up to 7 µg/kg; 250–500 µg *Repeat dose:* 3.5 µg/kg or 250 µg	90 seconds	5–10 minutes	• Caution when co-administered with other agents, reduce dose • Respiratory depression • Nausea and vomiting
Fentanyl (opioid)	*Bolus:* 0.5–1 µg/kg *Repeat:* Incremental boluses of 25–50 µg	2–5 minutes	45–60 minutes	• Caution when co-administered with other agents, reduce dose • Respiratory depression • Nausea and vomiting
Remifentanil (opioid)	*Bolus:* 0.25–0.1 µg/kg *Infusion:* 0.1–0.3 µg/kg/min	<90 seconds	6–10 minutes	• Caution when co-administered with other agents, reduce dose • Respiratory depression • Nausea and vomiting

Note: All doses are intravenous.
(GABA: gamma-aminobutyric acid; GI: gastrointestinal; TCI: target-controlled infusion; NMDA: N-methyl-D-aspartate)

OXYGEN SUPPLEMENTATION AND AIRWAY MANAGEMENT STRATEGIES TO MITIGATE HYPOXEMIA

Pharmacological sedative agents may cause respiratory impairment and upper airway obstruction, resulting in hypoxemia. During procedural sedation, oxygen desaturation seems to be the most predominant adverse event, followed by airway obstruction and apnea.[18] In the context of GE sedation, the definition of hypoxemia differs between studies, and the reported incidence varies between 15 and 21%.[19-22] The rate could be as high as 60% with advanced interventions such as ERCPs.[23] Higher ASA physical status, known or suspected sleep apnea, decreased cardiopulmonary reserve, obesity, and prolonged procedural duration are known risk factors for hypoxemia.[24,25] Sustained hypoxemia may precipitate periprocedural cardiac arrhythmias and myocardial ischemia.[26,27] In closed claims analysis, oxygenation/ventilation deficiency has been clearly demarcated as a marker of bad outcomes during procedural sedation for GE interventional procedures.[28,29] Optimum oxygenation/ventilation is best achieved with a thorough understanding of the pharmacokinetics of medications used for sedation, as well as by acknowledging both the strengths and limitations of oxygen delivery strategies.

OXYGEN DELIVERY DURING GASTROENTEROLOGICAL INTERVENTIONS

The shared airway during UGE interventions limits the applicability of oxygen delivery devices that preclude access to the oropharynx such as the simple face mask. Various approaches to oxygen delivery with less hindrance to the instrumentation of the oropharynx have been described in the literature and used in contemporary practice. These include standard nasal prongs with and without a CO_2 sampling port, oxygenating mouthguard, nasopharyngeal (NP) airway connected to either a Mapleson C, Bain's, or Jackson Rees pediatric circuits, and nasal positive pressure delivering device termed as SuperNO$_2$VA. All these strategies can be safely employed during colonoscopy, where a shared airway is not an issue. There are at least a couple of supralaryngeal airway devices specifically designed for UGE interventions, namely the Gastro-Laryngeal Tube (GLT) (G-LT, VBM Medizintechnik BmbH, Sulz, Germany) and the LMA®Gastro™ (Teleflex Medical, Athlone, Ireland).

Low-flow Devices

Sta ndard nasal prongs and simple face masks are low-flow oxygen delivery devices that allow maximum flow rates of 6 L/min and 15 L/min, respectively.[30] The FiO_2 is based on the inspiratory flow rate, usually between 0.3 and 0.6.[30,31] Some models of these devices come with an inbuilt CO_2 sampling port for capnography **(Figs. 1 and 2)**. The limitations of these devices are discussed in the subsequent sections.

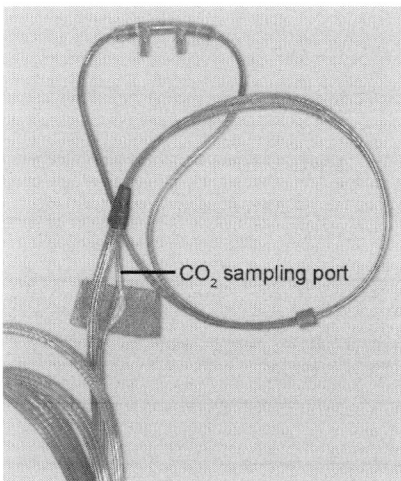

Fig. 1: Standard low-flow nasal cannula with CO_2 sampling port.

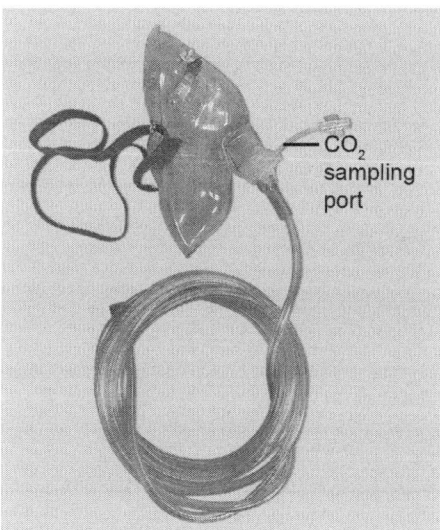

Fig. 2: Simple low-flow face mask with CO_2 sampling port.

Oxygenating Mouthguard

Oxygenating mouthguards with the ability to deliver oxygen to the mouth and nostrils are either used as a sole strategy or in conjunction with standard nasal prongs; they are routinely used at the authors' institution for patients at lower risk of hypoxemia. Models with an inbuilt CO_2 sampling port and a hydrophobic disk filter to prevent contamination are also commercially available **(Fig. 3)**.

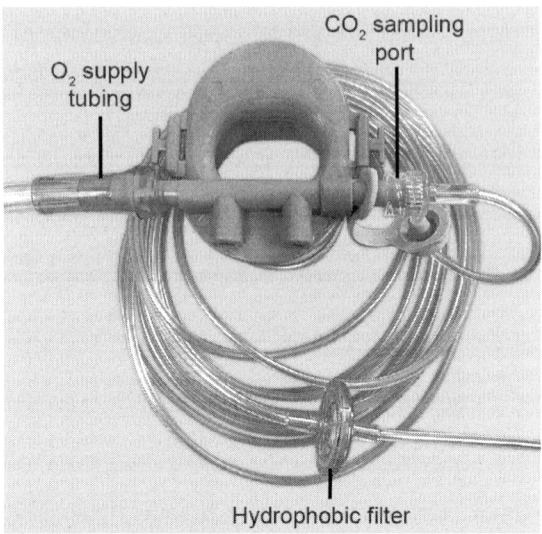

Fig. 3: Oxygenating mouthguard with CO_2 sampling port and a bacterial/viral filter.

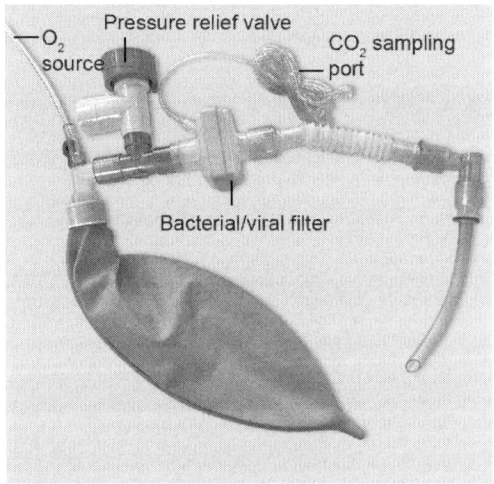

Fig. 4: Nasopharyngeal airway—Mapleson C assembly.

Nasopharyngeal Airway and Mapleson Circuit Assembly

An appropriately sized NP airway connected to a Mapleson C circuit with a 60 cm adjustable pressure relief valve using an endotracheal tube connector **(Fig. 4)** has been described in the North American literature **(Fig. 4)**.[32,33] The benefits claimed include provision of fraction of inspired oxygen (FiO_2) up to 1.0, some degree of continuous positive airway pressure (CPAP) generation being possible depending upon the extent to which the oral cavity is open, prolongation of the apnea time, improved airway patency with impending airway obstruction, provision for end-tidal CO_2 (ETCO$_2$) sampling.[33] The NP airway can either be inserted awake with adequate lubrication to the nostrils in cooperative patients or asleep after administering sedative agents. The application of vasoconstrictors may reduce the risk of bleeding. If inserting asleep, other ways of oxygen supplementation through a face mask or oxygenating mouthguards should be in place until its insertion.[32,33] Observational studies showed that this approach reduced hypoxemia in morbidly obese patients during EGD and ERCPs.[32,33] A low (8–10 L/min) and a high (12–15 L/min) flow rate have been described by the study authors.[32,33]

Other Mapleson circuit attachments such as the Bains and Jackson Rees commonly deliver FiO$_2$ up to 1.0 along with the aforementioned physiological benefits being achievable **(Figs. 5 and 6)**. Anecdotal information

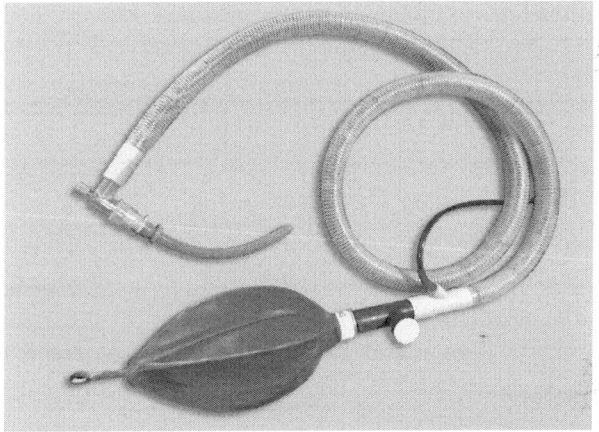

Fig. 5: Nasopharyngeal airway—Bain circuit assembly; note that a bacterial/viral filter in the assembly will reduce contamination.

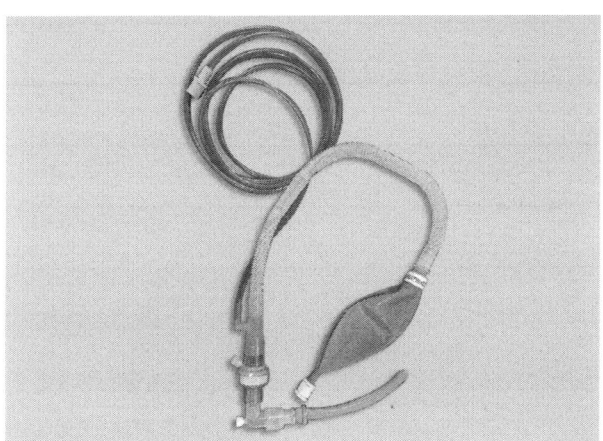

Fig. 6: Nasopharyngeal airway—Jackson-Rees circuit assembly.

suggests that the NP airway–Bains assembly with a flow rate of 6–8 L/min is a popular choice among anesthesiologists in the Indian subcontinent, where Mapleson C is not widely available. In thin-built individuals, a Jackson–Rees pediatric circuit offers a good alternative to Bains! Satisfactory ventilation and CO_2 clearance are possible through these NP attachments if the patency of the assembly is maintained without any kinks or mechanical obstruction.

SuperNO$_2$VA™

This device incorporates a sealed, nasal positive airway pressure mask with minimal dead space that can deliver higher fractions of FiO_2, along with titratable positive pressure up to 10 cmH_2O with flows up to 15 L/min when attached to a standard anesthesia machine or Mapleson circuit **(Fig. 7)**.[34] A CO_2 sampling line is embedded within the mask, and assisted ventilation, if required, is also feasible. Preliminary data suggest that the device may be more effective in reducing hypoxemia in GE interventions than low-flow nasal cannula oxygen delivery.[34,35]

Supralaryngeal Airway Devices

The GLT and the LMA®Gastro™ airway are commercially available supralaryngeal devices designed with distinct airway and endoscope channels. The principles of these devices are in congruence with a supraglottic airway devices and, hence, both require general anesthesia and adequate analgesia for insertion and maintenance. Both the devices enable spontaneous and assisted ventilation.

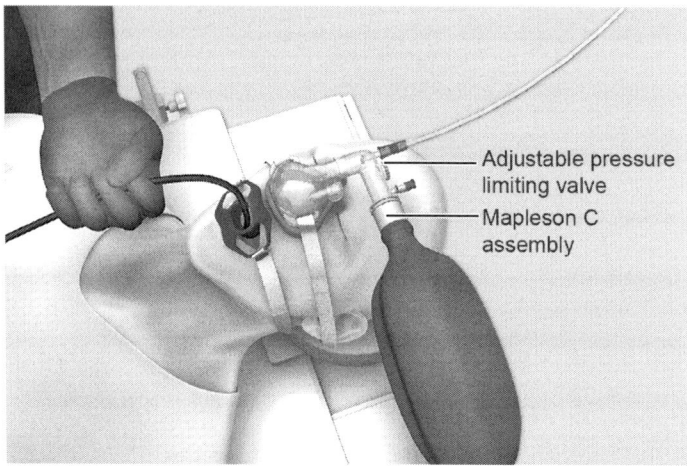

Fig. 7: SuperNO$_2$VA™ nasal mask.

Gastrolaryngeal Tube

The GLT has two interconnected inflatable cuffs, and the ventilation channel is located between the two cuffs **(Fig. 8)**.[36] It is supplied with an introducer to navigate the insertion and positioning of the distal tip well within the proximal esophagus. As such, more airway maneuvers may be required for its correct placement.[36] It has an internal diameter of 16 mm and enables passage of gastroscopes only up to 13.8 mm external diameter.[37] Further limitations include its presence as a single size and a minimum required body height of 155 cm for its deployment.[37]

LMA®Gastro™

In patients undergoing upper gastrointestinal endoscopy, the LMA®Gastro™ airway has proven clinical efficacy and yielded a high rate of endoscopy success, along with excellent airway insertion success rates.[38] The LMA®Gastro™ is designed exactly like a supraglottic airway device with an inflatable cuff and an endoscope channel with an internal diameter of 16 mm. The ventilation channel corresponds to the laryngeal inlet enclosing the inflatable cuff **(Fig. 9)**.[36,39] The manufacturers recommend medical-grade silicone spray lubrication inside the endoscope channel. It is presented in three sizes and can be used in patients weighing above 30 kg. All three sizes can accommodate gastroscopes up to 14-mm external diameter, thus facilitating most of the routinely performed GE interventions.[40] Design familiarity as a supraglottic airway, along with its flexible and curved design features, increases success rates of insertion.[41]

A recent randomized study comparing GLT and LMA®Gastro™ during ERCP showed that while the LMA Gastro had better ventilation capacity and

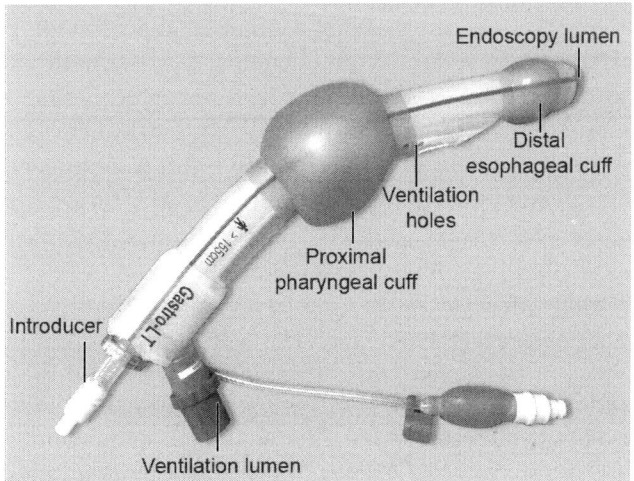

Fig. 8: Gastrolaryngeal tube.

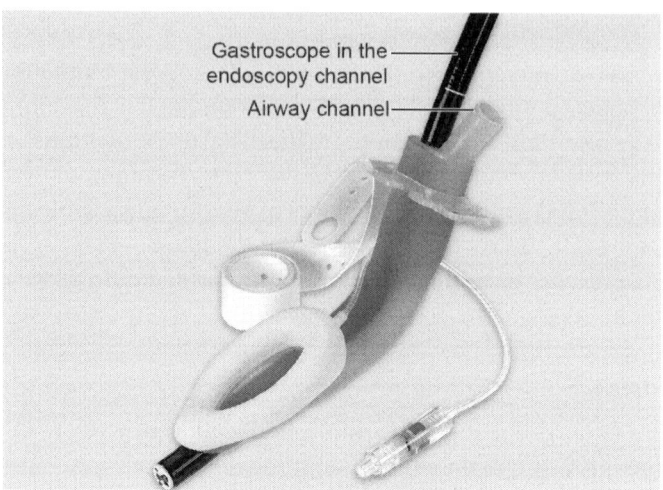

Fig. 9: LMA®Gastro™.

low complication rates, the GLT delivered a more satisfactory procedure performance.[36] The improved ventilation capacity with LMA®Gastro™ was attributed to lower leak rates and higher oropharyngeal leak pressures. Comparatively, the balloon-shaped proximal cuff of the GLT may reduce compliance with the oropharynx.[36] Mucosal damage and postprocedure sore throat were lower with LMA®Gastro™.[36] The anatomically configured design and flexible construction of LMA Gastro offer a smoother insertion compared to the wider-angle and stiff design structure of the GLT, the distal part of which needs to be maneuvered to the upper esophagus.[36] The study authors felt that more resistance might be encountered with the insertion and advancement of duodenoscopes through the LMA®Gastro™ given its narrow inner angle.[36]

An observational study by our group when the LMA®Gastro™ was introduced into practice showed that ventilation and successful procedure completion were achieved in 63 out of 64 ERCPs across a diverse case mix of low- and high-risk cases.[39] Occasionally, esophageal intubation with the duodenoscope may be difficult due to cervical osteophytes and/or thick cricopharyngeal muscle. Gastroenterologists who were part of our study felt that this difficulty was not encountered with LMA®Gastro™ albeit there was a lack of a comparative GLT group.[39] Successful airway and endoscopy outcomes have also been reported during GE interventions in the pediatric population weighing above 30 kg.[42]

A unique value proposition of the LMA®Gastro™ was appreciated during the early coronavirus disease 2019 (COVID-19) pandemic in Italy with a shortage of intensive care unit (ICU) beds. The device-benefited patients deemed to fail tracheal extubation after emergent/semiurgent gastroscopy procedures.[43] Similarly, LMA®Gastro™ is used in situations where tracheal intubation needs to be avoided in frail patients who have wished not to be ventilated and resuscitated. Yet, their clinical presentations warrant diagnostic or therapeutic UGE interventions that would otherwise require airway protection.

High-flow Nasal Oxygen

High-flow nasal oxygen (HFNO) has been recently adopted as an alternative approach to conventional oxygen delivery as it offers several distinct advantages.[44,45] These include ability to deliver FiO_2 up to 1.0 with flows up to 70 L/min, flows exceeding a patient's peak inspiratory flow rate, washing out anatomical dead space, and generating a flow-dependent positive airway pressure.[46]

Recent reviews have provided moderate certainty of evidence that HFNO reduces the risk of hypoxemia and increases minimum oxygen saturation (SpO_2) during GE procedural sedation.[47-49] Recent evidence supports the notion of employing this approach in high-risk cases such as those who are critically ill, have higher ASA physical status, obstructive sleep apnea, obesity, or during advanced GE interventions. Practitioners should be vigilant that the higher FiO_2 and the various physiologic benefits of HFNO may not mitigate hypoxemia due to drug-induced hypoventilation[50] or pulmonary shunt.[51,52] As the device setup and the consumables incur an additional cost, the use of HFNO should only be directed toward selected high-risk cases and universal adoption of this technique should be discouraged in both resource-rich as well as resource-deplete settings.

Mouth Breathing as a Caveat during Upper Gastroenterological Interventions

The effect of mouth breathing and its implications for inadequate oxygen delivery are poorly recognized. During procedural sedation with an open mouth, it has been shown that in most patients, the breathing pattern transforms from nasal to oral. This has significance while using low-flow oxygen delivery devices because room air entrainment and dead space rebreathing may potentially reduce the FiO_2. Assuming nasal breathing only, at nasal flow rates of 2–4 L/min, FiO_2 may reach 0.3–0.4 with a low-flow nasal cannula. The transformation to mouth breathing along with reduced minute ventilation has the potential to reduce FiO_2.

Conversely, FiO_2 dilution from room air is likely to be minimal with high-flow devices, and thus, a consistent FiO_2 is feasible.[53] Based on these, there is an argument in favor of delivering oxygen via both oral and nasal routes to improve oxygen delivery in procedures with an open mouth, such as gastroscopy and bronchoscopy, especially when low-flow devices are used.[53] A more recent multicenter trial by the authors' group revealed that the combination of low-flow nasal oxygen delivery and oxygenation via a mouthguard was as effective as HFNO in mitigating hypoxemia in high-risk patients undergoing ERCPs.[54] It should be noted, however, that a target-controlled infusion (TCI) of propofol was employed and that there is evidence in favor of using TCI propofol approaches over intermittent-bolus techniques to reduce hypoxemia during sedation for gastroscopy interventions.[55,56]

Certain limitations of HFNO with an open mouth are also worth reiterating. The positive airway pressure generated by HFNO is inconsistent with an open mouth, and it reaches only up to 1.7 cmH_2O with a flow rate of 50 L/min compared to 5.6 cmH_2O with a closed mouth.[57]

As the mouth is closed during colonoscopy, any airway device successfully used in the airway patency is maintained with an appropriate depth of sedation. Specific oxygen delivery approaches can be chosen based on the risk stratification: for instance, HFNO or $SuperNO_2VA$ for those at high risk of desaturation.

■ CONSIDERATIONS OF CAPNOGRAPHY MONITORING

The open mouth and the predominant mouth-breathing patterns observed during upper GE interventions have implications for capnography monitoring. The accuracy and efficacy of CO_2 monitoring are increased through sampling from oral routes instead of nasal routes. Some of the commercially available oxygenating mouthguards and standard nasal prongs have an inbuilt CO_2 sampling port **(Figs. 1 and 2)**. Newer models of the HFNO (Fisher and Paykel Healthcare, Auckland, New Zealand) cannula have a purpose-built CO_2 sampling attachment that can be directed either toward the nostrils or oral cavity **(Fig. 10)**. However, it should be acknowledged that the high-flow rates with HFNO may potentially dilute the expired CO_2.[58]

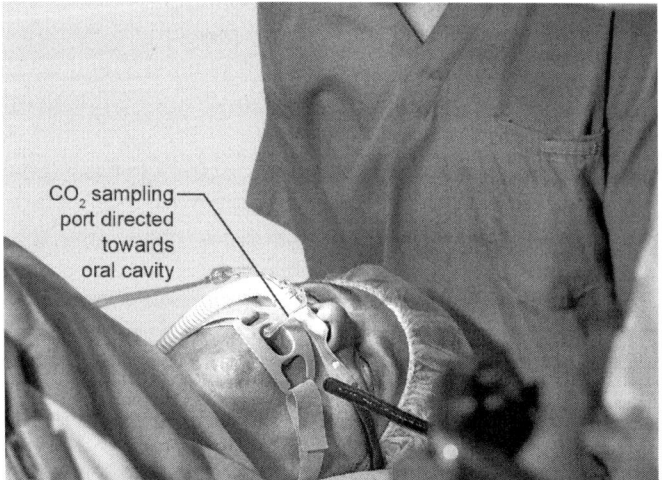

Fig. 10: High-flow nasal oxygen cannula with CO_2 sampling port.

International Governing bodies strongly recommend capnography monitoring during procedural sedation. The ASA Standards for Basic Anesthetic Monitoring state—"During moderate or deep sedation, the adequacy of ventilation shall be evaluated by continual observation of qualitative clinical signs and monitoring for the presence of exhaled carbon dioxide unless precluded or invalidated by the nature of the patient, procedure, or equipment".[59] In locations outside the OR, The Association of Anaesthetists of Great Britain and Ireland (AAGBI) Standards of Monitoring require an "end-tidal carbon dioxide monitor if the patient is sedated". The AAGBI Safety Statement insists—"Continuous capnography should be used for all patients undergoing moderate or deep sedation outside the operating theater".[60]

Therefore, it is imperative to use waveform capnography during sedation for GE interventions with an understanding that the low-amplitude waveform displayed is an indication of respiratory effort and not a reflection of CO_2 clearance. Various sources, including the authors, have utilized transcutaneous CO_2 in clinical trials to explore the efficacy of O_2 delivery devices/strategies in GE interventions.[45,54] Nonetheless, the CO_2 estimates should be interpreted with caution as there is a likelihood of bloodstream CO_2 absorption from CO_2 insufflation.

ASSESSMENT AND CONSIDERATIONS OF ASPIRATION RISK

The underlying risk of aspiration should be thoroughly evaluated before every procedure. Certain baseline and pathological conditions warrant an upper GE intervention may additionally increase the aspiration risk.[61] Such conditions include but are not limited to severe gastroesophageal reflux disease, indications for PEG insertion, upper gastrointestinal bleeding, achalasia, and dysphagia. Notably, patients with a pre-existing risk of aspiration may present for interventions that may further exacerbate the risk of aspiration. One such procedure is RIG insertion which demands up to 1,000 mL of air insufflation into the stomach.[62]

Aspiration risk should be assessed on a case-by-case basis, and practitioners should have a low threshold to embark on a GA technique with tracheal intubation in those deemed as having a high risk of aspiration.[61,63] It is not uncommon to encounter patients with significant baseline aspiration risk and impending tracheal extubation failure attributable to end-stage organ disease coupled with poor cardiopulmonary reserve, for example, those presenting for RIG insertion. In such scenarios, the risk and benefits of GA with tracheal intubation should be thoroughly explained to the patients, their caregivers, and proceduralists, and a shared decision should be taken. Performing the procedure only under local anesthetic infiltration may be the only safe option in such situations.

If residual gastric contents are noted during EGD, it should be immediately suctioned, and clear communication needs to be established between the anesthesiologists and the interventionalist to determine whether to proceed or abandon the procedure. This would depend upon the type (particulate vs. nonparticulate)[64] and volume of the contents, as well as the nature of the intervention intended. Airway protection with tracheal intubation may be required if there is a risk of airway soiling. Position changes along with colonic gas insufflation and application of external abdominal pressure to facilitate colonoscope navigation are some of the risk factors of aspiration during colonoscopy.[64] Anesthesiologists should be attentive during such occasions.

CONCLUSION

A structured approach for GE interventions has existed for many decades in the Western world. Once only available in large centers in the Indian subcontinent, this service is now being offered at many smaller regional centers with the assistance of anesthesiologists. As the number and complexity of cancer screening and other indications for GE interventions increases, the requirement for anesthesia services outside the operating is likely to grow. Originally, these suites were designed for ambulatory pathways with a rapid turnaround time. The environment and logistics in these areas are different from the traditional theater suites. Anesthesia providers should recognize these differences and play a key role in identifying areas of improvement. Quality improvement audits with closed cycles should be established, and new evidence-based approaches for airway management and pharmacological principles should be amenably embraced. A proper preprocedural risk stratification along with appropriate monitoring, early recognition, and management of adverse events, coupled with an improved understanding of oxygenation strategies and medications used for sedation will improve the outcome of GE interventions.

ACKNOWLEDGMENTS

We thank our colleague Dr Christine Hildyard for her valuable insights that helped us draft the segment on radiologically inserted gastrostomy tubes.

We extend our gratitude to our good friend Dr KC Venkatesh, anesthetist based at Coimbatore, Tamil Nadu, India for providing **Figures 5 and 6**.

Figure 3; Image Courtesy: Meditech Asia Pacific, Western Australia, Australia.

Figure 7; Vyaire Medical, New South Wales, Australia.

Figure 9; Image Courtesy: A/Professor Marcus Skinner, Royal Hobart Hospital, Tasmania, Australia.

Figure 10; Fisher and Paykel Health Services, Auckland, New Zealand.

REFERENCES

1. Kuzhively J, Pandit JJ. Anesthesia and airway management for gastrointestinal endoscopic procedures outside the operating room. Curr Opin Anesthesiol. 2019;32:517-22.
2. Lin OS, Weigel W. Nonoperating room anesthesia for gastrointestinal endoscopic procedures. Curr Opin Anesthesiol. 2018;31:486-91.
3. Shenbagaraj L, Thomas-Gibson S, Stebbing J, Broughton R, Dron M, Johnston D, et al. Endoscopy in 2017: a national survey of practice in the UK. Frontline Gastroenterol. 2019;10:7-15.
4. Tetzlaff JE. Practical considerations in the management of sedation for colonoscopy. Curr Opin Anesthesiol. 2016;29:512-8.
5. Leslie K, Allen M, Hessian E, Peyton PJ, Kasza J, Courtney A, et al. Safety of sedation for gastrointestinal endoscopy in a group of university-affiliated hospitals: a prospective cohort study. Br J Anaesth. 2017;118:90-9.
6. Early DS, Lightdale JR, Vargo JJ, Acosta RD, Chandrasekhara V, Chathadi KV, et al. Guidelines for sedation and anesthesia in GI endoscopy. Gastrointest Endosc. 2018;87:327-37.
7. Bechtold ML, Mir F, Puli SR, Nguyen DL. Optimizing bowel preparation for colonoscopy: a guide to enhance quality of visualization. Ann Gastroenterol. 2016;29:137.
8. Feagins LA. Management of anticoagulants and antiplatelet agents during colonoscopy. Am J Med. 2017;130:786-95.
9. Hochberg I, Segol O, Shental R, Shimoni P, Eldor R. Antihyperglycemic therapy during colonoscopy preparation: a review and suggestions for practical recommendations. United Eur Gastroenterol J. 2019;7:735-40.
10. Becker DE. Pharmacodynamic considerations for moderate and deep sedation. Anesthesia Prog. 2012;59:28.
11. Tobias JD, Leder M. Procedural sedation: a review of sedative agents, monitoring, and management of complications. Saudi J Anaesth. 2011;5:395.
12. Zacharias P, Mathew S, Mathews J, Somu A, Peethambaran M, Prashanth M, et al. Sedation practices in gastrointestinal endoscopy: a survey from southern India. Indian J Gastroenterol. 2018;37:164-8.
13. Kisilewicz M, Rosenberg H, Vaillancourt C. Remifentanil for procedural sedation: a systematic review of the literature. Emerg Med J. 2017;34:294-301.
14. José RJ, Shaefi S, Navani N. Sedation for flexible bronchoscopy: current and emerging evidence. Eur Res Rev. 2013;22:106-16.
15. Kaur M, Singh P. Current role of dexmedetomidine in clinical anesthesia and intensive care. Anesth Essays Res. 2011;5:128.
16. Becker DE. Pharmacokinetic considerations for moderate and deep sedation. Anesth Prog. 2011;58:166-73.
17. Muñoz-Fuentes D, Cabello-Montes JA, Herrera-Servin MA, Zavala-Castillo JC. Endoscopy anesthesia, team perspective. Revista médica del Hospital General de México. 2021;84:116-22.
18. Mason KP, Roback MG, Chrisp D, Sturzenbaum N, Freeman L, Gozal D, et al. Results from the adverse event sedation reporting tool: a global anthology of 7952 records derived from >160,000 procedural sedation encounters. J Clin Med. 2019;8:2087.

19. Corso R, Piraccini E, Agnoletti V, Lippi M, Buccioli M, Negro A, et al. Clinical use of the STOP-BANG questionnaire in patients undergoing sedation for endoscopic procedures. Minerva Anestesiol. 2012;78:109-10.
20. Althoff FC, Agnihotri A, Grabitz SD, Santer P, Nabel S, Tran T, et al. Outcomes after endoscopic retrograde cholangiopancreatography with general anaesthesia versus sedation. Br J Anaesth. 2021;126:191-200.
21. Smith ZL, Mullady DK, Lang GD, Das KK, Hovis RM, Patel RS, et al. A randomized controlled trial evaluating general endotracheal anesthesia versus monitored anesthesia care and the incidence of sedation-related adverse events during ERCP in high-risk patients. Gastrointest Endosc. 2019;89:855-62.
22. Fisher L, Fisher A, Thomson A. Cardiopulmonary complications of ERCP in older patients. Gastrointest Endosc. 2006;63:948-55.
23. Daskaya H, Uysal H, Çiftçi T, Baysal B, İdin K, Karaaslan K. Use of the gastro-laryngeal tube in endoscopic retrograde cholangiopancreatography cases under sedation/analgesia. Turk J Gastroenterol. 2016;27:246-51.
24. Sidhu R, Turnbull D, Newton M, Thomas-Gibson S, Sanders DS, Hebbar S, et al. Deep sedation and anaesthesia in complex gastrointestinal endoscopy: a joint position statement endorsed by the British Society of Gastroenterology (BSG), Joint Advisory Group (JAG) and Royal College of Anaesthetists (RCoA). Frontline Gastroenterol. 2019;10:141-7.
25. Hinkelbein J, Schmitz J, Lamperti M, Fuchs-Buder T. Procedural sedation outside the operating room. Curr Opin Anaesthesiol. 2020;33:533-8.
26. Holm C, Christensen M, Rasmussen V, Schulze S, Rosenberg J. Hypoxaemia and myocardial ischaemia during colonoscopy. Scand J Gastroenterol. 1998;33:769-72.
27. Johnston S, McKenna A, Tham T. Silent myocardial ischaemia during endoscopic retrograde cholangiopancreatography. Endoscopy. 2003;35:1039-42.
28. Metzner J, Posner KL, Domino KB. The risk and safety of anesthesia at remote locations: the US closed claims analysis. Curr Opin Anaesthesiol. 2009;22:502-8.
29. Woodward ZG, Urman RD, Domino KB. Safety of non-operating room anesthesia: a closed claims update. Anesthesiol Clin. 2017;35:569-81.
30. Bateman N, Leach R. Acute oxygen therapy. BMJ. 1998;317:798-801.
31. Singh V, Gupta P, Khatana S, Bhagol A. Supplemental oxygen therapy: important considerations in oral and maxillofacial surgery. Natl J Maxillofac Surg. 2011;2:10.
32. Goudra BG, Singh PM, Penugonda LC, Speck RM, Sinha AC. Significantly reduced hypoxemic events in morbidly obese patients undergoing gastrointestinal endoscopy: predictors and practice effect. J Anaesthesiol Clin Pharmacol. 2014;30:71.
33. Goudra BG, Singh PM, Sinha AC. Outpatient endoscopic retrograde cholangiopancreatography: safety and efficacy of anesthetic management with a natural airway in 653 consecutive procedures. Saudi J Anaesth. 2013;7:259.
34. Dimou F, Huynh S, Dakin G, Pomp A, Turnbull Z, Samuels JD, et al. Nasal positive pressure with the SuperNO2VA™ device decreases sedation-related hypoxemia during pre-bariatric surgery EGD. Surg Endosc. 2019;33:3828-32.
35. Bai Y, Xu Z, Chandrashekar M, St Jacques PJ, Liang Y, Jiang Y, et al. Comparison of a simplified nasal continuous positive airways pressure device with nasal cannula in obese patients undergoing colonoscopy during deep sedation: a randomised clinical trial. Eur J Anaesthesiol. 2019;36:633-40.

36. Uysal H, Senturk H, Calim M, Daskaya H, Guney IA, Karaaslan K. Comparison of LMA® gastro airway and gastro-laryngeal tube in endoscopic retrograde cholangiopancreatography: a prospective randomized observational trial. Minerva Anestesiol. 2021;87:987-96.
37. Gaitini L, Lavi A, Stermer E, Mora PC, Pott L, Vaida S. Gastro-Laryngeal Tube for endoscopic retrograde cholangiopancreatography: a preliminary report. Anaesthesia. 2010;65:1114-8.
38. Terblanche N, Middleton C, Choi-Lundberg D, Skinner M. Efficacy of a new dual channel laryngeal mask airway, the LMA® Gastro™ Airway, for upper gastrointestinal endoscopy: a prospective observational study. Br J Anaesth. 2018;120:353-60.
39. Tran A, Thiruvenkatarajan V, Wahba M, Currie J, Rajbhoj A, van Wijk R, et al. LMA® Gastro™ Airway for endoscopic retrograde cholangiopancreatography: a retrospective observational analysis. BMC Anesthesiol. 2020;20:1-7.
40. Goudra B, Gouda G, Mohinder P. Recent developments in drugs for GI endoscopy sedation. Dig Dis Sci. 2020;65:2781-8.
41. Schmutz A, Loeffler T, Schmidt A, Goebel U. LMA Gastro™ airway is feasible during upper gastrointestinal interventional endoscopic procedures in high-risk patients: a single-center observational study. BMC Anesthesiol. 2020;20:1-7.
42. Taylor CL, Wilson SR, Burgoyne LL, Endlich Y. LMA® Gastro™: a paediatric experience. Anaesth Intens Care. 2021;49:119-24.
43. Thiruvenkatarajan V, Lorenzetti M, Chung A, Wong CK, Currie J, Wahba M, et al. Airway Management Considerations for Upper Gastrointestinal Endoscopic Procedures in COVID-19 era. Dig Dis Sci. 2020;65:2739-42.
44. Lin Y, Zhang X, Li L, Wei M, Zhao B, Wang X, et al. High-flow nasal cannula oxygen therapy and hypoxia during gastroscopy with propofol sedation: a randomized multicenter clinical trial. Gastrointest Endosc. 2019;90:591-601.
45. Mazzeffi MA, Petrick KM, Magder L, Greenwald BD, Darwin P, Goldberg EM, et al. High-flow nasal cannula oxygen in patients having anesthesia for advanced esophagogastroduodenoscopy: HIFLOW-ENDO, a randomized clinical trial. Anesth Analg. 2021;132:743-51.
46. Gotera C, Lobato SD, Pinto T, Winck J. Clinical evidence on high flow oxygen therapy and active humidification in adults. Rev Port Pneumol. 2013;19:217-27.
47. Hung K-C, Chang Y-J, Chen I-W, Soong TC, Ho CN, Hsing CH, et al. Efficacy of high flow nasal oxygenation against hypoxemia in sedated patients receiving gastrointestinal endoscopic procedures: a systematic review and meta-analysis. J Clin Anesth. 2022;77:110651.
48. Doulberis M, Sampsonas F, Papaefthymiou A, Karamouzos V, Lagadinou M, Karampitsakos T, et al. High-flow versus conventional nasal cannula oxygen supplementation therapy and risk of hypoxia in gastrointestinal endoscopies: a systematic review and meta-analysis. Expert Rev Respir Med. 2022;16:323-32.
49. Zhang Y-X, He X-X, Chen Y-P, Yang S. The effectiveness of high-flow nasal cannula during sedated digestive endoscopy: a systematic review and meta-analysis. Eur J Med Res. 2022;27:1-11.
50. Douglas N, Ng I, Nazeem F, Lee K, Mezzavia P, Krieser R, et al. A randomised controlled trial comparing high-flow nasal oxygen with standard management for conscious sedation during bronchoscopy. Anaesthesia. 2018;73:169-76.

51. Sarkar M, Niranjan N, Banyal P. Mechanisms of hypoxemia. Lung India. 2017;34:47.
52. Goligher EC, Slutsky AS. Not just oxygen? Mechanisms of benefit from high-flow nasal cannula in hypoxemic respiratory failure. Am J Respir Crit Care Med. 2017;195(9):1128-31.
53. Hsu WC, Orr J, Lin SP, Yu L, Tsou MY, Westenskow DR, et al. Efficiency of oxygen delivery through different oxygen entrainment devices during sedation under low oxygen flow rate: a bench study. J Clin Monit Comput. 2018;32:519-25.
54. Thiruvenkatarajan V, Dharmalingam A, Arenas G, Wahba M, Liu WM, Zaw Y, et al. Effect of high-flow vs. low-flow nasal plus mouthguard oxygen therapy on hypoxaemia during sedation: a multicentre randomised controlled trial. Anaesthesia. 2022;77:46-53.
55. Chan WH, Chang SL, Lin CS, Chen MJ, Fan SZ. Target-controlled infusion of propofol versus intermittent bolus of a sedative cocktail regimen in deep sedation for gastrointestinal endoscopy: Comparison of cardiovascular and respiratory parameters. J Dig Dis. 2014;15:18-26.
56. Ndosi C, Mung'ayi V, Gisore E, Mir S. Effect of target controlled propofol infusion versus intermittent boluses during oesophagogastroduodenoscopy: a randomized controlled trial. Afr Health Sci. 2019;19:3136-45.
57. Parke RL, Eccleston ML, McGuinness SP. The effects of flow on airway pressure during nasal high-flow oxygen therapy. Respir Care. 2011;56:1151-5.
58. Greenland KB. A potential method for obtaining wave-form capnography during high flow nasal oxygen. Anaesth Intens Care. 2019;47:204-6.
59. Committee on Standards and Practice Parameters (CSPP), American Society of Anesthesiologists. (1986). Standards for basic anesthetic monitoring. [online] Available from https://www.asahq.org/standards-and-guidelines/standards-for-basic-anesthetic-monitoring. [Last accessed October, 2022].
60. Checketts M, Alladi R, Ferguson K, Gemmell L, Handy JM, Klein AA, et al. Recommendations for standards of monitoring during anaesthesia and recovery 2015: Association of Anaesthetists of Great Britain and Ireland. Anaesthesia. 2016;71:85-93.
61. Robinson M, Davidson A. Aspiration under anaesthesia: risk assessment and decision-making. Cont Edu Anaesth Crit Care Pain. 2014;14:171-5.
62. Karthikumar B, Keshava SN, Moses V, Chiramel GK, Ahmed M, Mammen S. Percutaneous gastrostomy placement by intervention radiology: techniques and outcome. Indian J Radiol Imaging. 2018;28:225-31.
63. Green S, Mason K, Krauss B. Pulmonary aspiration during procedural sedation: a comprehensive systematic review. Br J Anaesth. 2017;118:344-54.
64. Parker JD. Pulmonary aspiration during procedural sedation for colonoscopy resulting from positional change managed without oral endotracheal intubation. JA Clin Rep. 2020;6:1-4.

CHAPTER

17

Opioid-free Anesthesia with Friedberg's Triad

Barry L Friedberg

ABSTRACT

Opioid-free anesthesia (OFA) is the absence of opioid administration *during* anesthesia for surgery. Friedberg's triad is—(1) measure the brain, (2) preempt the pain, and (3) emetic drugs abstain. OFA with Friedberg's triad eliminates the persistent anesthesia problems of postoperative pain and postoperative nausea and vomiting (PONV). *Unlike* bolus propofol induction, processed electroencephalogram (pEEG) monitoring of incremental propofol induction maintains *temporalis, masseter, orbicularis oris, and genioglossus* muscle tone, preserving spontaneous ventilation and patent airways, eliminating the difficult airway, eliminating the "cannot ventilate, intubate" scenarios, identifying outliers (fragile and resistant), and reducing stress to both patients and their anesthesiologists.

Independent of body weight or age, fifty (50)-milligram intravenous (IV) ketamine (administered 2–3 minutes before skin incision, trocar punctures, or multiple local anesthetic injections) prevents the patient's brain from recognizing the surgeon's bodily invasion and precludes internal pain fibers going on "high alert". The ketamine dissociation deception is prolonged with subcutaneous tumescent analgesia.

Keywords: Friedberg's triad; Ketamine; Opioid-free anesthesia (OFA); Propofol; Processed electroencephalogram (pEEG) monitor.

KEY POINTS

- Opioid-free anesthesia eliminates persistent anesthesia problems such as postoperative pain and PONV.
- Friedberg's triad is one simplified pathway to OFA.
- Processed EEG monitoring is improved by the addition of real-time facial frontalis EMG.
- Postoperative pain is a function of intraoperative pain.
- OFA eliminates opioid-related adverse drug effects (ORADEs).

INTRODUCTION

Why abstain from opioids during anesthesia? Like the flat earth belief, a commonly held belief is—(1) surgery is painful, (2) opioids are "pain killers",

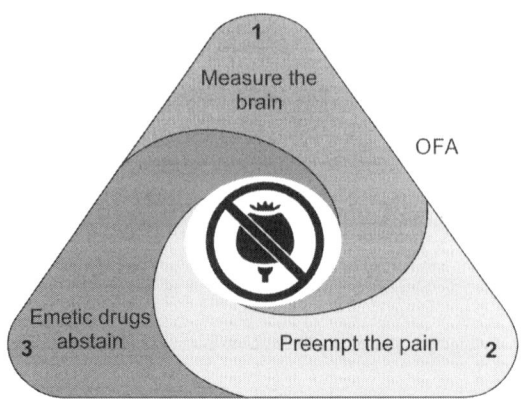

Fig. 1: Friedberg's Triad. (OFA: opioid-free anesthesia)

(3) therefore, all surgery requires the (judicious) use of opioids. However, if opioids effectively prevent pain *during* surgery, why do patients continue to require opioid rescue *after surgery*? A recent meta-analysis of 23 studies in 1,304 patients compared opioid inclusive care (OIC) to opioid-free anesthesia (OFA) and concluded that OIC failed to reduce postoperative pain but *increased* PONV.[1] PONV has been validated as patients' number one outcome to avoid.[2] However, anesthesiologists believe pain is the number one outcome to avoid.[3]

Why is there such a disparity between what patients and anesthesiologists believe the most important outcome to avoid is? When patients sign a surgical consent, they expect some pain associated with a scalpel cut. Skin cuts are common nonsurgical experiences associated with pain but *not* emesis, gagging on the endotracheal tube, or nausea.[2] Patients still do not desire to have pain, but, surprisingly, it is not their number one priority.

Pain and PONV remain the two most common reasons for unexpected admission after day surgery. Friedberg published a 0.6% PONV rate in an Apfel-defined high-risk group *without* antiemetics.[4] Later, there were zero pain or PONV hospital admissions over 20 years for more than 4,000 processed electroencephalogram (pEEG) monitored, opioid-free, propofol *then* ketamine elective cosmetic surgery outpatients[5] **(Fig. 1)**. All patients had commercial insurance. Hospital admission was never required. Most patients were discharged directly home 1 hour postoperatively and required no professional aftercare providers. No opioid addicts or opioid overdose deaths occurred.

■ FRIEDBERG'S TRIAD 1.0: MEASURE THE BRAIN

All things in moderation, nothing in excess.
–2,500-year-old Greek stone inscription

If you cannot measure it, you cannot improve it.
–Lord Kelvin

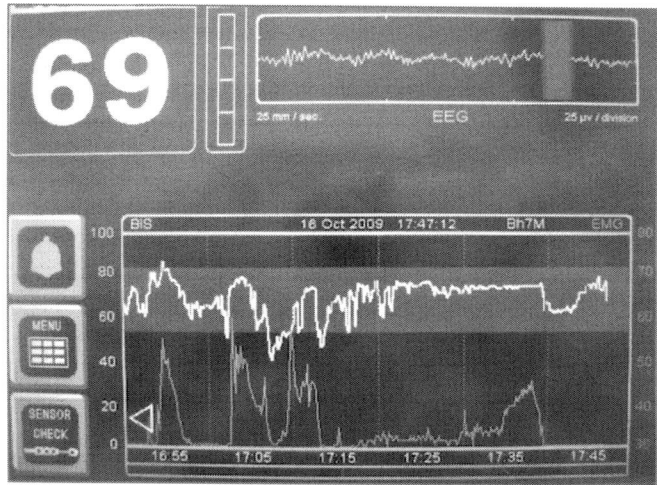

Fig. 2: Free-standing Bispectral (BIS™) index monitor.

That which anesthetizes least anesthetizes best.
–Charles Laurito

pEEG monitoring with bispectral (BIS) and facial frontalis electromyogram (EMG)... processing takes time BIS/EMG and propofol management... Less is more.
–Mies van der Rohe

Airway management... If it ain't broke, don't fix it.
–English proverb

- Non-purposeful vs. purposeful movement... "too light" vs. "more local".
- Analgesia monitors... answer or enigma.
- Minimal sedation.
- General Anesthesia (GA) considered.
- Pre-pEEG... a qualitative pathway.
- pEEG monitoring with BIS™ and facial *frontalis* electromyogram (EMG)... processing takes time.

The brain is the target organ of anesthetics.[6] Anesthesia may be the sum of hypnosis plus analgesia. "Amnesia" is implied in hypnosis. "Analgesia" to provide sufficient muscle relaxation to imbricate the rectus muscle sheath for abdominoplasty or dissect the pectoralis muscle from the chest wall for augmentation mammoplasty is implied.

Monitors such as the Bispectral (BIS™) index can only measure the *hypnosis* portion of anesthesia, not analgesia **(Fig. 2)**. The BIS index values have no units **(Table 1)**. The left to right sweep of the vital signs monitors displays real-time, non-cortical information such as electrocardiogram (EKG), oxygen saturation (SpO_2), and end-tidal carbon dioxide ($EtCO_2$). Anesthesiologists make clinical decisions based on real-time information.

TABLE 1: BIS™ index values.

1.	98–100	Awake
2.	60–75	Moderate-to-deep sedation
3.	45–60	Hypnosis compatible with GA
4.	<45	Over medicated

(BIS: bispectral; GA: general anesthesia)

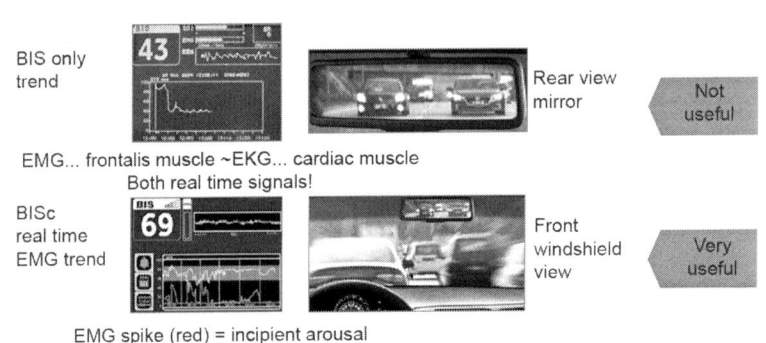

Fig. 3: Why is BIS™ not used more often? (BIS: bispectral; EKG: electrocardiogram; EMG: electromyography)

Processing a BIS™ value takes time, specifically 15–30 seconds. Setting the facial *frontalis* electromyogram (EMG) as a secondary trend to BIS provides useful, real-time information.

The frustrating delay in BIS™ information has discouraged many anesthesiologists from using the device **(Fig. 3)**. However, trending the lower trend provides real-time EMG of the facial *frontalis* muscle. EMG is as real-time a trend as the EKG of the cardiac muscle. EMG spikes are not readily observed when neuromuscular-blocking agents (NMBAs) are used in general anesthesia (GA). *Responding to EMG trending is useful with the increased popularity of ultrasound-guided regional anesthesia (UGRA) and spontaneously breathing patients.*

Nonpurposeful vs. Purposeful Movement... "Too Light" vs. "More Local":

Immobility in response to noxious stimulation is called the dissociative effect.[7] Dissociation reflects N-methyl-D-aspartate (NMDA) receptor saturation.[8] In the author's 26-year experience with >6,000 patients weighing between 30 and 145 kg, immobility for multiple local analgesia injections was produced with the same 50-mg ketamine dose **(Fig. 4)**. Patients aged between 7 and 94 years of age also remained immobile with the same 50-mg ketamine dose. As opposed to the traditional 0.5 mg/kg dose, the effective NMDA receptor saturating ketamine dose does *not* appear to vary with weight or age.[9]

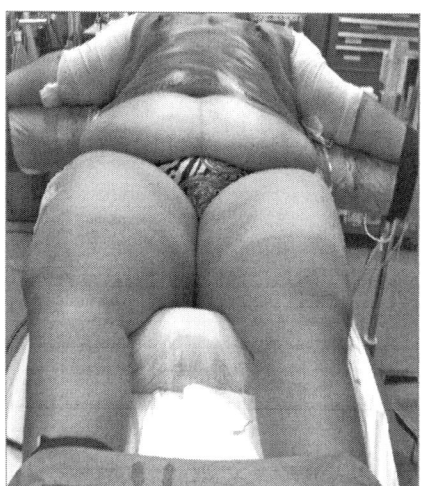

Fig. 4: 145-kg patient rendered immobile with 50-mg ketamine.

One common ketamine preparation is 50 mg per cc. The simplicity, convenience, and efficacy argue for a 1-cc ketamine dose to provide immobility for skin incision, trocar punctures, or multiple local anesthetic injections.

Electromyogram spikes signal incipient arousal.[10] Arousal precedes nociception.[11] By responding to EMG with the same alacrity reserved for heart rate (HR) or blood pressure (BP) changes with sufficient additional propofol to "drive" the EMG spike back to baseline, arousal is prevented. Simply stated, when the EMG goes up, the propofol goes in, representing the best BIS/EMG use. *Preventing arousal prevents nociception.*[11] *When prompt EMG spike response was followed, perturbations in HR and BP were minimal.*[11] There is a 15–30-second interval between an EMG spike and BIS value change. Do not give so much propofol so quickly to prevent loss of spontaneous ventilation. Take advantage of the 15–30 second delay when considering how quickly one attempts to decrease the EMG spike. A recall is not determined by a single BIS value but by 3–5 minutes' duration of an elevated, greater than 78 BIS value or the area under the BIS trend curve.

As opposed to being totally awake or minimally sedated, many patients prefer a greater degree of consciousness alteration during their surgery. To what degree must patients be medicated to assure hypnosis and amnesia and good operating conditions for the surgeon? Numb patients tend to remain immobile during surgery. Since a decapitated chicken still moves, a brain is not necessary to produce movement. How can one demonstrate to the surgeon that most patient movement under sedation is nonpurposeful and unrelated to awareness with recall? Propofol titrated to 60 < BIS < 75 with baseline EMG defines moderate to deep sedation *with* amnesia **(Fig. 2)**. This level of propofol sedation, along with *adequate* local analgesia, provides GA-like operating conditions for the surgeon and amnesia for the patient.

What is the surgeon's dilemma? Why are so many reluctant to reinject the immediate area of dissection with patient movement? Having injected the operative field with a lidocaine/epinephrine solution, the surgeon observes vasoconstriction and believes vasoconstriction guarantees adequate analgesia if the patient moves under IV sedation. The surgeon commonly perceives movement as inadequate sedation and demands "deeper" anesthesia. The anesthesiologist not uncommonly responds to the surgeon's demand with "more local", setting the stage for a contest of wills that may not beneficial to the patient. Since nociception activation in the spinal cord and brain persists even under deep GA, the problem of nonpurposeful patient movement will not be satisfactorily resolved by acquiescing to the surgeon's demand for deeper sedation.[12] Patient movement under moderate-to-deep sedation *without EMG spike* defines the *nonpurposeful* movement **(Fig. 2)**. 98-99% of nonpurposeful movement is eliminated with additional local analgesia in the immediate dissection area.[11]

BIS/EMG and propofol management...Less is More.
–Mies van der Rohe

A Medfusion 2010i infusion pump was used for propofol titration **(Fig. 5)**. The initial infusion *rate* was set at 25 µg per kg per min, and the initial *bolus* was set at 50 µg per kg. Repeated, sequential 50 µg per kg propofol boluses were administered until a decrease in real-time EMG was observed. The real-time EMG trend will decrease before the 15-30 seconds delayed BIS value. Most patients achieved a BIS^{TM} value of <75 but >60 *with* baseline EMG in <3 minutes (*https://lnkd.in/gAnPtSD*). EMG above baseline values artificially elevates BIS values. True BIS values are seen only when EMG activity is at baseline on free-standing units or 26-30 on plugin modules. With induction,

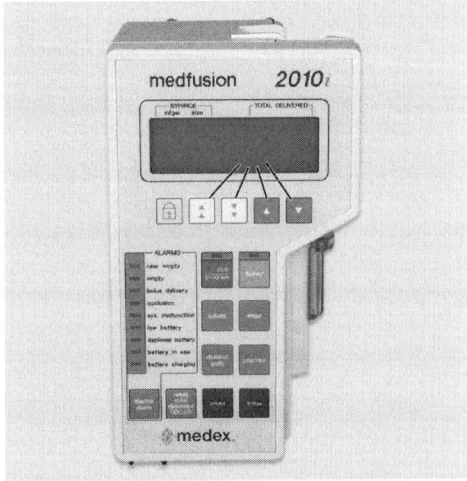

Fig. 5: Medfusion 2010i infusion pump.

once the EMG trend falls to baseline (or 26–30), *but* the BIS value continues to decrease below 60, *decrease* the base rate to that which maintains the BIS level above 60 but below 75. Conversely, if the BIS level remains above 75 with a baseline EMG, *increase* the base infusion rate and consider increasing the base rate and increase the bolus to 75 or 100 µg per kg to decrease the BIS below 75 but above 60.

Directly measuring cortical propofol response and incremental induction revealed a *one hundred-fold variation* in propofol rates to achieve the *same numerical level* of moderate-to-deep sedation.[11] Specifically, average patients achieved 60 < BIS < 75 with baseline EMG at 25–50 µg per kg per minute of propofol. Fragile patients took as little as 2 µg per kg per min. Resistant patients required as much as 200 µg per kg per min.[11]

Airway management... If it ain't broke, don't fix it. —English proverb:
Why try to avoid instrumenting the airway? Cosmetic surgery patients are prone to complain, whether the complaint was a painful intravenous (IV) start or a sore throat. Routinely instrumenting the airway produces more sore throat complaints than not doing so. Can this practice be safe? Based on 26-years' experience in >6,000 patients without hypoxemic insult or aspiration, yes. Induction of elective surgery cases is different than responding to prolapsed umbilical cords or ruptured aneurysms. The only "emergency" is the one created from bolus inductions.

Incremental propofol induction preserves the *temporalis, masseter, orbicularis oris,* and *genioglossus* muscle tone. Rather than routinely inserting an airway after a bolus induction, the degree of airway management is *progressively* determined by the patient's response to incremental induction **(Box 1)**. The increased time required beyond bolus induction is recaptured by time not spent on chin lifting, positive pressure ventilation, airway insertion, or precipitating with a "difficult" airway. Over 26 years of experience with >6,000 incrementally induced patients, approximately two-thirds required *no artificial airways* on induction or maintenance! Initially, one-third were placed in the rhytidectomy (facelift) position with chin up, and head rotated laterally. The lateral rotation adds a vector of force on the *genioglossus* beyond that the chin lift provides. If the airway was still not patent, about another one-third of patients required the addition of an unheated IV bag under the shoulders to increase the force of extension on the *genioglossus* **(Fig. 6)**.

BOX 1: Progressive airway management c̄ incremental propofol induction.

1. Rhytidectomy (facelift) position... chin up, head rotated laterally
2. Rhytidectomy + unheated IV bag under shoulders
3. Nasal airway
4. LMA

(IV: intravenous; LMA: laryngeal mask airway)

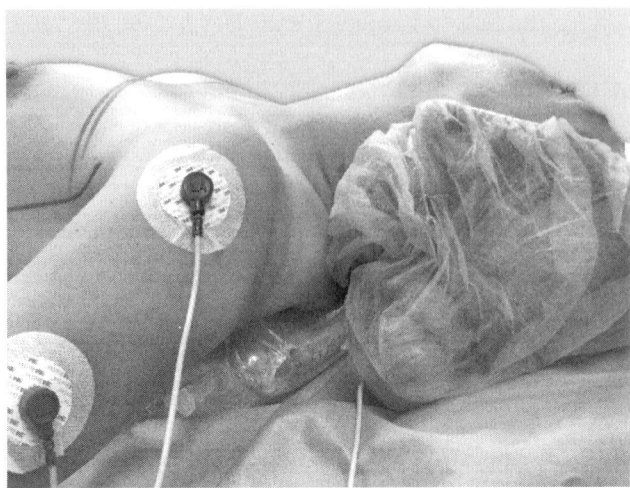

Fig. 6: Rhytidectomy position plus unheated IV bag under patient's shoulders. (IV: intravenous)

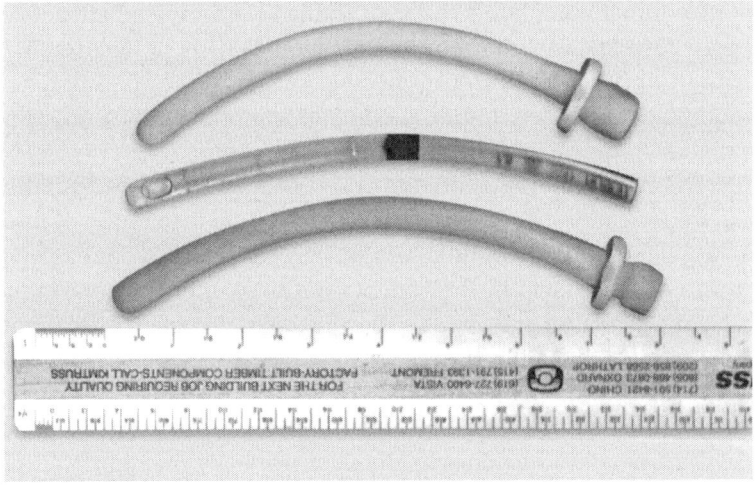

Fig. 7: Nasal airways.

If passive airway maneuvers were inadequate to provide a patent airway, about another one-third patients required nasal airways that tend to produce less cough response than oral airways **(Fig. 9)**. Very small percentage of remaining patients ultimately did require an laryngeal mask airway (LMA) to maintain airway patency. Surprisingly, even with obstructive sleep apnea patients or those with short mandibles and thick tongues, few required more aggressive airway management with incremental induction. Only for rhinoplasties did Friedberg routinely insert a flexible LMA taped to the chin, providing a direct visual access line for the surgeon **(Fig. 8)**.

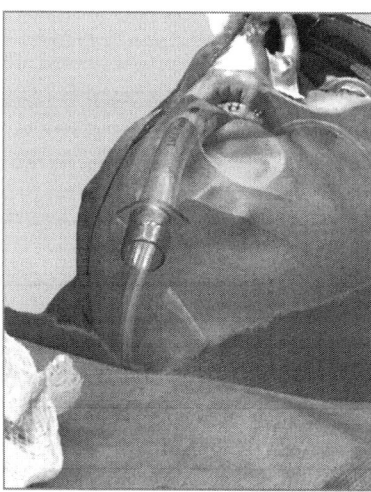

Fig. 8: Open rhinoplasty with LMA not oral endotracheal tube.
(LMA: laryngeal mask airway)

Analgesia monitors... answer or enigma:

Recently, two monitors—namely, analgesia nociception index (ANI™, MDoloris) and nociception level (NOL™, Medasense)—have become available, *purporting* to reflect analgesia, or lack thereof, by analyzing the balance between sympathetic and parasympathetic tone in the HR. Awareness is a cortical function. Changes in HR and BP are notoriously unreliable signs of awareness under anesthesia.[13] ANI and NOL information is derived from *peripheral* HR signals, not cortical input. Like awareness, nociception is also a *cortical* function and may not be specifically reflected in HR variation. Neither ANI nor NOL has been validated in Level-I randomized controlled trials (RCTs) or large-scale clinical trials. If either, or both, of these devices deliver on their promise, patients' pain management under GA with NMBs might be well served.

Minimal sedation:

All cosmetic surgery cases can be performed under local only analgesia. Recently, some plastic surgeons have advocated administering 30 μg sublingual sufentanil lozenges (SSLs) instead of having an anesthesiologist provide sedation.[14] Sufentanil has a 6–9-hour half-life and is 5–10 times more potent than fentanyl. A 30-μg SSL dose is equivalent to 300-μg fentanyl. Even if only 50% of the administered sublingual dose is absorbed, 150 μg is >100 μg fentanyl and, therefore, no longer a short-acting opioid. The short action of fentanyl is based on redistribution, not metabolism. Given the black box respiratory depression sufentanil warning, this drug may be best monitored by anesthesiologists in a medically supervised healthcare setting.[15]

GA considered:

Why not the convenience of GA? The expense of an anesthesia machine equipped with exhaust gas scavenging must be borne. Isoflurane, sevoflurane, desflurane, as well as succinylcholine are malignant hyperthermia (MH) triggers. Although MH is rare, it has happened (*https://abcnews.go.com/GMA/Parenting/story?id=4520099* or *https://tinyurl.com/2p93rvbp*). Any facility using MH triggers must be prepared to treat MH with a dantrolene loading dose of 2.5 mg/kg.[16] Time-consuming MH drills must be scheduled with the same frequency as cardiac arrest or "Code Blue" drills. Friedberg was never asked to be involved in any of these drills and cannot comment on whether they were being performed in offices using GA. Dantrolene has a 3-year shelf life and must be replaced regularly. As with crash cart medications, dantrolene expiration dates may not always be properly monitored. A newer dantrolene preparation (Ryanodex™) is reported to be much faster to prepare and requires less volume in an emergency MH crisis. For many office facilities, the expense of providing GA may be greater than the caseload warrants. The rare risk of MH is unacceptable in patients having surgery *without* medical indication, i.e., elective cosmetic procedures.

Pre-pEEG... a qualitative pathway:

Beginning 1992 through 1998, office-based surgery and anesthesia were unregulated in California. Most offices did not have anesthesia machines, much fewer machines with ventilators. Faced with the choice of manually ventilating a paralyzed patient for a 4-hour body surgery case or the impractical manual ventilation for a 4-hour facial surgery case, the virtue of preserving spontaneous ventilation became obvious. These offices were equipped with crash carts, defibrillators, oxygen, Ambu™ bags, airways, and suction. Vital signs monitors varied widely. To keep a consistent monitoring environment, Friedberg purchased his Propaq™ monitor [EKG, noninvasive arterial blood pressure (NIABP), and SpO_2] when providing anesthesia for different surgeons' offices. The BIS monitor was acquired in 1997. In response to requests for "the numbers", an infusion pump was incorporated in 2002 **(Fig. 5)**.

A 50-cc IV bag was used and injected with two 20-cc propofol ampules (10 mg per cc), resulting in approximately 5 mg per cc propofol. The bag was then spiked with 60 drops per cc IV set (i.e., minidrip, microdrip, or pedidrip). Each small drop equaled approximately 74-µg propofol. The initial drip rate was set to approximate the patient's HR then adjusted upward or downward according to patient response.

Pre-pEEG monitoring, propofol was titrated to maintain spontaneous ventilation with a patent airway, $94 < SpO_2 < 96$ and loss of lid reflex (LLR) and loss of verbal response (i.e., no response to "Are you awake?").[4] Spontaneous ventilation and patent airway were difficult to maintain in pharmacologically fragile patients until the initial 5 mg per cc concentration was additionally diluted to approximately 2.5 mg per cc. Other patients were so resistant to achieve LLR that undiluted, 10 mg per cc propofol was required. Incipient emergence was defined by the resumption of swallowing.[4]

FRIEDBERG'S TRIAD 2.0 PREEMPT THE PAIN

An ounce of prevention is worth a pound of cure.

–Ben Franklin

- Opioid-free, preemptive analgesia
- Ketamine dosing
- Ketamine-associated laryngospasm
- Tumescent analgesia.

Opioid-free, Preemptive Analgesia

The brain cannot process information it has not received (**Fig. 9**). The dissociative effect of ketamine means no incoming, noxious information goes above the tentorium.[6] Following the establishment of a stable CNS propofol level (*https://lnkd.in/gAnPtSD*), a 50-mg ketamine dose was administered 2–3 minutes before multiple local anesthetic injections.[4] Ketamine is an NMDA receptor-blocking agent.[8] The dissociative effect or immobility to noxious stimulation reflects NMDA receptor *saturation*. Beginning in 1992 through 2018, in more than 6,000 opioid-free patients, 50-mg ketamine dose produced 10–20 minutes' immobility to multiple local injections in patients weighing between 30 and 145 kg. The largest patient immobilized is pictured (**Fig. 4**). Patients ages 7 to 94 remained immobile with the same 50-mg ketamine dose.[11] The number of NMDA receptors does not appear to vary with body weight or age. Immobility reflects NMDA receptor *saturation*, not merely blocking an indeterminate number of receptors.[11] Failure to block NMDA receptors is why preemptive analgesia fails with opioids or inhalation anesthetics alone. The absence *of EMG spikes* with multiple local anesthetic

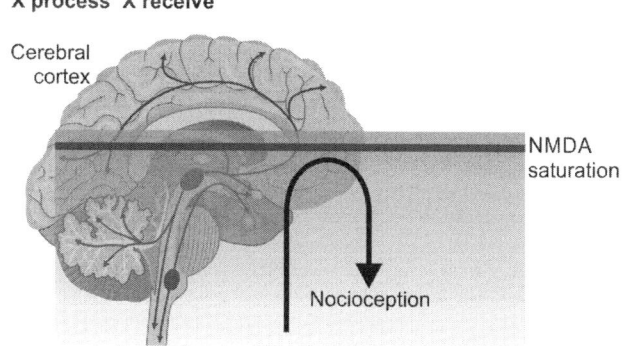

Fig. 9: Brain cannot process information not received. (NMDA: N-methyl-D-aspartate)
Source: Friedberg BL. Propofol-ketamine technique, dissociative anesthesia for office surgery: a five-year review of 1,264 cases. Aesth Plast Surg. 1999;23:70-4.

injections is *prima facie* evidence of NMDA receptor saturation (dissociation) and the beginning of opioid-free, preemptive analgesia. The 50-mg ketamine dose prevents the patient's brain from recognizing the surgeon's bodily invasion with local anesthesia injection and precludes internal pain fibers on high alert.

Ketamine Dosing

Hypnotic propofol doses prevent ketamine hallucinations.[17] Nearly three decades of clinical experience confirmed this early observation.[18] An informal survey of 1,000 of the author's propofol ketamine cases revealed that 80% were done with one or two 50-mg ketamine doses. Any "virgin" surgical filed injection requires a 50-mg ketamine dose to produce immobility. Even a 4-hour abdominoplasty case only required the initial 50-mg ketamine dose to inject the initial 2.5 liters of tumescent analgesia into the anterior abdominal wall (see *https://tinyurl.com/yjw88n8m*). The reason a second 50 mg ketamine dose was required was that the surgeon feared loss of vasoconstriction and analgesia if both sides of the face were injected at the same time. As more experience was gained, surgeons became comfortable injecting both sides of the face *without* observing the loss of either vasoconstriction or analgesia. *Only* a 50-mg ketamine dose was administered for these 4–6-hour cases. Aggregate ketamine doses >200 mg resulted in delayed emergence and discharge. No ketamine should be administered in the last 20 minutes of a case or emergence, possibly with horizontal nystagmus and PONV. Late ketamine doses may also delay discharge.[18]

Tumescent Analgesia

After an incremental propofol induction/maintenance with multiple, sequential 50-μg per kg doses and 25-μg per kg per min base infusion rate (*shorturl.at/buHPV*), a 50-mg ketamine dose, subcutaneous tumescent analgesia was administered by the author's surgeons.[4] The basic tumescent anesthesia formula is 500 mg plain lidocaine, 1 mg epinephrine in 1,000 cc lactated ringers (LR), or normal saline solution (NSS). Klein described his "regional anesthesia" for the regions in which he intended to perform liposuction.[19] He published 35 mg per kg of ultra-dilute (0.05%) lidocaine as safe for liposuction and 28 mg per kg *without* liposuction.[20] Ostad et al. later published up to 55 mg per kg as safe for liposuction.[21] When Coldiron's review compared 4 years of reported liposuction deaths in Florida between dermatologists' tumescent anesthesia and plastic surgeons' GA; tumescent anesthesia had fewer fatalities.[22] Liposuction limits in California are not to exceed 5,000 cc of tumescent fluid. Florida limits are not to exceed 4,000 cc. Complication rates increase when these limits are not adhered to. Tumescent analgesia has also been administered for rhytidectomies, mammoplasties, and abdominoplasties.

Caution: There is an increased risk of local anesthetic toxicity for anesthesiologists using IV lidocaine infusions and *concomitant* tumescent analgesia.

Local anesthesia administered *after* ketamine dissociation *prolongs* the initial ketamine dissociation or cortical deception. What level of analgesia is effective for cosmetic surgeries beyond liposuction? For rhinoplasty and blepharoplasty surgeries, analgesia with 0.5–1% lidocaine with 1:100,000 epinephrine often proved inadequate. Small volumes of 2% lidocaine with 1:100,000 epinephrine provided more consistent analgesia. Facial resurfacing cases were performed with facial nerve blocks after the ketamine was administered. Compared to body cosmetic surgeries, the relatively small amounts of 2% lidocaine with epinephrine for rhinoplasty and blepharoplasty make local anesthetic toxicity unlikely. Pre-emergence, postoperative infiltration of the supraorbital ridge with 0.25% bupivacaine effectively prevented postoperative headache complaints after brow lifts. Postoperative abdominoplasty analgesia was supplemented with 50 cc 0.25% bupivacaine sprayed, not injected, onto the field or the drains retrograde after closure. Total bupivacaine <50 cc 0.25% or 125 mg is safe. Concomitant augmentation mammoplasty and abdominoplasty postoperative analgesia were provided by diluting the 50 cc 0.25% bupivacaine to 100 cc and injecting 20 cc in each breast pocket while reserving 60 cc for the abdomen either in entirety before closure or retrograde injecting the bilateral drains after closure. This dilution provides good analgesia and has not resulted in toxic events in the author's experience.

Ketamine-associated Laryngospasm

Caution: Ketamine-associated laryngospasm is a very rare but distressing event.[23] It is often triggered by secretions contacting the vocal cords. To minimize ketamine-associated secretions, glycopyrrolate 0.2 mg IV was always administered before propofol induction **(Box 2)**. Glycopyrrolate is preferred over atropine. Atropine causes more tachycardia than glycopyrrolate. No hypertension or tachycardia was observed after the initial ketamine dose on numerous occasions when the surgeon failed to inject local anesthesia promptly. The surgeon's lidocaine/epinephrine injections also frequently produce tachycardia, successfully treated with 10-mg IV labetalol.

BOX 2: Opioid-related adverse drug effects (ORADEs).

- Postoperative nausea and vomiting (PONV)
- Respiratory depression/obstruction
- Aspiration/pneumonia/death
- Sedation/prolonged emergence/discharge
- Cognitive dysfunction ("brain fog")
- Urinary retention
- Ileus/constipation

Unexplained tachycardia is often the only sign of an MH event. Neither propofol nor ketamine is an MH trigger. The vocal cords are completely closed with ketamine-associated laryngospasm. The typical "crowing" of partially closed cords is absent. A cough or sneeze is the only prodrome. Larson's maneuver, i.e., anterior jaw thrust with positive pressure ventilation, does not satisfactorily resolve this uncommon type of laryngospasm. Lidocaine 1 mg per pound or 2 mg per kg reliably resolves this spasm.[23]

■ FRIEDBERG'S TRIAD 3.0 EMETIC DRUGS ABSTAIN

As long as emetogenic (opioids) are part of the anesthetic regimen, the use of antiemetics is of limited utility.

–Christian Apfel

If you want patients to stop throwing up, stop giving them drugs that make them sick to their stomachs.

–Chris Pollock

Opioids are the problem, not the answer.

Opioids invariably create opioid-related adverse drug effects (ORADES) **(Box 3)**. A large *hospital-based* study concluded, "Opioid-related adverse drug events were common among patients undergoing hospital-based invasive procedures and were associated with significantly worse clinical and cost outcomes". Hospital-acquired harm from ORADEs in the surgical patient population is an important opportunity for health systems to improve patient safety and reduce cost".[24] Another hospital-based study concluded the risk of only one ORADE included a 55% increased length of stay, 47% increased cost, 36% increased 30-day readmission rate, and 3.6 times increased mortality risk.[25] The clinical and economic effects of ORADES are even less acceptable in the modern era of increasing *outpatient*, minimally invasive surgery cases.

A commonly held belief is that opioids mitigate pain during and *after* surgery. A meta-analysis of 23 studies comparing OIC to OFA concluded that OIC did not reduce postoperative care but increased PONV.[1] PONV

BOX 3: Clinical pathway.

- Glycopyrrolate 0.2 mg IV
- Propofol titrated to BIS <75 c baseline EMG
- Ketamine 50 mg IV
- Dexamethasone 10 mg IV
- Local anesthesia by a surgeon
- Ketorolac 30 mg IV 30–45 minutes preclosure (optional)

Rx Laryngospasm… stat IV lidocaine 1 mg per pound with cough or sneeze.
Brow lift: Pre-closure…supraorbital ridge infiltration c 0.25 bupivacaine
Abdominoplasty… 50 cc 0.25% bupivacaine sprayed onto the field or injected up drains after closure

(EMG: electromyography; IV: intravenous)

is patients' number one outcome to avoid after surgery![2] Many believe eliminating opioids from the anesthesia regimen will expose patients to postoperative pain. While trying to ascertain if hypnotic doses of propofol prevent ketamine hallucinations, the author observed his first 50 opioid-free propofol ketamine cases emerge *without* pain.[26] The subcutaneous local analgesia injection by the surgeon *after* the ketamine *but* preincision was a probable explanation patient emerging without pain. Opioid avoidance was a probable explanation for the near-total absence of PONV. Consensus PONV guidelines call for one antiemetic maneuver for every PONV risk.[27] Apfel-defined high PONV risk factors were nonsmoking females with PONV or motion sickness histories having emetogenic (cosmetic) surgery.[28] Friedberg published a 0.6% PONV rate in 1,264 Apfel-defined, high PONV risk, opioid-free, cosmetic surgery patients *without* antiemetics.[4] Apfel cited this paper in his PONV chapter and favorably compared Friedberg's 0.6% PONV rate to Paul White's 7% PONV rate.[29]

■ CHALLENGING CASES

How can one perform a rhytidectomy of brow lift with a BIS™ sensor on the forehead? Unless foreign bodies such as cheek implants or brow fixation screws are used, neither procedure is sterile. If the surgeon is concerned, the sensor should only be prepped with a dabbing motion. Vigorous scrubbing will dissolve the adhesive and cause the failure of sensor adhesion. Nicanor Isse is one of three American plastic surgeons credited with developing the endoscopic brow lift **(Fig. 10)**.

In Isse's Newport Beach and Burbank, California offices, Friedberg used a BIS™ monitor on every brow lift and rhytidectomy patient without a single

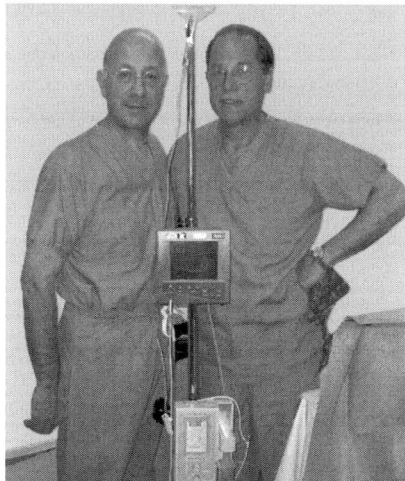

Fig. 10: Doctors Nicanor Isse (left) and Barry Friedberg (right).

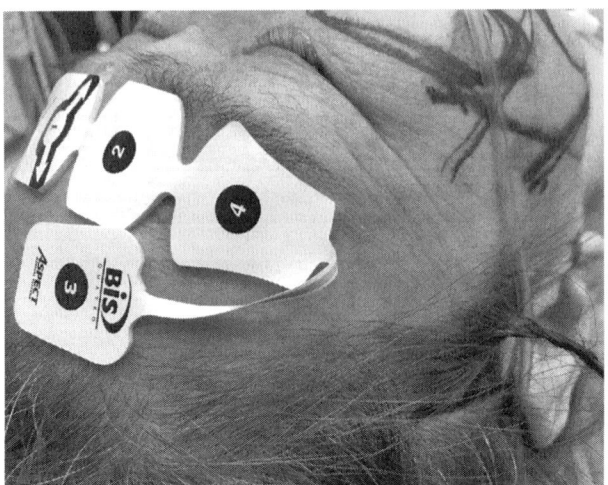

Fig. 11: Alternative BIS™ #3 Quatro sensor placement.
(BIS: bispectral)

surgical site infection between 1999 through 2004. For rhytidectomies, the #3 BIS Quatro sensor can alternatively be placed on either the forehead or the temple area to avoid the pre-auricular incision **(Fig. 11)**. For brow lift patients, only during the relatively brief interval when the forehead flap is completely elevated from the skull does the loss of contact cause the BIS™ transiently fail to provide a BIS or EMG value. Otherwise, during the closure, the flap contacts the skull, and BIS/EMG data transmission resumes.

CONCLUSION

Opioid-free anesthesia propofol ketamine sedation guided by Friedberg's triad has advantages over either local only or GA plus local, especially in remote settings such as office-based surgery suites. Patients do not hear, feel, or remember their surgery. Patient satisfaction is high. For the surgeon, the operative field approximates GA conditions without the greater pharmacologic trespass, need for an anesthesia machine, scavenging, MH risk, or dantrolene. The persistent anesthesia problems of pain and PONV are virtually eliminated. Ketamine hallucination fears are eliminated with hypnotic levels of propofol. BIS™/EMG monitored cortical response introduces the scientific practice of reproducibility across the hundred-fold variation in propofol requirement at the same numerical sedation level. BIS™/EMG monitoring transformed the original qualitative propofol ketamine sedation into a *reproducible*, quantitative paradigm. BIS™/EMG monitoring also objectively assuages surgeons' awareness fears and resolves the dilemma of "too light" versus "more local" that prevents more elective cosmetic surgery being performed with IV sedation.

Disclosure: No financial interest to disclose.

REFERENCES

1. Frauenknecht J Kirkham KR, Jacot-Guillarmod A, Albrecht E. Analgesic impact of intra-operative opioids vs. opioid-free anaesthesia, a systematic review and meta-analysis. Anaesthesia. 2019;74(5):651-62.
2. Macario A, Weinger M, Carney S, Kim A. Which clinical anesthesia outcomes are important to avoid? The perspective of patients. Anesth Analg. 1999;89:652-8.
3. Macario A, Weinger M, Truong P, Lee M. Which clinical anesthesia outcomes are both common and important to avoid? The perspective of a panel of expert anesthesiologists. Anesth Analg. 1999;88:1085.
4. Friedberg BL. Propofol-ketamine technique, dissociative anesthesia for office surgery: a five-year review of 1,264 cases. Aesth Plast Surg. 1999;23:70-4.
5. Friedberg BL. BIS monitoring transformed opioid-free propofol ketamine anesthesia from art to science for ambulatory cosmetic surgery. Aesth Plast Surg. 2020;44:2308-11.
6. Friedberg BL. (2005). Brain is target organ for anesthesia. Anesthesia Patient Safety Foundation Newsletter. [online] Available from https://www.apsf.org/article/brain-is-target-organ-for-anesthesia/. [Last accessed October, 2022].
7. Pender JW. Dissociative anesthesia. JAMA. 1971;215:1126-30.
8. Zorumski CF, Izumi Y, Mennerick S. Ketamine: NMDA receptors and beyond. J Neurosci. 2016;36:11158-64.
9. Friedberg BL. Can Friedberg's Triad solve persistent anesthesia problems? Over-medication, pain management, postoperative nausea and vomiting. Plast Reconstr Surg Global Open. 2017;5:e1527-734.
10. American Society of Anesthesiologists Task Force on Intraoperative Awareness. Practice advisory for intraoperative awareness and brain function monitoring. Anesthesiol. 2006;104:847-64.
11. Friedberg BL. Tríada de Friedberg, un camino hacia la anestesia libre de opioides y mejores resultados/Friedberg's Triad, a pathway to opioid free anesthesia (OFA) and better outcomes. [online] Available from https://www.mpainjournal.com/friedberg%E2%80%99s-triad-a-pathway-to-opioid-free-anesthesia-ofa-and-better-outcomes95. [Last accessed October, 2022].
12. Lichtner G, Auksztulewicz R, Velten H, Mavrodis D, Scheel M, Blankenburg F, et al. Nociceptive activation in the spinal cord & brain persists DURING deep general anesthesia. Br J Anaesth. 2018;121:291-302.
13. Domino KB, Posner Kl, Caplan RA, Cheney FW. Awareness under anesthesia: a closed claim analysis. Anesthesiology. 1999;90:1053-61.
14. Seify H. Awake plastic surgery procedures: the use of a sufentanil sublingual tablet to improve patient experience. Aesth Surg J Open Forum. 2022;4:ojab056.
15. Mikaela L, Kislevitz ML, Coleman J. Commentary on: awake plastic surgery procedures: the use of a sufentanil sublingual tablet to improve patient experience. Aesth Surg J Open Forum. 2022;4:ojac003.
16. MHAUS. How much dantrolene should be kept on hand? [online] Available from https://www.mhaus.org/faqs/how-much-dantrolene-should-be-kept-on-hand/. [Last accessed October, 2022].
17. Friedberg BL. Hypnotic doses of propofol block ketamine induced hallucinations. Plast Reconstr Surg. 1993;91:196.
18. Friedberg BL. Ketamine hallucination and dose limits rebutted. Transl Perioper Pain Med. 2020;7:170.

19. Klein JA. Tumescent technique for regional anesthesia permits lidocaine doses of 35 mg/kg for liposuction. J Dermatol Surg Oncol. 1990;16:248-63.
20. Klein JA, Jeske DR. Estimated maximal safe dosages of tumescent lidocaine. Anesth Analg. 2016;122(5):1350-9.
21. Ostad A, Kageyama N, Moy RL. Tumescent anesthesia with a lidocaine dose of 55 mg/kg is safe for liposuction. Dermatol Surg. 1996;22:921-7.
22. Coldiron B, Fisher AH, Adelman E, Yelverton CB, Balkrishnan R, Feldman MA, et al. Adverse event reporting: lessons learned from 4 years of Florida office data. Dermatol Surg. 2005;31:1079-92.
23. Friedberg BL. Ketamine associated laryngospasm during processed EEG monitored propofol sedation. Transl Perioper Pain Med. 2020;7:291-3.
24. Shafi S, Collinsworth AW, Copeland LA, Ogola GO, Qiu T, Kouznetsova M, et al. Association of opioid-related adverse drug events with clinical and cost outcomes among surgical patients in a large integrated health care delivery system. JAMA Surg. 2018;153:757-63.
25. Kessler ER, Shah M, Grushkus SK, Raju A. Opioid-related adverse events and their impact on clinical and economic outcomes. Pharmacother. 2013;33:383-91.
26. Friedberg BL. Propofol-ketamine technique. Aesth Plast Surg. 1993;17:297-300.
27. Gan TJ, Belani KG, Bergese S, Chung F, Diemunsch P, Habib A, et al. Fourth consensus guidelines for the management of postoperative nausea and vomiting. Anesth Analg. 2020;131:411-48.
28. Apfel CC, Korttila K, Abdalla M, Kerger H, Turan A, Vedder I, et al. IMPACT investigators. A factorial trial of six interventions for the prevention of postoperative nausea and vomiting. N Engl J Med. 2004;350:2441-51.
29. Apfel CC. Postoperative nausea and vomiting ch. in Miller's Anesthesia, 7th edition. Philadelphia, PA: Elsevier; 2010. p. 2743.

CHAPTER 18

Environmental and Occupational Considerations of Anesthesia

Parli Raghavan Ravi, Rajini Kausalya, Basavaraju Karan

ABSTRACT

The deleterious effects of climate change on health continue to increase. Inhaled anesthetics are exceptionally strong global warming potential (GWP) and may pose considerable environmental risks. Within the field of anesthesia, the potential to reduce harmful environmental effects of volatiles can be briefly summarized as follows: Stop or avoid the use of nitrous oxide (N_2O) and desflurane, consider the use of total intravenous or local-regional anesthesia, invest in the development of new technologies to minimize volatile anesthetics consumption, scavenging systems, and destruction of waste gas. Further, the balance between the prevention of infection and environmental hazards caused by the use of disposables and nondisposable items has to be perfectly balanced to ensure there is no undesirable environmental effect. With the increasingly precarious work relationship associated with the lack of knowledge of occupational hazards, anesthesiologists become vulnerable; therefore, knowledge of occupational hazards and means of prevention is important for safeguarding anesthesiologists' health.

Keywords: Environment; Greenhouse gases (GHG); Global warming potential (GWP); Inhaled anesthetics; Lifecycle assessment; Occupational health hazards.

KEY POINTS

- The conduct of anesthesia does cause many deleterious effects on the environment, which need to be reduced or minimized.
- Total intravenous anesthesia appears to have a slight edge over the use of inhalational anesthetic agents in reducing the environmental pollution.
- Among the volatile anesthetic agents used, desflurane has the longest gas atmospheric lifetime and thus causes maximum harm to the environment.
- Lifecycle assessment (LCA) is a purely scientific method for analyzing the "cradle to grave" environmental "footprint" associated with medical products used in diagnosing and managing cases.
- Low-flow anesthesia, effective vapor capture condensation and destruction, total intravenous anesthesia, and waste prevention strategies

(avoid, reduce, reuse, recycle, and reprocess) are some effective strategies to reduce the environmental pollution caused in the operating theater.
- Standard precautions (SPs) include the appropriate application and use of handwashing, personal protective equipment (PPE), and respiratory hygiene/cough etiquette. This can prevent infectious exposure of anesthesiologists directly or indirectly.
- Workplace stress in anesthesia is a real issue, and a multipronged strategy should be used to reduce it. The effect of radiation on anesthesia personnel working in such areas should be continuously monitored.

INTRODUCTION

The climate crisis is the largest, prolonged, and most disastrous threat to global health, which can affect and harm human life. If anesthesiology was a country, it would have been the fifth largest polluter in the world. Due to the greenhouse gas (GHG) emissions, the temperature of the planet has been rapidly increasing since the times of the industrial revolution.[1] The Intergovernmental Panel on Climate Change (IPCC) Special Report gave us less than a decade to dramatically reduce our GHG emissions to limit the increase in global temperatures to 1.5°C and thus try to limit the climate change-related public health disasters.[2] The Hippocratic oath to "first do no harm" guides physician practice, yet the healthcare itself pollutes and harms public health. If global healthcare was a country, it would be the fifth largest carbon emitter on the planet. Sustainable healthcare requires balancing patient outcomes with economic, environmental, and social costs. Much of the environmental emissions generated by healthcare are indirect or embodied in upstream manufacturing of products and energy that support healthcare facilities.[3] In the infancy of the sustainability movement, efforts tended to focus on highly visible endeavors such as solid waste recycling efforts and carbon emissions reductions. The work environment also poses unique risks to anesthesiologists, which can have a detrimental effect on the individual's health. Anesthetists are in a unique position of authority and responsibility to make valuable contributions in the transition to sustainable healthcare and hence, reduce the burden of disease caused by environmental pollution and reduce the harm caused by them.[4]

EARTH ATMOSPHERE

The atmospheric divisions of earth are troposphere, stratosphere, and mesosphere. The majority of the ozone (about 80%) is in the stratosphere, which limits the transmission of potentially harmful ultraviolet rays. This is somewhere between 20,000 and 30,000 meters. Troposphere which makes the most of the earth atmosphere has almost all the water vapor.[5,6]

EARTH'S ENERGY EXPENDITURE

Earth remains energy neutral. For this, the incoming solar radiation energy of about 340–350 Wm^{-2} is neutralized by the reflected solar radiation and the outgoing infrared radiation. There is a atmospheric window of about 10–14 micrometer where there is little absorption of infrared takes place by the water vapor or GHG. But outside these frequencies, there is a possibility of water vapor and GHG absorbing and reemitting the infrared radiations, and thus tilting the balance of net energy toward gain of energy for Earth[6] (Figs. 1 and 2).

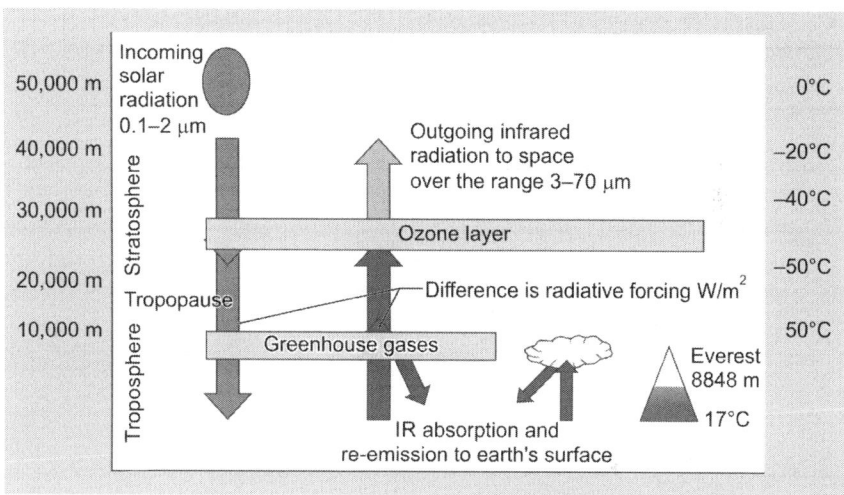

Fig. 1: Earth energy expenditure. (IR: infrared)

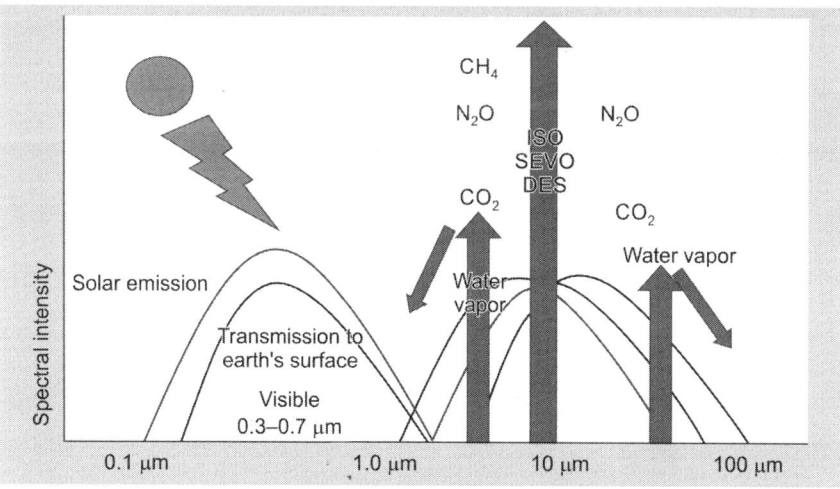

Fig. 2: Clinical chemistry of volatiles and environment. (CH$_4$: methane; CO$_2$: carbon dioxide; DES: desflurane; ISO: isoflurane; N$_2$O: nitrous oxide; SEVO: sevoflurane)

TERMINOLOGY AND DEFINITIONS[2,7,8]

Intergovernmental Panel on Climate Change (IPCC) has given following definitions: These are desirable to understand before evaluating environmental energy data.
- "Radiative forcing is a term to describe the change in irradiance (incoming solar-outgoing IR) at the tropopause (Wm^{-2}). The accepted value for total radiative forcing was + Wm^{-2} in 2.88".
- "Radiative efficiency is the change in irradiance per ppb of a particular 2014 compound ($Wm^{-2}ppb^{-1}$) and depends on the strength and position of the compound's IR absorption bands".
- "The global warming potential (GWP) of a GHG is taken to be over the 100-year time horizon (GWP100), which depends on the radiative efficiency and the atmospheric life. By convention, the GWP100 for CO_2 is 1".
- "Carbon footprint is the total GHG emissions caused directly and indirectly by a person, organization, event, or product".
- "Carbon dioxide equivalency (CO_2e) is a quantity that describes, for a given mixture and amount of GHG, the amount of CO_2 that would have the same GWP when measured over a specified timescale (generally, 100 years). CO_2e reflects the time-integrated radiative forcing of several emissions or rate of GHG emissions that flow into the atmosphere—rather than the instantaneous value of the radiative forcing of the concentration of GHGs in the atmosphere".

MONTREAL PROTOCOL FOR OZONE LAYER

The catastrophic effect of chlorofluorocarbons on ozone layer, by releasing stratospheric chlorine-containing compounds (chlorofluorocarbons or CFCs) such as CFCl3 (CFC-11) undergo photolysis with the liberation of chlorine atoms, each capable of catalyzing the destruction of up to 100,000 molecules of ozone. In 1987, the use of CFCs was universally banned. Hydrochlorofluorocarbons contain proportionately less chlorine, which lowers the ozone depletion potential and has been introduced as an alternative to chlorofluorocarbons.[9]

KYOTO PROTOCOL

In 1997, the UN Framework Convention on Climate Change set binding obligations to reduce the emission of GHG, which is known as the Kyoto Protocol. China, India, and other developing countries were exempt from the requirements of the Kyoto Protocol because they were not the main contributors to the GHG emissions during the industrialization period that is believed to be causing today's climate change. Perfluorocarbons, HFCs, carbon dioxide, nitrous oxide, and methane are some of the gasses, whose emission is controlled under this protocol.[10]

Nitrous Oxide

Since the lifespan of the nitrous oxide in the stratosphere is quite long, apart from its global warming effect, it causes the destruction of ozone layer due to phylogenetically generated oxygen molecule. Nitrous oxide accounts for almost 4% of the total emissions.[12]

Halogenated Anesthetic Agents

The halogenated inhalational anesthetic agents typically absorb infrared radiations within 5-10 μm and thus contribute to the global warming. Sevoflurane appears to have the smallest and least GWP100 in comparison to desflurane, which has the highest GWP100. It is postulated that vaporization of a bottle of desflurane can generate about 1,000 kg of carbon dioxide. However, since neither sevoflurane nor desflurane has chloride component they do not contribute to ozone depletion. Isoflurane has a negligible effect on ozone depletion as it has a chloride component.[5]

CLIMATE CHEMISTRY AND INHALED ANESTHESIA AGENTS

The two factors which decide the ability of gas to contribute to the warming of environment, better defined as GWP, are the radiative efficiency and gas atmospheric lifetime (GAL). GAL is always measured as a time constant, t3/4 to 99% initial concentration.[13] All the halogenated anesthetic ethers have similar radiative efficiency with the exception of sevoflurane, which has about 30% less. The alkane halothane has half of sevoflurane's radiative efficiency. The GAL of a volatile agent depends upon the how rapid it is broken down by the OH radical. Due to this, the GAL of all the volatiles is different. The carbon strength of C-F bond being the highest, the atmospheric lifetime of the desflurane is highest. It is almost five times that of sevoflurane.[14-16] The GWP is the prime reason for longevity of the volatile gases rather than its radiative efficiency. The GWP100 of desflurane is 254,021 (1 g desflurane has the same GWP as 2,540 g CO_2), sevoflurane 1,302,125, isoflurane 51,025, and N_2O approximately 265.[13]

GLOBAL WARMING AND INHALATION ANESTHETIC AGENTS

It is postulated that the combine warming effects of all the anesthetic agents used can fire up a coal-based fire power station and are equivalent to roughly one hundredth of CO_2 that will be released from the current fossil fuel consumption of the earth.[15]

Lifecycle Assessment

The lifecycle assessment (LCA) of a product is defined as scientific method of evaluating the carbon footprint of an equipment from its origins from the raw material to the process of manufacturing, packaging, transporting, using till the time it is disposed of. The international organization for standardization has laid down four phases for LCA:[16]

- The first phase describes the objective and aim of the LCA and it is referred to as functional unit. For example, if one opens an entire spinal analgesia pack and only uses the plastic tray, entire pack must be considered as the functional unit and the components are to be accounted for.
- Second, the cataloging of each material and its environment emissions are considered as lifecycle inventories (LCIs).[17,18] It gives the understanding that how much a particular material contributes to the environmental emissions and at what phase of the lifecycle of the equipment will that emission occur the maximum. The most frequently reported environmental impact category is CO_2e apart from some other categories such as air, water, and LCIs are used to understand how much those materials contribute to environmental emissions and where in the lifecycle of a particular product or process those emissions occur. CO_2e emissions are the most reported environmental impact category; however, other categories exist, including energy use, air, water, and soil pollutants, ozone depletion and others.
- Third, assessment of lifecycle impact[19] compares the relative advantage and disadvantage of the equipment in interest to assess the environmental impact based on one environmental impact category to the another (for example, the comparing the equipment for relative advantage of CO_2e emissions to water and terrestrial pollution).
- Fourth, it is imperative to interpret the result for the decision makers as implementation of environment friendly processes are to be implemented. For example, there is always a geographic and variations in the CO_2 intensity of electricity generation (g CO_2e/kW h generated) from one region to another.[20] In certain regions, for example, coal is used to produce energy instead of renewable sources. Such countries (China, Australia, etc.) will have more CO_2 intensity of power generation.

Several types of LCAs are there, but only two have relevance to healthcare systems:
- *Process-based LCAs:* This is usually used when the data input is not complicated and the products are easily defined and are comparable[21] (e.g., reusable vs. disposable equipment). For example, there can be healthcare analyses of disposable and reusable airway devices such as LMAs wherein the weights, compositions, and actual use of such items are focused in detail.

Environmentally extended economic input/output:[22] These are usually used when the data input is large. They estimate the environmental cost of the material, after directly measured inputs and comparing them with the LCI databases of emissions of those materials.

Lifecycle assessment in anesthesia: The first relevant lifecycle assessment for any equipment was done by Dettenkofer and colleagues[16] bought out the intrinsic tension between infection prevention and environmental care. There are very few studies done on emissions produced by medical devices, various surgical techniques, pharmacy, or other healthcare services. Whereas there is no doubt that the CO_2e emissions of disposables largely depend upon the source of production of electricity, there is a similar concern of equivalent emissions from use of reusable items as they undergo repeated cleaning.[23,24] The calculation of ecological footprint will depend upon the number of times the item is reused, the method and frequency of cleaning, the level of cleaning (low-level or high-level disinfection), the method of sterilization and waste disposal.[25]

There have been contrasting studies with respect of carbon footprints generated by the reusable and single use medical equipments. In one of the studies in Australia, it was reported that the carbon footprints of reusable equipment were similar or higher in comparison to similar single-use equipment. This was in contrast to a study in US, which found that the carbon footprints of reusable were only two-thirds to the single-use equipment. One study found that reusable blood pressure cuffs were 40 times environmentally preferable to disposable cuffs[19] Sherman and colleagues[26] in their study assessed the lifecycle and GWP of inhaled anesthetics and compared it with the lifecycle of propofol. They deduced that the GWP of inhaled anesthetics is almost four times that of the lifecycle of propofol.

From the environmental perspective, total intravenous anesthesia (TIVA) is always preferable to inhaled anesthetics (especially desflurane and N_2O). Parvatker and colleagues[27] further estimated CO_2e emissions for the API of 20 common anesthetic/critical care drugs, finding an average of 340 g CO_2e/g API. A study found that the primary source of CO_2e emissions in morphine manufacture was steam sterilization and drug packaging rather than the morphine API.[28] Multiple studies have shown that if desflurane is used, then the CO_2e emissions generated by anesthesia itself are more than CO_2e emissions of all surgical equipment and OR-associated energy, including from heating, ventilation, and air conditioning (HVAC). It is strongly suggested that changing the source of energy from the coal to renewables will drastically reduce the carbon footprints.[29-32]

STRATEGIES TO REDUCE ENVIRONMENTAL HAZARDS IN ANESTHESIA

Reducing Environmental Contamination by Inhalation Anesthesia Agents inside the Operation Theater

The anesthetic vapors are metabolized to a minimum and, hence, are exhaled predominantly unchanged, which in spite of effective scavenging systems lands up in the environment. Therefore, there should be multiple strategies to reduce the OT pollution and thus the environmental pollution. Few of the strategies are enumerated below:

Low-flow/very low-flow anesthesia: Low-flow anesthesia is defined as flow rates of 1 L/min. Very low-flow anesthesia is defined as flow rates of 500 mL/min. The OT pollution drastically reduces by using low-flow anesthesia.[12]

Vapor Capture Condensation and Destruction

There are various devices built that can condense the exhaled gases from the scavenging systems thus reducing the atmospheric discharge of these gases to minimum. Various methods, which are used for such, include fractional distillation or catalytic conversion of the gases.[33,34] Ensuring good and effective seal with airway devices, use of pediatric cuffed tubes, and avoiding frequent disconnections of anesthesia circuit and machine are few other strategies to reduce the OT pollution.

Total IV Anesthesia

Total intravenous anesthesia as well as use conduct of anesthesia with regional anesthesia completely avoids the volatile gas agents and, hence, eliminates the complete possibility of GHG emissions. However, they still exert a certain burden on the environment because of the process of manufacture, transport, and delivery.

The complete metabolism of propofol ensures that only trace amount of the drug reaches the environment and minimum impact is seen. However, the syringe, which is discarded, is toxic and remains in the environment for a long time and pollutes the aquatic environment. Hence, the remaining propofol with the syringe should be incinerated.

WASTE PREVENTION: AVOID, REDUCE, REUSE, RECYCLE, AND REPROCESS

Anesthesia produces almost 30% of the waste generated in the OT. Waste generation seems like an inevitable outcome of treating patients. It is imperative to follow the waste hierarchy (reduce, reuse, and recycle) and adopting waste prevention programs such as "Choosing Wisely"[35] **(Table 1)** initiative that seeks to maintain/improve clinical care while

TABLE 1: Research base for the environmental impact of anesthesia and intensive care.

Anesthetic activity	Evidence and uncertainties
Gases: Use gases with low GWP	• Avoid the use of nitrous oxide and desflurane if not required for a particular indication • Use low- to very low-flow anesthesia • Use of TIVA and regional anesthesia to be encouraged • Propofol has certain environmental impact but less in comparison to volatile agents
Plastic syringes: Avoid excessive use	Use minimum number of syringes. Keep the emergency equipment unopened, but within the reach
OT dress Use reusables	Use of laundered OT dresses, hats, and shoes
Energy consumption	Anesthesia machines to be turned off along with scavenging and suction. The HVAC system also to be put on optimal mode after out of hours
Anesthesia circuits	Weekly change of anesthesia circuit, until unless for specific situation demand so
Surgical OT dress	They have lower carbon footprint if reused or recycled
Anesthetic drugs tray	Reusable has a lower footprint and economically cheaper
Laryngeal mask airway	Reusables have lesser carbon footprints than single use
Anesthesia equipment	Reusable facemasks, circuits, and laryngoscope blades have lesser carbon footprint
Washing of anesthesia equipment	The washable reusable equipment's use higher amount of water than manufacturing of single use equipment
Donation	Donation of equipment's to third world countries will lead to social, financial, and environmental benefits

(GWP: global warming potential; HVAC: heating, ventilation, and air conditioning; LCA: lifecycle assessment; LMA: laryngeal mask airway; TIVA: total intravenous anesthesia)

promoting rational resource use such as reducing unnecessary investigations and medications can significantly reduce the environmental footprint of healthcare[36,37] (but basins, gowns, and drapes) remain in. It is postulated in multiple studies that return to reusable and laundered surgical gowns, hats, and dedicated theater footwear will reduce the amount of single-use clothing while maintaining infection control standards.[36,37] If all the above three measures are not possible then recycling should be considered. Roughly, one-fourth of the OT waste can be recycled. If 1 ton of the mixed plastics is recycled then it can generate roughly 5,774 kWh of energy (enough to power an average household for 6 months) or can be equivalent to almost 17 barrels of oil or can save 30 cubic yards of precious earth from landfill.[38,39] Medical device reprocessing, or "remanufacturing", is defined as the cleaning and packaging of a single-use equipment for reuse, which may save money and reduce emissions from manufacture. The workplace carbon footprint is based on the energy and infrastructure. If workplace efficiency is improved, it will reduce the cost of energy and waste generation thus reducing the overall carbon footprint.[40]

EDUCATION AND ADVOCACY

Educational publications such as anesthesia journals and scientific articles can play an important role in advocating the effect of anesthesia gases on climate change and atmosphere. There has to be a strong link between the environmental and social pillars for sustainable development without compromising the environmental sustainability. The three pillars, plane, people, and profit, have to be imperatively looked into before planning any long-term goals and growth of healthcare infrastructure.[16,41,42]

GLOBAL CONSENSUS STATEMENT FROM THE WORLD FEDERATION OF ANESTHESIOLOGISTS ON ENVIRONMENTAL PROTECTION[16]

The World Federation of Anesthesiologists released the consensus statement on environmentally sustainable anesthesia and stressed seven key principles to reduce the environmental burden. These seven principles are enumerated below:

Anesthesia providers should:
1. Minimize the environmental impact of their clinical practice.
2. Use clinically safe, environmentally preferable medications and equipment.
3. Minimize the overuse/waste of medications, equipment, energy, and water.
4. Incorporate environmental sustainability principles within formal anesthesia education.
5. Embed environmental sustainability principles within anesthesia research and quality improvement programs.
6. Lead environmental sustainability activity within their healthcare organizations.
7. Collaborate with industry to improve environmental sustainability.

OTHER ENVIRONMENTAL HAZARDS EXPOSURE TO ANESTHESIOLOGIST

Infectious Exposure

Anesthesiologists are prone to infections from hospital staff and patients because of more effective antimicrobial agents resulting in more resistant microbes. There is more significant risk of viral infection to an anesthesiologist. The most common mode of transmission is through respiratory route, and followed by hand-to-hand transmission. The most effective strategy is hand wash in preventing transmission of infection. Viral infections such as hepatitis B and influenza can be prevented with immunization. Transmission of blood-borne infections can be prevented with mechanical barriers. According to recent recommendations from the Centers for Disease Control and Prevention (CDC) preemployment screening, immunization, infection control practices, postexposure treatment, and work restrictions for infected personnel should be followed in the respective health organization.[43]

Standard Precautions

Standard precautions (SPs) are practiced to prevent airborne, droplet, and contact transmission of infections to medical personnel as recommended by CDC. SP includes hand washing, use of personal protective equipment (PPE), and respiratory hygiene/cough etiquette. Application of plain or antibacterial soap with water and the use of alcohol-based gels without water is gold standard for hand hygiene.

Specific transmission-based precautions should be used in addition to SP in infected patients or suspected infectious patients.[43,44]

Environmental factors: Negative pressure rooms, high-efficiency particulate air (HEPA) filtration, frequent air exchange rates, and ultraviolet irradiation of air in the upper portion of a room or air ducts are the additional safety measures to prevent airborne infectious particles in hospitals.[44]

Needlestick and sharps safety: Routine use of needle-less devices (e.g., stopcocks, needle-less access ports, and valves) and needle products with needlestick protection safety features helps in reducing the risk of sharp object injuries to healthcare personnel. Recapping and detaching needle from syringes should be avoided unless such action is required by a specific procedure or has no feasible alternative.[45]

Vaccine-preventable illness: The CDC recommends that all healthcare personnel should be vaccinated against vaccine-preventable diseases to reduce the risk of occupational exposure and transmission of these diseases as per CDC advisory committee.[43,46]

Transmission-based Precautions

Modes of transmission: An infectious agent may be transmitted from its natural reservoir to a susceptible host in different ways:
- *Direct:*
  - Direct contact
  - Droplet spread

- *Indirect:*
  - Airborne
  - Vector borne.

Transmission-based precautions are the second tier of basic infection control and are to be used in addition to SPs for patients who may be infected or colonized with certain infectious agents for which additional precautions are needed to prevent infection transmission.

SUBSTANCE USE, ABUSE, AND ADDICTION

Abuse implies the use of a substance despite negative consequences. Addiction is characterized by continued abuse despite attempts to curtail use, the need for increasing doses, physical dependence (withdrawal occurring in the absence of the substance), and increasing energy expended seeking the substance. The most common substance misused by anesthesia personnel has traditionally been opioids. There has been an increase in the abuse of other drugs, including propofol, ketamine, and remifentanil, as well as volatile anesthetics.[47]

Early recognition of addiction is critical for implementing life-saving interventions. Efforts must be made on multiple fronts to decrease this tragic occupational hazard, including education, controlled substance accounting, and systems of discovery, treatment, and recovery.[47,48]

Workplace Stress

The nature of work is changing at whirlwind speed. Perhaps now more than ever before, job stress poses a threat to the health of workers and, in turn, to the health organizations. Job stress results when the requirements of the job do not match the capabilities, resources, and needs of the anesthesiologist. Job stress can lead to poor work performance, which have a huge impact on the safety of patients and anesthesiologist's health and family lives.[48]

Early detection and treatment in symptomatic cases are essential. Treatment should aim for significant changes in lifestyle modifications, quality of life, and search for better work opportunities.

Burnout Syndrome

Burnout is a state of emotional, physical, and mental *exhaustion* caused by excessive and prolonged stress. Burnout affects the quality of life, professional performance, drug abuse, suicidal ideation, and psychiatric disorders.[48]

Measures should be taken on three fronts—personal, team, and institutional levels.
- Individual prevention is accomplished by control of potential stressor factors, enhancing knowledge, taking up hobbies, changing eating and sleeping habits, spend quality time with family and friends.
- Colleagues in the team who addresses first should make an early diagnosis.

- Colleagues can lend a help and share workload and provide psychological support.
- Conduct occupational health programs that include mental health and counseling for healthcare personnel.
- The health organizations must devise plans for early recognition and diagnosis who are at risk and provide psychological support and treatment in symptomatic cases.[48,49]

RADIATION

Anesthesiologists are exposed to radiations on regular basis from ionizing and nonionizing electromagnetic radiation. Well-documented consequences of radiation exposure include DNA damage, cell death, and organ injury. Ionizing radiation has enough energy to create both free radicals and ionized molecules in tissues by driving electrons completely out of their stable orbitals. If the radiation exposure is severe enough, tissues may be destroyed, or chromosomal changes may cause malignant growth. Nonionizing radiation causes damage to tissues that may result from the heat produced by the absorbed radiation.[49]

Ionizing Radiation: X-rays

Ionizing radiation interacts with cells; it can cause damage to the cells and genetic material.

The recommended annual limit is 5 rems and for pregnant or lactating workers, it should not exceed a monthly limit of 0.5 rem. Preventative strategies include limiting the intensity and exposure time, maintaining distance from the source of the radiation, and using shields to minimize the risk of radiation-induced injury.[50]

Nonionizing Radiation: Lasers

A surgical laser produces intense, focused electromagnetic radiation to cut or destroy tissues. The laser is potentially unsafe because of its intensity and the matter released from tissues during treatment. Eye injuries are the greatest risk to personnel working near lasers. Protective eyewear filters out the radiation produced by a specific type of laser while still permitting vision.[51]

SURGICAL SMOKE

During surgical procedures that use a laser or electrosurgical unit, the thermal destruction of tissue creates a smoke byproduct. The surgical smoke contains toxic gases and vapors such as benzene, hydrogen cyanide, formaldehyde, bioaerosols, dead and live cellular material (including blood fragments), and viruses. NIOSH research has shown that airborne contaminants generated by these surgical devices can be effectively controlled. Two control methods are recommended: portable smoke evacuators and room suction systems.[52]

CONCLUSION

The conduct of anesthesia itself generates a multitude of factors that cause environmental pollution and its consequences. There are multiple ways to mitigate it. Newer technologies in the future should address the need for environmentally stable and sustainable drugs and processes to ensure minimum harm to the ecological balance caused by the administration of anesthesia. There is a requirement to maintain a delicate balance between developing newer medical technology and the environmental hazards it creates. All newer technologies and drugs being developed should be environment friendly.

The practice of anesthesia puts the clinician in unique yet stressful conditions. Anesthesiologists work in an extremely stressful environment, wherein decision delays in even seconds can be catastrophic. This creates a lot of work-related pressure among anesthesiologists leading to many problems. Long, unpredictable working hours are a common norm in anesthesia, and hence the adverse toll of it on personal and professional life is tremendous. The working environment is also prone to subject them to hostile organisms. The recent COVID pandemic was an example of the risks to which anesthesiologists are subjected. There should be mechanisms both at the personal level and organizational level to ensure that these effects are minimized.

REFERENCES

1. National Aeronautics and Space Administration (NASA). (2018). Vital signs of the planet fourth warmest year in continued warming trend, according to NASA, NOAA. [online] Available from https://climate.nasa.gov/news/2841/2018-fourth-warmest-year-in-continued-warming-trend-according-to-nasa-noaa/. [Last accessed October, 2022].
2. Intergovernmental Panel on Climate Change. (2018). Global warming of 1.5°C: an IPCC special report on the impacts of global warming of 1.5°C over pre-industrial levels and related global greenhouse gas emission pathways. In: the context of strengthening the global response to the threat of climate change, sustainable development, and efforts to eradicate poverty. [online] Available from https://www.ipcc.ch/sr15/. [Last accessed October, 2022].
3. NHS England. (2017). NHS Sustainable Development Unit study report. [online] Available from https://www.england.nhs.uk/greenernhs/whats-already-happening/sustainable-development-unit-archive/ [Last accessed October, 2022]
4. American Society of Anesthesiologists. (2020). Greening the operating room and perioperative arena: environmental sustainability for anesthesia practice. [online] Available from https://www.asahq.org/about-asa/governance-and-committees/asa-committees/environmental-sustainability/greening-the-operating-room [Last accessed October, 2022].
5. Australia and New Zealand College of Anaesthetists. (2019). Statement on environmental sustainability in anaesthesia and pain medicine practice. PS64. https://www.anzca.edu.au/resources/professional-documents/standards-(1)/ps64-statementon-environmental-sustainability-in.aspx. [Last accessed October, 2022].

6. World Meteorological Organization. (2021). WMO Greenhouse Gas Bulletin: The state of greenhouse gases in the atmosphere based on global observations. [online] Available https://reliefweb.int/report/world/wmo-greenhouse-gas-bulletin-state-greenhouse-gases-atmosphere-based-global-2. [Last accessed October, 2022]
7. Chen G, Laane J, Wheeler SE, Zhang Z. Greenhouse gas molecules: a mathematical perspective. Not Am Math Soc. 2011;58:1421-34.
8. Petty G. A first course in atmospheric radiation. Madison, WI: Sundog Publishing; 2006.
9. The United Nations Environment. Environmental rights and governance. Montreal Protocol. [online] Available from https://www.unenvironment.org/ozonaction/who-weare/about-montreal-protocol. [Last accessed October 2022].
10. United Nations Framework Convention on Climate Change. (2016). The Paris agreement. [online] Available from https://unfccc.int/process-and-meetings/the-parisagreement/the-paris-agreement. [Last accessed October, 2022].
11. Charlesworth M, Swinton F. Anaesthetic gases, climate change, and sustainable practice. Lancet Planet Health. 2017 Sep;1(6):e216-e217. doi: 10.1016/S2542-5196(17)30040-2. Epub 2017 Jun 16. PMID: 29851604.
12. Muret J, Fernandes TD, Gerlach H, Imberger G, Jornvall H, Lawson C, et al. Environmental impacts of nitrous oxide: no laughing matter!. Br J Anaesth. 2019;123:e481-2.
13. White S, Shelton CL. Abandoning inhalational anaesthesia. Anaesthesia. 2020;75:451-4.
14. https://noharm-europe.org/sites/default/files/documents-files/5250/2017-11_RCoA_slides_JMT_Pierce.pdf.
15. Linden-Snders A, Nielsen N, Bentzer P. Klimateffekterna fran anestesinkan minska [Climate footprint of halogenated inhalation anesthetics]. Lakartidningen. 2019;116:FR9L (Swedish).
16. McGain F, Muret J, Lawson C, Sherman JD. Environmental sustainability in anaesthesia and critical care. Br J Anaesth. 2020;125(5):680-92.
17. European Environment Agency. EU greenhouse gas inventory. [online] Available from https://www.eea.europa.eu/themes/climate/eu-greenhouse-gas-inventory. [Last accessed October 2022].
18. Ecoinvent Centre. (2015). Ecoinvent d the world's most consistent & transparent life cycle inventory database. [online] Available from https://ecoinvent.org/the-ecoinvent-database. [Last accessed October 2022].
19. Sanchez SA, Eckelman MJ, Sherman JD. Environmental and economic comparison of reusable and disposable blood pressure cuffs in multiple clinical settings. Resour Conserv Recycl. 2020;155:104643.
20. Malik A, Lenzen M, McAlister S, McGain F. The carbon footprint of Australian health care. Lancet Planet Health. 2018;2:e27-35.
21. McAlister S, Barratt AL, Bell KJ, McGain F. The carbon footprint of pathology testing. Med J Aust. 2020;212:377-82.
22. Eckelman MJ, Sherman JD, MacNeill AJ. Life cycle environmental emissions and health damages from the Canadian healthcare system: an economic-environmental-epidemiological analysis. PLoS Med. 2018;15:e1002623.

23. Dettenkofer M, Kümmerer K, Schuster A, Mühlich M, Scherrer M, Daschner FD. Environmental auditing in hospitals: approach and implementation in a university hospital. J Hosp Infect. 1997;36:17-22.
24. McGain F, Story D, Lim T, McAlister S. Financial and environmental costs of reusable and single-use anaesthetic equipment. Br J Anaesth. 2017;118:862-9.
25. MacNeill AJ, Hopf H, Khanuja A, Alizamir S, Bilec M, Eckelman MJ, et al. Transforming the medical device industry: road map to a circular economy. Health Affairs. 2020;39:2088-97.
26. Sherman JD, LAt Raibley, Eckelman MJ. Life cycle assessment and costing methods for device procurement: comparing reusable and single-use disposable laryngoscopes. Anesth Analg. 2018;127:434-43.
27. Parvatker AG, Tunceroglu H, Sherman JD, Coish P, Anastas P, Zimmerman JB, et al. Cradle-to-gate greenhouse gas emissions for twenty anesthetic active pharmaceutical ingredients based on process scale-up and process design calculations. ACS Sustain Chem Eng. 2019;7:6580-91.
28. McAlister S, Ou Y, Neff E, Hapgood K, Story D, Mealey P, McGain F. The Environmental footprint of morphine: a life cycle assessment from opium poppy farming to the packaged drug. BMJ Open. 2016 Oct 21;6(10):e013302. doi: 10.1136/bmjopen-2016-013302. PMID: 27798031; PMCID: PMC5093647.
29. Sherman J, Le C, Lamers V, Eckelman M. Life cycle greenhouse gas emissions of anesthetic drugs. Anesth Analg. 2012;114:1086-90.
30. Sherman JD, Barrick B. Total intravenous anesthetic versus inhaled anesthetic: pick your poison. Anesth Analg. 2019;128:13-5.
31. Jensen A, Petersen P. Energy efficiency in hospitals and laboratories. Proc of ECEE, 2011 France: Summer Study Toulon; 2011; 5-10.
32. Axelrod D, Bell C, Feldman J. Greening the operating room and perioperative arena: environmental sustainability for anesthesia practice. Schaumburg, IL: American Society of Anaesthesiologists; 2015. [online] Available from https://www.asahq.org/about-asa/governance-and-committees/asa-committees/environmental-sustainability/greening-the-operating-room. [Last accessed October 2022].
33. Hass SA, Andersen ST, Andersen MPS, Nielsen OJ. Atmospheric chemistry of methoxyflurane ($CH_3OCF_2CHCl_2$): kinetics of the gas-phase reactions with OH radicals, Cl atoms and O3. Chem Phys Lett. 2019;722:119-23.
34. Grand View Research. Market Analysis report. Inhalational anaesthesia market size share & trends analysis report by application (induction, maintenance), by product (Sevoflurane, Isoflurane, Desflurane), by region, and segment forecasts, 2019-2025. [online] Available from https://www.grandviewresearch.com/industry-analysis/inhalation-anesthesia-market. [Last accessed October 2022].
35. The Sustainable Development Unit, UK. (2014). Identifying high greenhouse gas intensity prescription items for NHS in England. [online] Available from https://www.fph.org.uk/media/3126/k9-fph-sig-nhs-carbon-footprint-final.pdf. [Last accessed October 2022].
36. Thiel CL, Schehlein E, Ravilla T, Ravindran RD, Robin AL, Saeedi OJ, et al. Cataract surgery and environmental sustainability: waste and lifecycle assessment of phacoemulsification at a private healthcare facility. J Cataract Refract Surg. 2017;43:1391-8.
37. Healthcare Plastics Recycling Council. (2019). Telling the story: how to effectively communicate your hospital recycling program's successes and lessons learned.

[online] Available from https://www.hprc.org/resources/communicating-your-hospital-recycling-program-successes-and-lessons-learned/. [Last accessed October, 2022].
38. The Vinyl Council of Australia. (2012). PVC recovery in hospitals. [online] Available from https://www.vinyl.org.au/pvc-recycling-in-hospitals. [Last accessed October, 2022].
39. Wyssusek KH, Foong WM, Steel C, Gillespie BM. The gold in garbage: implementing a waste segregation and recycling initiative. AORN J. 2016;103:316. e1-8.
40. McGain F, Story D, Lim T, McAlister S. Response to 'Healthcare and ecological economics at a crossroads'. Br J Ananesth. 2017;119:1057-8.
41. Association of Anaesthetists RCoA, College of Anaesthetists of Ireland. (2017). Joint environmental policy statement. [online] Available from https://anaesthetists.org/Portals/0/PDFs/Environment/Joint%20Environmental%20Policy%20Statement%20-%20FINAL.pdf?ver=2019-05-12-081735-747. [Last accessed October, 2022].
42. Australian and New Zealand College of Anaesthetists. (2019). Statement on environmental sustainability in anaesthesia and pain medicine practice, 2019. [online] Available from http://www.anzca.edu.au/documents/ps64-statement-on-environmental-sustainability-in.pdf. [Last accessed October 2022].
43. Siegel JD, Rhinehart E, Jackson M, Chiarello L; Health Care Infection Control Practices Advisory Committee. (2007). Guideline for isolation precautions: preventing transmission of infectious agents in health care settings. Am J Infect Control. 2007;35(10 Suppl 2):S65-164.
44. Sehulster L, Chinn RYW. Guidelines for environmental infection control in health-care facilities: recommendations of CDC and the healthcare infection control practices advisory committee (HICPAC). MMWR Recomm Rep. 2003;52(RR-10):1-43.
45. U.S. Department of Labor. Occupational Safety and Health Administration: Occupational Exposure to Bloodborne Pathogens; Needlestick and Other Sharps Injuries; Final Rule: (29 CFR, Part 1910). Washington, DC: U.S. Department of Labor: 2001.
46. Centers for disease control and prevention. Immunization of healthcare personnel. MMWR. 2011;60(7):2-29.
47. Barash, Paul G. Clinical Anesthesia, 8th edition. Philadelphia, PA: Wolters Kluwer Health/Lippincott Williams & Wilkins; 2017.
48. Occupational Well-being in Anesthesiologists. In: Duval Neto GF (Ed). Rio de Janeiro: Brazilian Society of Anesthesiology; 2014. p. 286.
49. Ronald MD. Miller's Anesthesia, 9th edition. Philadelphia, PA: Churchill Livingstone/Elsevier; 2020.
50. Jackson SH. The role of stress in anesthetists' health and well-being. Acta Anaesthesiol Scand. 1999;43(6):583-602.
51. Calabrese G: Guía de Prevención y Protección de los Riesgos Profesionales del Anestesiólogo. Anest Analg Rean Dic. 2006;20(2):4-40.
52. Occupational Safety and Health Administration, United States Department of Labor. Maximum Permissible Dose Equivalent for Occupational Exposure. [online] Available from http://www.osha.gov/SLTC/radiationionizing/intrtoionizinglionizingattachmentsix.html. [Last accessed October 2022].

CHAPTER

19

Enhanced Surgical Recovery Programs and Cancer Outcomes

Anoushka Afonso, Vijaya Gottumukkala

ABSTRACT

Globally, cancer is the second leading cause of death after cardiovascular diseases. As perioperative physicians, we will encounter a growing demand for anesthesia services for perioperative and periprocedural care during the patient's cancer journey. Despite significant advances in biological and targeted therapies for cancer care, surgery will continue to be a mainstay strategy for reducing tumor burden, particularly for solid tumors. Anesthesiologists should be well informed on the immediate and long-term systemic effects of cancer therapies (organ toxicities) and their effects on nutrition, fatigue, anemia, and physical deconditioning, all of which could influence surgical recovery and long-term outcomes. Recovery after surgery is of utmost importance for cancer patients as decreased cancer recurrence and improved survival occurs in patients who return to complete their planned adjuvant cancer treatment earlier than later.

Keywords: Cancer; Enhanced surgical recovery programs (ESRPs); Perioperative outcomes; Return to intended oncologic therapy (RIOT).

KEY POINTS

- Cancer is among the leading causes of death worldwide.
- Surgery is a mainstay strategy for reducing tumor burden, particularly for solid tumors.
- The goals of care for the surgical patient must be a margin-free resection, along with care pathways to minimize complications and enhance functional recovery.
- Enhanced surgical recovery programs facilitate earlier return to planned adjuvant therapies and improved cancer outcomes.

INTRODUCTION

Globally, cancer is the second leading cause of death in the developed world.[1,2] It is estimated that up to 50% of in-patient admissions worldwide are for a diagnosis of cancer.[3] As cancer prevalence increases over time, an even larger number of cancer patients will need anesthesia services for perioperative and periprocedural care. Despite significant advances in cancer care, surgery will continue to be a mainstay strategy for reducing tumor burden, particularly for solid tumors. Frequently chemoradiation therapies are administered before surgical resection as neoadjuvant therapy or after the surgical resection as adjuvant therapies to minimize the risk of locoregional or distant metastasis and prolong disease-free survival. In addition to routine presurgical evaluation and optimization, patients with cancer need special perioperative considerations. These relate to evaluating and optimizing the anatomic and physiological effects of cancer on specific organ function, paraneoplastic effects of cancer, and the systemic effects of cancer therapies. Anesthesia providers should, therefore, be cognizant of immediate and long-term systemic effects of cancer therapies (organ toxicities) and the effects of chemoradiation on nutrition, fatigue, anemia, and physical deconditioning, all of which could influence the recovery profile after major surgery.

To optimize surgical care and enhance oncological outcomes, multidisciplinary programs should be implemented in the perioperative care continuum to minimize symptom burden, enhance functional recovery, and minimize preventable postoperative complications. These coordinated multidisciplinary care pathways and principles of care aimed to enhance the functional recovery of the surgical patient are the enhanced surgical recovery programs (ESRPs) **(Fig. 1)**. ESRP focuses on minimizing the neuroinflammatory signaling (stress) response to surgical trauma through minimal access surgery when indicated, utilizing procedure-specific multimodal opioid-sparing strategies, minimizing periprocedural

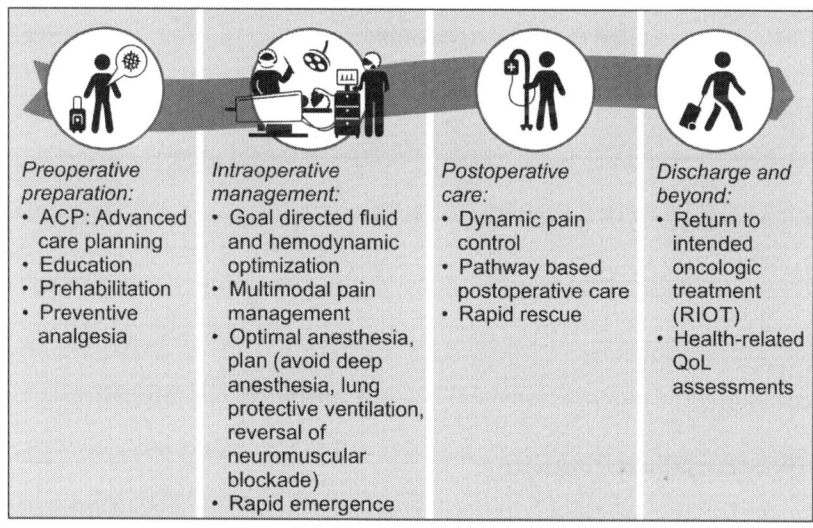

Fig. 1: Enhanced recovery of cancer care.

oxygen debt, providing optimal anesthesia care with an emphasis on rapid emergence, utilizing lung protective ventilatory strategies, and ensuring complete reversal from neuromuscular blockade. In addition, the postoperative phase demands a focused approach to safely implement early drinking, eating, and ambulating measures. An important postoperative component of enhanced recovery principles is procedure-specific pathway-based care and institution of monitoring systems for rapid rescue from postoperative complications.[4] The enhanced recovery pathways, therefore, have specific elements of care in the preoperative, intraoperative, postoperative, and postdischarge phases of surgical practice. Adherence to the key elements in each phase of care is vital to improve outcomes for surgical patients. Gustafsson et al. indicated a dose–response relationship between enhanced recovery after surgery (ERAS) protocol adherence and clinical outcomes after major colorectal surgery.[5]

While earlier recovery to baseline function without major postoperative complications is important for any surgical patient population, this is particularly relevant for patients with cancer as frequently adjuvant therapies are part of the cancer care plan for many diseases. In pancreatic,[6] thoracic,[7] and breast cancer,[8] there is a correlation between postoperative complications, timely delivery of adjuvant therapies, and survival. Delaying adjuvant therapies after a successful ablative surgery lead to a worse prognosis. Common causes for delayed adjuvant therapies are postoperative complications, postoperative fatigue, and poor general physical condition (a general measure of recovery after major surgery). One of the major goals for surgical patients with cancer should, therefore, be earlier functional recovery after surgery to get back to their intended oncologic therapy. Thus, every enhanced recovery protocol implemented for cancer patients should consider the stage of the disease, overall prognosis, appropriateness of care for maintaining the quality of life (QoL) and ability to withstand the treatment plan, risks associated with therapies, and patient's wishes for overall goals of care.

PREOPERATIVE PREPARATION

In addition to routine presurgical evaluation and medical optimization of comorbidities, surgical patients with cancer have certain special considerations. The critical components encompass preoperative care of patients with cancer are advanced care planning, patient education, prehabilitation, anemia management, and nutritional optimization.

Advanced Care Planning

Cancer treatments frequently utilize an exorbitant number of resources, particularly during advanced stage disease with little to no chance for a cure, and often at the expense of adding meaningful years with an acceptable QoL that meets the patient's wishes. This is also true during end-of-life care, with increased hospitalization rates, intensive care unit stays, several emergency department visits in the last month of life, and consistently high rates of terminal hospitalizations.[9] Unfortunately, approximately 25–30% of terminally ill cancer patients will die in the hospital rather than at home with their families.[9]

Unlike noncancer conditions, functional decline is an innate characteristic of cancer's trajectory. Preoperative period is a critical phase in which patients can benefit from advanced care planning (ACP) and early introduction of palliative care principles for symptom management and psychosocial behavior management.[9,10] Professional oncologic organizations such as the National Comprehensive Care Network (NCCN) and the American Society of Clinical Oncology (ASCO) have long emphasized the importance of ACP in providing optimal palliative care.[9,11] Shahrokni et al. demonstrated that in oncogeriatric patients (aged ≥75 years), the comprehensive geriatric assessment (CGA) deficits were strongly associated with 6-month mortality, whereas the ASA classification was not.[12] Additionally, measuring frailty in older cancer patients can potentially identify those with an increased risk of treatment complications. Data from 20 studies with over 2,900 older cancer patients reported a frailty prevalence of 42% (range 6–86%). Frailty is independently associated with increased postoperative mortality [HR: 2.67, 95% confidence interval (CI): 1.08–6.62], along with increasing treatment-related complications (OR: 4.86, 95% CI: 2.19–10.78).[13] Accurate evaluation of risk for perioperative complications, along with discussion about the available treatment options, including the prognosis after surgery concerning the expected QoL, should form the mainstay of informed choice and consent. This exercise will form the foundation for shared decision-making and ACP, fulfilling patients' choices, expectations, and goals for care.

Education

A well-designed preoperative education program sets the stage for patient empowerment and improved outcomes through the oncologic perioperative journey. Usually, preoperative education begins in the surgical office, continues through the preadmission clinic and testing, and is emphasized during the preadmission phase on the day of surgery when these patients and families come into the hospital. Additionally, it is important to provide patients and families with a detailed understanding of their surgical procedure, so there are clear expectations and anticipation for potential events that could happen during the perioperative period. Setting patient expectations regarding pain management, ambulation, and resuming oral intake can pave the way for accelerated recovery. It has been demonstrated that perioperative education is associated with decreased anxiety, better postoperative outcomes, and improved patient and family satisfaction.[4] Providing patients with appropriate educational materials that they can read and instructions that are written in clear, simple language can also facilitate clear learning.[4] Pereira et al. showed 104 patients that an empathic patient-centered approach could reduce preoperative anxiety and increase surgical recovery and patient satisfaction.[14]

Prehabilitation

In addition to optimizing the nutritional status of the cancer patient, prehabilitation strategies should be implemented during the preoperative period to decrease the psychological and physiological stress associated with surgery.[15] Cancer prehabilitation is "a process during the continuum of care that occurs between the time of cancer diagnosis and the beginning of acute treatment, which includes physical and psychological assessments to establish a baseline functional level, identify modifiable impairments, and provide targeted interventions to improve patient's health to reduce the incidence and the severity of current and future impairments".[16] Prehabilitation programs implementing an effective exercise regimen before surgery have demonstrated a faster return to functional baseline status.[15,17] Exercise capacity is a strong marker for health status and is associated with increased functional status and decreased morbidity and mortality.[18] Because delays in cancer treatment can lead to poor outcomes, the timing of prehabilitation implementation as it relates to the anticipated date of surgery is critical when building an exercise regimen.[16] As little as 3 weeks before surgery may be sufficient to build up physiological reserves, which can further improve surgical outcomes.[15] Additionally, the integration of neoadjuvant radiation therapy and chemotherapy expands the window in which exercise prehabilitation can be implemented.[4,15] Prehabilitation also provides psychological benefits to cancer patients, as it gives them a sense of control over their state of health and thereby decreases anxiety.[17] Psychological interventions should also be implemented in the prehabilitation landscape to address any psychiatric disturbances (i.e., depression, anxiety, etc.) and provide psychosocial support,[16] as a cancer diagnosis can be particularly burdensome mentally and emotionally.

Cancer patients who undergo neoadjuvant chemotherapy often have a decline in overall physical fitness, which is associated with the worst outcome after surgery.[19] Preoperative exercise training may have an important benefit for surgical outcome and recovery after surgery in cancer patients.[20] Licker and colleagues demonstrated that high-interval training (HIT) resulted in "significant improvement in aerobic performances, but failed to reduce early complications after lung cancer resection".[21] Objective measures of physical fitness such as cardiopulmonary exercise testing (CPET) have shown an association between decreased exercise capacity and postoperative morbidity.[22] The effect of exercise on cancer patients was evaluated by Loughney and colleagues.[23] They showed acceptable adherence rates and safety with preoperative exercise regimens in patients scheduled for neoadjuvant chemotherapy and surgery. The concept of the "dual hit" of neoadjuvant chemotherapy and surgery was explored in the context of preoperative exercise training. Larger randomized controlled trials are necessary to truly evaluate the effect of preoperative exercise programs in different cancer populations.

Wijeysundera and colleagues[24] did an elegant multicenter international prospective trial comparing preoperative subjective assessment with alternative markers of fitness, such as CPET, serum N-terminal pro-B-type natriuretic peptide (NT pro-BNP), and Duke Activity Status Index (DASI) questionnaire scores, for predicting death or complications after major elective noncardiac surgery. They included 1,404 patients in the study, with 28 (2%) having died or suffering from a myocardial infarction within 30 days of surgery. Subjective assessment of preoperative functional capacity consistently performed poorly and did not predict postoperative myocardial complications, while the simple DASI questionnaire was associated with the improved prediction.

Anemia Management

Preoperative anemia in cancer patients is prevalent and associated with a higher risk factor for perioperative transfusion, increased morbidity, and poor oncological outcomes.[25] The pathophysiology of anemia in the cancer patient is multifactorial, including nutritional deficiencies, anemia of chronic disease, and marrow suppression due to cancer and chemotherapeutic agents that affect red blood cell production. Surgical recovery in cancer patients can be improved with interventions for treatable anemia in the preoperative period. For example, Munoz et al.[26] describe a patient blood management strategy that involves a multidisciplinary multimodal individualized approach for addressing perioperative anemia in the colorectal cancer patient population. Treating anemia early and aggressively in colorectal patients allows for optimization of preoperative hemoglobin, which reduces the transfusion risk and improves overall outcomes.[26] Iron therapy, erythropoiesis-stimulating agents when indicated, and active blood management protocols should be routine practice. Follow-up in the postoperative period is vital as patients often receive adjuvant chemotherapy and radiotherapy. For the long-term success of blood management programs, technology integration, as well as patient and clinician educational programs, is critical for implementation and sustainability.

Nutrition

Nutritional optimization is important to increase anabolism and minimize the catabolic state in the postoperative period. Malnourished surgical patients benefit from perioperative nutrition. Klek S et al. and colleagues aimed to assess the clinical significance of route and type of nutritional support (enteral, parenteral, standard, or immunomodulating) in the perioperative setting of malnourished cancer patients with comparable results.[27] However, another prospective randomized trial that implemented the administration of a supplemented enteral formula during the perioperative period reported a significant difference in reducing postoperative infections and length of stay in cancer patients undergoing surgery.[28] A double-blinded randomized control trial, which provided a more comprehensive prehabilitation program with nutritional counseling, whey protein intake, exercise, and psychological care interventions initiated 4 weeks prior for patients undergoing colorectal resection showed a clinically meaningful improvement in functional walking capacity.[29] Optimizing functional capacity and minimizing complications are the cornerstone of most enhanced recovery programs.

Optimizing the Nutritional Status of a Cancer Patient before Surgery

In high-risk patients, objective perioperative nutritional screening should be used to assess a cancer patient's nutritional status.[18] Adequate tests that can be used to evaluate nutritional status before surgery include the nutritional risk indicator (NRI), the patient-generated subjective-global-assessment (PG-SGA), and nutritional risk screening tests such as Reilly's NRS.[4] Each of these tests provides a scoring system that categorizes the nutritional status of the patient, which can then be used as a guideline to triage and implement proper preoperative nutrition protocols. Malnutrition is a risk factor for increased mortality, complications, costs, and readmission,[4,30] as well as decreased functional status and reduced QoL.[9,31] Malnutrition and subsequent weight loss in cancer may be related to a combination of factors including undernutrition, cancer catabolism, and inflammation, which can further lead to cachexia and sarcopenia.[30] Furthermore, there is an increased risk of gradual nutritional decline during the perioperative period; thus, it is imperative to decrease the deleterious metabolic effects of oncological treatments by correcting for nutritional deficiencies.[30] When managing the nutritional status of a cancer patient before surgery, strategies should be implemented that avoid decreasing insulin resistance, prevent negative protein balance, and modulate the immune system.[18] Additionally, when determining the proper nutritional intervention necessary for treating the cancer patient, it should be determined if a patient's cancer therapy is high-risk or low-risk with regards with its impact on the patient's nutritional status.[32] Utilizing both the patient's baseline nutritional status and the risk of nutritional deterioration associated with their treatment regimen, nutritional intervention can be determined for those who fall below the threshold for adequate preoperative nutrition.[32]

For those deemed malnourished before surgery, nutritional supplementation should be implemented 5–7 days before surgery via enteral or total parenteral nutrition as an alternative, if needed.[4,18,33] However, total parenteral nutrition should be implemented 7–10 days before surgery.[33] Enteral feeding is preferred to total parental feeding, however, as it has lower risk of complications and reduced length of stay for patients that are critically ill.[18] In addition to properly correcting for any nutritional deficiencies before surgery, there are key steps that should be taken immediately before surgery to optimize recovery. Patients should receive liberal hydration with an intake of clear liquids up to 2 hours before scheduled arrival for surgery. Rather than fasting before surgery, patients should consume clear carbohydrate beverages to allow for the replication of normal metabolic responses and place the patient in a fed state before surgery.[4,33] This method can decrease the body's metabolic stress response to surgery, thereby decreasing the risk of postoperative complications.[4,33] Furthermore, a carbohydrate drink may decrease protein loss by placing patients in an anabolic state.[18] As cancer patients mostly have a low immune function, immune supplementation is intended to improve the immune status of these patients. However, guidelines that referred to specific immune nutrients (fish oils and glutamine), as well as vitamin C, have not been adequately cited or studied. Given that there is cancer-related inflammation and cachexia in our patients, an investigation into anti-inflammatory and immune-enhancing interventions could be the next focus of research from a cancer standpoint.

One must also balance the heterogeneity in nutrition guidelines with their cancer patients. Zhao and colleagues demonstrated that the quality of the nutrition care guidelines was highly variable for cancer patients.[34] Upon further analyses, heterogeneity was due to insufficient attention to nutrition risk screening, differences in nutritional assessment recommendations, immune nutrient support, and lack of high-quality research on energy and nitrogen demand.

INTRAOPERATIVE MANAGEMENT

Postoperative Nausea and Vomiting Prophylaxis

As stated by Wesmiller et al., postoperative nausea and vomiting (PONV) has a large impact on the overall health of breast cancer patients and is related to significant morbidity (dehydration, wound dehiscence, pain, and immobility).[35] In women with breast cancer, PONV has a significant impact on both the well-being and health of these women. In addition, PONV is also related to significant morbidities such as immobility and dehydration, to name a few.[36] PONV should also be addressed vigilantly in the cancer patient population during the preoperative period to minimize its potential effects. After surgery, as many as 80% of women with early stage breast cancer experience PONV.[35,37] PONV prophylaxis before surgery is recommended rather than reactively treating and addressing PONV as it occurs.[4] A risk assessment of PONV can be conducted using the Apfel score.[4] The Apfel score evaluates the risk of PONV by using female gender, nonsmoking status, history of PONV, and administration of postoperative opioids as predictive measures.[4,37] Because prophylaxis for PONV is expensive, it is important to identify those at a higher risk and provide them with targeted prophylaxis.[38] Low-risk patients should not receive prophylaxis for PONV unless the surgery is emetogenic.[38] However, for those that are at moderate-to-high risk for PONV, combination therapy that targets more than one type of receptor may be more effective than single therapy for prophylaxis.

For surgeries that are at high risk for PONV, such as gynecological, laparoscopic, head and neck, intra-abdominal, and breast procedures, as well as those that are of longer duration, PONV prophylaxis should be administered regardless of Apfel score.[38] In the context of cancer patients, preoperative psychological factors can intensify the severity of PONV in patients with breast cancer.[35,39] Despite the use of multiple antiemetic agents, almost 30% of women after breast cancer surgery had experienced nausea, with 10% having both nausea and vomiting.[35]

Fluid Management and Hemodynamic Optimization

Fluid management of the patient should be optimized throughout the perioperative period with the goal of a euvolemic, hydrated state before surgery.[40] For the cancer patient, preoperative radiation and chemotherapy can cause treatment-related diarrhea, leading to dehydration and fluid depletion.[41] Radiation can cause increased intestinal motility, while chemotherapy causes damage to the intestinal mucosa—leading to decreased absorption.[41] Prolonged fasting and bowel preparations should be avoided, as they may lead to dehydration before surgery.[40] Thus, it is important to ensure that the surgical cancer patient is optimized throughout the perioperative period. Perioperative goal-directed fluid therapy (GDFT) is "the concept of using indices of continuous blood flow and/or tissue oxygen saturation to optimize end-organ function."[4] Monitoring dynamic flow indices can be used to predict the hemodynamic effects of fluid administration to optimize oxygen delivery to tissues.[18] GDFT should be customized to patients' surgical risk, vascular access, monitoring needs, and the operating context to optimize hemodynamic stability.[4,40,42] During surgery, fluid administration should be carefully adjusted to reduce perioperative organ dysfunction and restore tissue perfusion and cellular oxygenation.[4] Intraoperative fluid management should aim to maintain euvolemia and minimize excess salt and water through low-crystalloid therapy and fluid boluses (when necessary) to replace blood/fluid loss and maintain intravascular volume.[40] GDFT may decrease major complications, length of stay, and improve outcomes.[4,40] However, in a recent meta-analysis in noncardiac surgical patients, GDFT does have a questionable benefit over standard care as it relates to postoperative mortality, length of intensive care unit (ICU) stay, and length of hospital stay.[43] However, the incidence of all complications, including wound infection, abdominal complications, and postoperative hypotension, is reduced.[43] There is no evidence of benefit for using crystalloid or hydroxyethyl starch (HES) for colorectal cancer surgery for GDFT, despite a lower 24-hour fluid balance with HES.[43,44] In addition, results from a pragmatic international trial showed that among patients at increased risk for complications during major abdominal surgery, a restrictive fluid group was not associated with a high rate of disability-free survival than a liberal fluid regimen but was associated with a higher rate of acute kidney injury (8.6 vs. 5.0%; $p < 0.001$).[45] And, in a randomized trial of high-risk patients undergoing major gastrointestinal surgery,[46] use of cardiac output-guided hemodynamic therapy algorithm compared with usual care did not reduce the composite outcome of complications and 30-day mortality. We must consider the results from both the trials above as we apply optimal fluid management for our cancer patients.

Salmasi and colleagues[47] showed that mean arterial pressure (MAP) below absolute thresholds of 65 mm Hg or relative thresholds of 20% were progressively related to myocardial and kidney injury. At any given threshold, prolonged exposure to hypotension was associated with increased odds of myocardial and kidney injury. Furthermore, there were no clinically important interactions between preoperative blood pressures and the relationship between hypotension and myocardial or kidney injury at intraoperative mean arterial blood pressures over 65 mm Hg. The authors concluded that anesthetic management could thus be based on intraoperative blood pressures without regard to preoperative systolic blood pressure. A recent review on preoperative hypertension mentioned that most of the data about perioperative blood pressure management are based on epidemiological data rather than randomized controlled trials, hence, that it may not be appropriate to defer anesthesia and surgery in a patient with mild or moderate hypertension. The anesthesiologist shares the responsibility to ensure that a patient with persistently elevated blood pressure during preassessment is referred for further management before or after surgery as appropriate.[48] To minimize oxygen debt, optimal management of fluid therapy, cardiac index (stroke volume), perfusion pressure, and anemia indices must be considered in totality and not in isolation.

Multimodal Pain Management

Because pain can prolong recovery time and delay discharge, it is important to optimize pain management throughout the perioperative period.[49] Multimodal analgesia is a key element of the ERAS pathway that is defined as "the use of more than one modality of pain control to achieve effective analgesia while reducing opioid-related side effects".[49] The concept of a multimodal analgesic plan allows us to improve postoperative analgesia and reduce the incidence of any opioid-related effects. Multimodal pain management consists of the combinatory use of analgesics with different modes of action to minimize side effects and maximize analgesic effects.[50] Multiple agents that act at different receptors within the central and peripheral nervous system to improve pain control should be utilized intraoperatively and postoperatively. Nonopioid analgesics include nonsteroidal anti-inflammatory drugs (NSAIDs), acetaminophen, paracetamol, α-2 agonists, ketamine, gabapentin-type drugs, dexamethasone, neuraxial/regional techniques using local anesthetics, hypnosis, and acupuncture. Ultimately, multimodal analgesia serves to minimize the postsurgical length of stay, accelerate recovery, and improve outcomes.[49] Pain management strategies should be carefully planned, initiated before incision, tailored precisely to patient-specific considerations, and geared toward the surgical procedure the patient is undergoing. This careful selection of pain management can allow for the best outcomes for cancer patients.[2] Because pain secondary to cancer is a common occurrence due to the pathophysiology of cancer and therapeutic interventions,[2] anesthesiologists must take cancer pain into account when planning an analgesic regimen for their cancer patients. Additionally, surgical interventions for cancer therapies are complex—adequate analgesia should be administered that allows for improved functionality to allow patients to return to chemotherapy and radiation therapy expeditiously.[2] Analgesic plans should aim for early mobilization, decreased perioperative complications, and improved quality care, in addition to lowering pain in the cancer patient.[50] In addition, controversy exists around perioperative opioids and cancer recurrence. Currently, there is no level 1 evidence that opioids influence the perioperative period. Recent meta-analysis[51] showed no conclusive evidence to avoid the use of opioids to reduce the risk of recurrence in colorectal cancer. Stress reduction and optimal pain control for our surgical cancer patients should be the goal, with opioids for rescue if needed.

Avoiding Hypothermia

Avoiding hypothermia is also part of the optimal anesthetic plan for cancer patients undergoing an enhanced recovery protocol. Enhanced recovery programs emphasize the need for maintenance of normothermia, as perioperative hypothermia is associated with poor outcomes that could be preventable. Perioperative hypothermia causes impaired pharmacodynamics, surgical site infections, coagulopathy, increased transfusion requirements, thermal discomfort, prolonged recovery, and prolonged duration of hospitalization. Measurement of central core temperature, maintaining normothermia, and consequent warming of patients in the perioperative period are, therefore, essential.[52] In the NICE (National Institute for Health and Clinical Excellence) guidelines,[53] there is acceptable evidence showing a significant dependence of surgical wound infection and incidence of morbid cardiac events on the incident of inadvertent perioperative hypothermia (IPH). In addition, a complete reversal of neuromuscular blockade and lung-protective ventilation strategies are strategies in an optimal anesthesia plan for ERAS for cancer patients.

POSTOPERATIVE CARE

Pain Management Maintenance

In postoperative care during the perioperative period, continued effective pain management, complication-free recovery, reduced symptom burden, and enhanced QoL should be emphasized for the cancer patient. Postsurgically, major physiological changes can occur, which can delay recovery.[4] Pain, in particular, can amplify these physiologic changes, thereby increasing the time to restoration to baseline function.[54] Similar to intraoperative multimodal pain management strategies, this approach should be also utilized postoperatively.[49] Postoperative analgesia should focus on maximizing the pharmacologic benefits while minimizing side effects to allow for enhanced recovery and functional restoration to ultimately improve outcomes.[4,49]

Postsurgical Complications and Return to Intended Oncological Therapies

The concept of return to intended oncological therapies (RIOTs) was introduced by Kim and colleagues[55] as a novel metric to measure and monitor perioperative interventions impact functional recovery in cancer patients. RIOT has two components: whether the patient did or did not initiate intended oncologic therapies after surgery and the time between surgery and initiation of these therapies.[56] When RIOT was introduced into the enhanced recovery pathways, the team noted significant practice change management. For example, in colon cancer patients with metastases to the liver, the identified RIOT rate was 75%. During the introduction of ERP in the liver surgery department, the RIOT rate increased to 95%.[57] Merkow et al. analyzed the American College of Surgeons National Surgical Quality Improvement Program and the National Cancer Database from

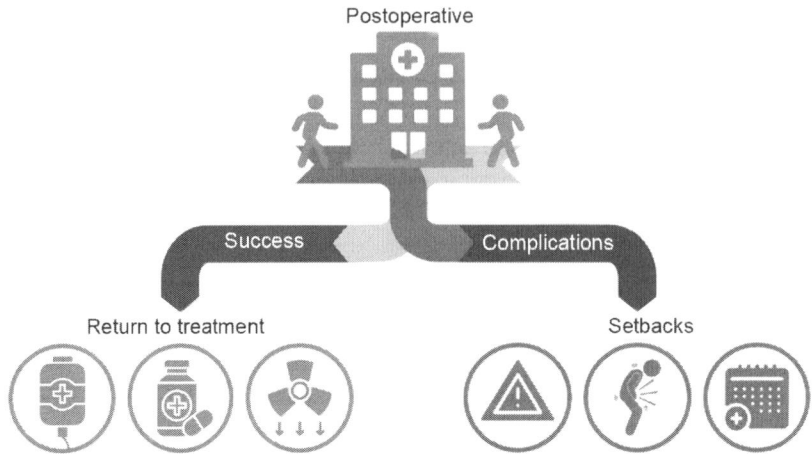

Fig. 2: Return to intended oncologic treatment (RIOT).

2006 to 2009. It showed that 61.8% of the patients who did not experience complications after pancreatic resection for stages I-III adenocarcinoma received adjuvant chemotherapy.[58] Patients with no complications had a median time of 52 days to adjuvant chemotherapy, and patients with complications such as deep surgical-site infections had a median time of 70 days to adjuvant chemotherapy. Breast cancer overall survival is dependent on both completion and amount of adjuvant chemotherapy. If a delay is >12 weeks, recurrent free survival and overall survival are adversely affected.[8] The survival rate of cancer patients undergoing surgical procedures is highly dependent on the biology of the tumor, comorbidities associated with cancer, effects of cancer and cancer therapies on QoL and functionality, and the impact of surgery on recovery.[56] Implementation of an enhanced recovery protocol was associated with receiving on-time adjuvant chemotherapy, defined by ≤8 weeks postoperatively, in a colorectal cohort of 363 patients.[59] In the nonsmall cell lung cancer patient, enhanced recovery after thoracic surgery is associated with improved adjuvant chemotherapy completion.[60] Enhanced recovery pathways can potentially allow for a more rapid recovery and shortened time to patient oncologic therapy, which has a meaningful impact on survival **(Fig. 2)**.

Health-related Quality of Life Assessment

After discharge, patient recovery and health QoL measures are an increasingly valuable component in the landscape of ERAS.[4] While morbidity and mortality serve as markers for surgical outcomes, health-related QoL should be incorporated in the overall postoperative assessment of the cancer patient.[61] Health-related QoL assessment is a subjective measure answered by the patient that is used to determine how the patient's health state affects their QoL through the evaluation of various health domains.[62] Additionally, health-related QoL is a multidimensional measure that encompasses psychological, social, and physical well-being.[61] Each of these measures should be globally assessed in the cancer patient to allow for the optimization of treatment and overall well-being.[61] The assessment of the QoL for cancer patients can evaluate complications and side effects,[61] both of which can have deleterious effects on functional recovery. Additionally, QoL assessments can help to determine the most appropriate surgical procedure[61] that incorporates the needs of the cancer patient and the goals of the surgical oncologist. In the case of palliative care, it is especially important to consider the impact that surgical procedures may have on a cancer patient's QoL. The treatment of cancer patients can be rather complex[63]—often utilizing chemotherapy or radiation in addition to surgery as treatment modalities. While this multifactorial approach may serve as a curative treatment, the morbidities associated with these therapies can lead to a decreased QoL. The prospect of a cure may make toxicity associated with cancer treatment acceptable and tolerable.[62] However, for cancer patients with a decreased probability of cure, these adverse side effects may be less acceptable.[62] Thus, it is important to assess the QoL measures to ensure that the patient has the best possible QoL in the postsurgical setting.

■ CONCLUSION

Enhanced surgical recovery programs for cancer patients should encompass the risks associated with the grade and stage of the disease, treatment regimens, and planned surgical procedures to allow for optimization of patient outcomes in the perioperative setting and beyond. Additionally, cancer patients who recover without complications after surgery can, in turn, return to their intended therapy expeditiously with improved outcomes.

Disclaimer: This submission is a modification of the work by the authors submitted for publication in a textbook titled "Perioperative Care of the Cancer Patient", Elsevier Publications, 2022.[64]

■ REFERENCES

1. Siegel RL, Miller KD, Jemal A. Cancer Statistics, 2017. CA: a cancer journal for clinicians. 2017;67(1):7-30.
2. Popat K, McQueen K, Feeley TW. The global burden of cancer. Best Pract Res Clin Anaesthesiol. 2013;27(4):399-408.
3. Rose J, Weiser TG, Hider P, Wilson L, Gruen RL, Bickler SW. Estimated need for surgery worldwide based on prevalence of diseases: a modelling strategy for the WHO Global Health Estimate. Lancet Glob Health. 2015;3 Suppl 2:S13-20.
4. Gan TJM, Thacker JK, MD, Miller TM, Scott MJM, Holubar SDM. Enhanced Recovery for major abdominopelvic surgery. First ed: Professional Communications, Inc.; 2016.

5. Gustafsson UO, Hausel J, Thorell A, et al. Adherence to the enhanced recovery after surgery protocol and outcomes after colorectal cancer surgery. Arch Surg. 2011;146(5):571-7.
6. Wu W, He J, Cameron JL, et al. The impact of postoperative complications on the administration of adjuvant therapy following pancreaticoduodenectomy for adenocarcinoma. Ann Surg Oncol. 2014;21(9):2873-81.
7. Salazar MC, Rosen JE, Wang Z, et al. Association of delayed adjuvant chemotherapy with survival after lung cancer surgery. JAMA Oncol. 2017;3(5):610-19.
8. Lohrisch C, Paltiel C, Gelmon K, et al. Impact on survival of time from definitive surgery to initiation of adjuvant chemotherapy for early-stage breast cancer. J Clin Oncol. 2006;24(30):4888-94.
9. Narang AK, Wright AA, Nicholas LH. Trends in advance care planning in patients with cancer: results from a national longitudinal survey. JAMA Oncol. 2015;1(5):601-8.
10. Teno JM, Weitzen S, Fennell ML, Mor V. Dying trajectory in the last year of life: does cancer trajectory fit other diseases? J Palliat Med. 2001;4(4):457-64.
11. Levy MH, Weinstein SM, Carducci MA, Panel NPCPG. NCCN: palliative care. Cancer Control. 2001;8(6 Suppl 2):66-71.
12. Shahrokni A, Vishnevsky BM, Jang B, et al. Geriatric Assessment, Not ASA physical status, is associated with 6-month postoperative survival in patients with cancer aged ≥75 years. Journal of the National Comprehensive Cancer Network : JNCCN. 2019;17(6):687-94.
13. Handforth C, Clegg A, Young C, et al. The prevalence and outcomes of frailty in older cancer patients: a systematic review. Annals of oncology: official journal of the European Society for Medical Oncology. 2015;26(6):1091-1101.
14. Pereira L, Figueiredo-Braga M, Carvalho IP. Preoperative anxiety in ambulatory surgery: the impact of an empathic patient-centered approach on psychological and clinical outcomes. Patient education and counseling. 2016;99(5):733-38.
15. West MA, Wischmeyer PE, Grocott MPW. Prehabilitation and nutritional support to improve perioperative outcomes. Curr Anesthesiol Rep. 2017;7(4):340-49.
16. Silver JK, Baima J. Cancer prehabilitation: an opportunity to decrease treatment-related morbidity, increase cancer treatment options, and improve physical and psychological health outcomes. Am J Phys Med Rehabil. 2013;92(8):715-27.
17. Santa Mina D, Brahmbhatt P, Lopez C, et al. The case for prehabilitation prior to breast cancer treatment. PM R. 2017;9(9S2):S305-16.
18. Ericksen LM, MEng, Miller TEMC, FRCA, Mythen M, MBBS MD, FRCA, FFICM, FCAI (Hon), Gan TJM, MBA, MHS, FRCA. Enhanced surgical recovery: from principles to standard of care. Annual Congress of Enhanced Recovery Perioperative Medicine; 2017; Washington, DC.
19. Lakoski SG, Eves ND, Douglas PS, Jones LW. Exercise rehabilitation in patients with cancer. Nat Rev Clin Oncol. 2012;9(5):288-96.
20. Valkenet K, Trappenburg JC, Schippers CC, et al. Feasibility of exercise training in cancer patients scheduled for elective gastrointestinal surgery. Dig Surg. 2016;33(5):439-47.
21. Licker M, Karenovics W, Diaper J, et al. Short-term preoperative high-intensity interval training in patients awaiting lung cancer surgery: a randomized controlled trial. J Thorac Oncol. 2017;12(2):323-33.

22. Jack S, West MA, Raw D, et al. The effect of neoadjuvant chemotherapy on physical fitness and survival in patients undergoing oesophagogastric cancer surgery. Eur J Surg Oncol. 2014;40(10):1313-20.
23. Loughney L, West MA, Kemp GJ, Grocott MP, Jack S. Exercise intervention in people with cancer undergoing neoadjuvant cancer treatment and surgery: a systematic review. Eur J Surg Oncol. 2016;42(1):28-38.
24. Wijeysundera DN, Pearse RM, Shulman MA, et al. Assessment of functional capacity before major non-cardiac surgery: an international, prospective cohort study. Lancet (London, England). 2018;391(10140):2631-40.
25. Diaz-Cambronero O, Matoses-Jaen S, Garcia-Claudio N, Garcia-Gregorio N, Molins-Espinosa J. [Preoperative management of anemia in oncologic surgery]. Rev Esp Anestesiol Reanim. 2015;62 (Suppl 1):45-51.
26. Munoz M, Gomez-Ramirez S, Martin-Montanez E, Auerbach M. Perioperative anemia management in colorectal cancer patients: a pragmatic approach. World J Gastroenterol. 2014;20(8):1972-85.
27. Klek S, Sierzega M, Szybinski P, et al. Perioperative nutrition in malnourished surgical cancer patients: a prospective, randomized, controlled clinical trial. Clin Nutr. 2011;30(6):708-13.
28. Braga M, Gianotti L, Radaelli G, et al. Perioperative immunonutrition in patients undergoing cancer surgery: results of a randomized double-blind phase 3 trial. Arch Surg. 1999;134(4):428-33.
29. Gillis C, Loiselle SE, Fiore JF, Jr., et al. Prehabilitation with whey protein supplementation on perioperative functional exercise capacity in patients undergoing colorectal resection for cancer: a pilot double-blinded randomized placebo-controlled trial. J Acad Nutr Diet. 2016;116(5): 802-12.
30. Sandrucci S, Beets G, Braga M, Dejong K, Demartines N. Perioperative nutrition and enhanced recovery after surgery in gastrointestinal cancer patients: a position paper by the ESSO task force in collaboration with the ERAS society (ERAS coalition). Eur J Surg Oncol. 2018.
31. Bozzetti F. Nutritional support of the oncology patient. Crit Rev Oncol Hematol. 2013;87(2):172-200.
32. Ottery FD. Definition of standardized nutritional assessment and interventional pathways in oncology. Nutrition. 1996;12(1 Suppl):S15-19.
33. Gupta R, Gan TJ. Preoperative nutrition and prehabilitation. Anesthesiol Clin. 2016;34(1):143-53.
34. Zhao XH, Yang T, Ma XD, et al. Heterogeneity of nutrition care procedures in nutrition guidelines for cancer patients. Clin Nutr. 2020;39(6):1692-704
35. Wesmiller SW, Sereika SM, Bender CM, et al. Exploring the multifactorial nature of postoperative nausea and vomiting in women following surgery for breast cancer. Auton Neurosci. 2017;202:102-7.
36. Murphy MJ, Hooper VD, Sullivan E, Clifford T, Apfel CC. Identification of risk factors for postoperative nausea and vomiting in the perianesthesia adult patient. J Perianesth Nurs. 2006;21(6):377-84.
37. Gan TJ, Diemunsch P, Habib AS, et al. Consensus guidelines for the management of postoperative nausea and vomiting. Anesth Analg. 2014;118(1):85-113.
38. Habib AS, Gan TJ. Evidence-based management of postoperative nausea and vomiting: a review. Can J Anaesth. 2004;51(4):326-41.

39. Montgomery GH, Schnur JB, Erblich J, Diefenbach MA, Bovbjerg DH. Presurgery psychological factors predict pain, nausea, and fatigue one week after breast cancer surgery. J Pain Symptom Manage. 2010;39(6):1043-52.
40. Miller TE, Roche AM, Mythen M. Fluid management and goal-directed therapy as an adjunct to Enhanced Recovery After Surgery (ERAS). Can J Anaesth. 2015;62(2):158-68.
41. Shaw C, Taylor L. Treatment-related diarrhea in patients with cancer. Clin J Oncol Nurs. 2012;16(4):413-17.
42. Colantonio L, Claroni C, Fabrizi L, et al. A randomized trial of goal directed vs. standard fluid therapy in cytoreductive surgery with hyperthermic intraperitoneal chemotherapy. J Gastrointest Surg. 2015;19(4):722-9.
43. Som A, Maitra S, Bhattacharjee S, Baidya DK. Goal-directed fluid therapy decreases postoperative morbidity but not mortality in major non-cardiac surgery: a meta-analysis and trial sequential analysis of randomized controlled trials. J Anesth. 2017;31(1):66-81.
44. Yates DR, Davies SJ, Milner HE, Wilson RJ. Crystalloid or colloid for goal-directed fluid therapy in colorectal surgery. Br J Anaesth. 2014;112(2):281-9.
45. Myles PS, Bellomo R, Corcoran T, et al. Restrictive versus liberal fluid therapy for major abdominal surgery. The New England journal of medicine. 2018;378(24):2263-74.
46. Pearse RM, Harrison DA, MacDonald N, et al. Effect of a perioperative, cardiac output-guided hemodynamic therapy algorithm on outcomes following major gastrointestinal surgery: a randomized clinical trial and systematic review. JAMA. 2014;311(21):2181-90.
47. Salmasi V, Maheshwari K, Yang D, et al. Relationship between intraoperative hypotension, defined by either reduction from baseline or absolute thresholds, and acute kidney and myocardial injury after noncardiac surgery: a retrospective cohort analysis. Anesthesiology. 2017;126(1):47-65.
48. Howell SJ. Preoperative hypertension. Curr Anesthesiol Rep. 2018;8(1):25-31.
49. Tan M, Law LS, Gan TJ. Optimizing pain management to facilitate Enhanced Recovery After Surgery pathways. Can J Anaesth. 2015;62(2):203-18.
50. Jakobsson JG. Pain management in ambulatory surgery: a review. Pharmaceuticals (Basel). 2014;7(8):850-65.
51. Diaz-Cambronero O, Mazzinari G, Cata JP. Perioperative opioids and colorectal cancer recurrence: a systematic review of the literature. Pain Management. 2018;8(5):353-61.
52. Ruetzler K, Kurz A. Consequences of perioperative hypothermia. Handbook of Clinical Neurology. 2018;157:687-97.
53. National Collaborating Centre for Nursing and Supportive Care (UK). The Management of Inadvertent Perioperative Hypothermia in Adults. In: National Institute for Health and Clinical Excellence: Guidance. London: Royal College of Nursing (UK); 2008.
54. Kehlet H. Multimodal approach to control postoperative pathophysiology and rehabilitation. Br J Anaesth. 1997;78(5):606-17.
55. Kim BJ, Caudle AS, Gottumukkala V, Aloia TA. The impact of postoperative complications on a timely return to intended oncologic therapy (RIOT): the role of enhanced recovery in the cancer journey. Int Anesthesiol Clin. 2016;54(4):e33-46.

56. Aloia TA, Zimmitti G, Conrad C, Gottumukalla V, Kopetz S, Vauthey JN. Return to intended oncologic treatment (RIOT): a novel metric for evaluating the quality of oncosurgical therapy for malignancy. J Surg Oncol. 2014;110(2):107-14.
57. Day RW, Cleeland CS, Wang XS, et al. Patient-reported outcomes accurately measure the value of an enhanced recovery program in liver surgery. J Am Coll Surg. 2015;221(6):1023-1030, e1021-22.
58. Merkow RP, Bilimoria KY, Tomlinson JS, et al. Postoperative complications reduce adjuvant chemotherapy use in resectable pancreatic cancer. Ann Surg. 2014;260(2):372-7.
59. Hassinger TE, Mehaffey JH, Martin AN, et al. Implementation of an enhanced recovery protocol is associated with on-time initiation of adjuvant chemotherapy in colorectal cancer. Diseases of the colon and rectum. 2019;62(11):1305-15.
60. Nelson DB, Mehran RJ, Mitchell KG, et al. Enhanced recovery after thoracic surgery is associated with improved adjuvant chemotherapy completion for non-small cell lung cancer. The Journal of Thoracic and Cardiovascular Surgery. 2019;158(1):279-286.e271.
61. Langenhoff BS, Krabbe PF, Wobbes T, Ruers TJ. Quality of life as an outcome measure in surgical oncology. Br J Surg. 2001;88(5):643-52.
62. Darling GE. Quality of life in patients with esophageal cancer. Thorac Surg Clin. 2013;23(4):569-75.
63. Breeze J, Rennie A, Dawson D, et al. Patient-reported quality of life outcomes following treatment for oral cancer. Int J Oral Maxillofac Surg. 2018;47(3):296-301.
64. Afonso AM, Gottumukkala NR. V. 54—Enhanced Surgical Recovery and Cancer. In: Hagberg C, Gottumukkala V, Riedel B, Nates J, Buggy D (Eds). Perioperative Care of the Cancer Patient. New Delhi: Elsevier; 2023. pp. 557-65.

CHAPTER

20

Perioperative Surgical Homes

Rashmi Datta

ABSTRACT

The present perioperative care service is fragmented, costly and neither evidence-based nor patient-centered. The perioperative surgical home (PSH) is a newly developed perioperative care system which extends care. It is an anesthesiologist-led, multidisciplinary team which provides consistent, coordinated, and integrated care throughout the entire perioperative period, from the time of decision to operate till 30 days postdischarge phase. Several evidence-driven perioperative strategies for reducing postoperative complications and shortening hospital stay are adapted to each specific hospital situation as per the local environment and patient characteristics, rather than strictly applying strategies as was with the "Enhanced Recovery from Surgery" protocols. The expected metrics include improved operational efficiencies, decreased resource utilization, a reduction in length of stay and readmission, and a decrease in complications and mortality-resulting in a better patient experience of care. It is also a good hospital business model.

Keywords: Perioperative period; Enhanced recovery from surgery; Perioperative surgical homes; Enhanced recovery from surgery protocols.

KEY POINTS

- The perioperative period consists of three stages—preoperative, intraoperative, and postoperative, extending from the time the decision to perform the procedure was taken to 30 days postdischarge.
- Each stage has been traditionally fragmented into nearly water-tight "silos". This led to a poorly coordinated approach to patient management between the stages with suboptimal communication of the surgical team with the patient.
- Following the implementation and validation of Enhanced Recovery after Surgery protocols, the concept of Patient-centered Medical Home was introduced to provide a multidimensional safe and high-quality solution for managing chronic illness and multimorbidity.
- Extending this approach to another area which was fragmented with multiple teams involved around a patient, a "Perioperative Surgical

Home" concept was introduced. In this novel concept, a personalized and coordinated care is proposed where physician-led multidisciplinary teams steer the patient throughout the entire surgical period.
- Currently, the full range of perioperative care is not covered by any one specialty. Surgeons are often well conversant with the nuances of perioperative medical preparation. Management of various problems associated with anesthesia is usually beyond the scope of training of surgical specialties. Physicians are not well versant with the anesthetic or surgical procedures or the possible complications that can occur. They are also not familiar with acute postoperative pain management.
- The special and extensive training assists the anesthesiologists to acquire core knowledge and procedural skills ranging from preoperative preparation, intraoperative anesthetic management, and postoperative pain management. Hence, they are best suited to function as the team leader.
- There is evidence that implementation of PSH leads to improved outcomes of patients, healthcare provider, and healthcare system as well as decreases complications and cost. However, there is a paucity of strong evidence and more high-powered studies are needed to validate the concept.

INTRODUCTION

The perioperative period of any invasive surgical, diagnostic, or therapeutic procedure is arbitrarily considered to be starting from the time the need for the procedure is determined to the time the patient is discharged from the acute-care facility to 30 days after surgery. This also includes a period after discharge from the hospital. Traditionally, this period had been fragmented into three stages, (1) the preoperative stage, (2) operative stage, and (3) the postoperative stage. The preoperative stage was arbitrarily subdivided into preoperative assessment and stabilization of existing comorbidities stage and hospital admission stage. The operative stage consisted of the anesthetic induction, surgery, and anesthetic recovery stages. The postoperative stage during hospitalization also had two periods, i.e., the nonambulatory phase which included walking with assistance and the walking, ambulatory phase **(Flowchart 1)**.[1,2]

While each "stage" had basic standards of training, laid out procedures and protocols, these stages were nearly water-tight "silos". The patient was exposed to different teams in each stage and in busy hospitals there was no overlapping of these teams. The team doing the preoperative assessment was not always the team giving anesthesia or the postoperative pain management. This led to a poorly coordinated approach to patient management between the stages with suboptimal communication of the surgical team with the

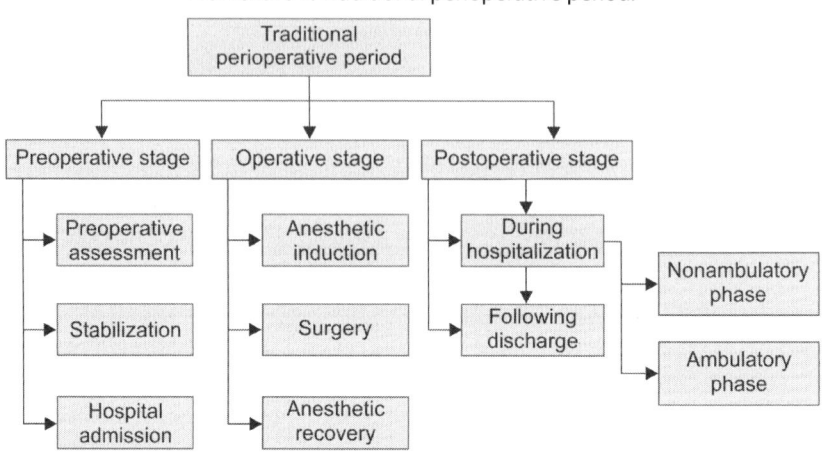

Flowchart 1: Traditional perioperative period.

patient. Due to different specialists with individualized plan of management, there was a tendency of variability in the management of same diseases between patients.[1,3-5]

Additionally, the demand for healthcare has now outstripping the available resources. This has prompted deliberations on the economic costs of healthcare. Hospitals across the world now focusing on finding ways to deliver higher quality care at lower cost. "Pay for volume" system of hospital management is inexorably and relentlessly transforming into a "pay for value" system. With increasing demand on limited healthcare resources and increased case complexity, the need for a re-look at the perioperative period management has risen.[4,6-9]

TRADITIONAL PERIOPERATIVE MANAGEMENT

Traditionally, the perioperative management of a patient starts with a referral from a primary healthcare provider to a surgeon.[1,2,9] After assessment, the various surgical and nonsurgical options are discussed with the patient. In case surgery is advised and based on the medical complexity, patients are referred to preoperative assessment clinics (PACs). In these clinics, apart from the anesthesiologist, internal medicine and other specialists examine the patients and perioperative medical risks including cardiac risks are discussed with the patient and he/she is advised for optimization of his clinical conditions.[2-4,10]

The timing of the PAC visit is also crucial. Both early and late optimization cause a proclivity for increased rate of complications, longer lengths of hospital stay, an increased incidence of readmissions, and high costs. In case the PAC visit is scheduled shortly before the surgical procedure, there may not be sufficient time to optimize attenuable risk factors. A time lapse between optimization of the comorbidities and the surgery may occur due to outpatient waiting lists before surgery. Although waiting lists are inevitable and can help in rationing scarce resources, prolonged waiting is clearly undesirable as it threatens the equity and timeliness of healthcare provision. There may also be deterioration of clinical outcomes or spontaneous resolution of symptoms in the waiting period. The former can cause the patient to resort to alternative level of care while the latter may make the patient question the original decision to perform the procedure. Both lead to patient dissatisfaction.[11-13]

Additionally, different teams address different problems. The discussions of risks and benefits of preoperative optimization of risk factors as well as the surgical procedures as happen in different clinics and different times with different teams. This often results in suboptimal communication between the patient and the various specialists, which forestalls an informed decision-making process.[1,4,14]

The recovery from surgery can be divided into three phases: an immediate or postanesthetic phase, an intermediate phase, encompassing the hospitalization period, and a convalescent phase. During the first two phases, care is principally directed at maintenance of homeostasis, treatment of pain, and prevention and early detection of complications. The convalescent phase is a transition period from the time of hospital discharge to full recovery. Postoperative management of patients requires careful attention, equal to that of the technical skill and focus required of surgery. Patient and family education on the potential side effects and complications of the procedure is a critical component of a successful postoperative course.[2,5,15-17] While the life expectancy of the general population has increased, so has the prevalence of coexisting chronic diseases. Hence, in the postoperative period due to multiple comorbidities, there is an increasing need for complex and avant-garde postoperative care. On the other hand, the number of sufficient and well-trained surgeons has not increased to meet these demands. The dependence on less trained, junior, relatively inexperienced doctors to man the wards, postoperative care has become increasingly neglected. Also with the working hours of interns and residents being enforced in accordance with labor laws, hospitals are facing a drop in workforce in the wards, especially in the night staff.[3,18]

There has been a widespread international paradigm shift from the current physician-centric care to a new perioperative service system for surgical patient care. This is based on a multidisciplinary team with vertical and horizontal pathway integration with coordination between the various stages of the traditional system patient. The model aims to reduce the cost of surgical care while maintaining or even increasing the quality of patient care.[1,10]

■ EVOLUTION OF THE CONCEPT

In the 1990s, Kehlet *et al.* hypothesized that the physiological stress response and the resultant organ dysfunction following surgery was a key factor in

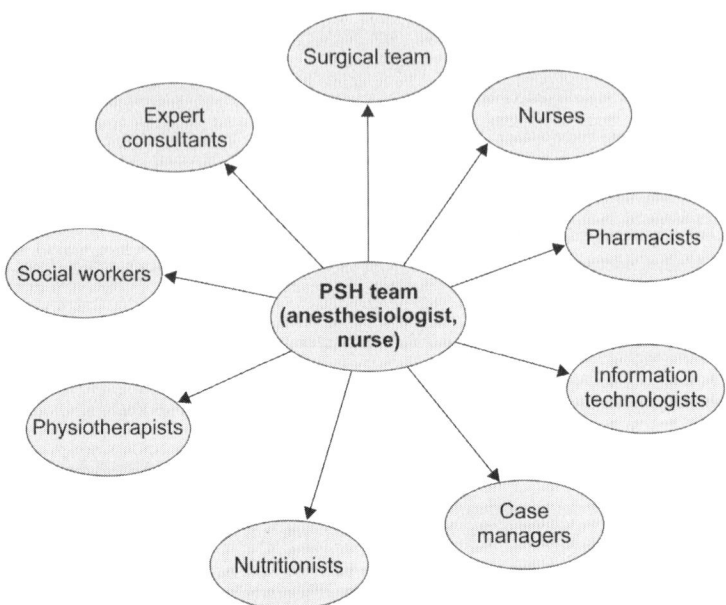

Fig. 1: The perioperative surgical hometeam (PSH).

postoperative morbidity. The authors proposed that if a multidisciplinary team delivered a series of evidence-based interventions to mitigate the perioperative physiological stress response and preserve anabolic homeostasis it would help in early recovery. These suggested interventions or protocols covered all aspects ranging from preadmission to the preoperative, intraoperative, and the postoperative periods in a synergistic and coordinated fashion, rather than acting in isolation and were named as "Enhanced Recovery After Surgery (ERAS)" protocols **(Fig. 1).**[19-21] Following the foundation of the ERAS society in 2010, guidelines and ERAS protocols have been successfully in place in many specialties in more than 25 countries worldwide.[8,14,15,22,23]

The Patient-centered Medical Home (PCMH) model was one of the general practitioner-led chronic care models that was introduced to provide a multidimensional safe, high-quality solution for managing chronic illness and multimorbidity. The key elements of this enhanced primary care model were clinical decision-support tools, evidence-based care, shared decision-making, performance measurement, and population health management. This model demonstrated both an improvement in patient satisfaction and in the quality of care.[24,25]

The Perioperative Surgical Home (PSH, sometimes referred to as POSH) model was initially developed by the American Society of Anesthesiologists (ASA). This engirdled the entire perioperative period, starting from the deliberation of a surgical procedure to postoperative recovery. After this the patient returned to the care of the PCMH. It was defined as "a patient-centered and physician-led multidisciplinary and team-based system of coordinated care that guides the patient throughout the entire surgical experience".[8] A smooth and logical transition from the PCMH to the PSH and back to the PCMH with continuous care between the two resulted in reduced visits to the emergency medicine department and hospital admissions.[3-5,26,27]

Redundant and nonessential preoperative testing leads to delay in perioperative care. A fragmentary perioperative care system can cause a variability of care and absence of proper communication. This can also increase occurrence of errors and complications. The PSH model treats the entire perioperative care as a continuous spectrum rather than separate, disjunctive preoperative, intraoperative, postoperative, and postdischarge episodes. All aspects of perioperative care are managed by one team from the time that the decision for surgery is made by the patient and the surgeon up to 30 days after discharge.[5,27,28]

The Perioperative Surgical Home has adapted the *Lean Six Sigma processes*. Conceptually, the perioperative period could be compared to a car production line where standardization of all perioperative procedures could remove waste and inefficiency and improve outcomes and patient satisfaction. The car industry was revolutionized by a synergized managerial concept adopted by Toyota. "Lean Six Sigma" is a method that relies on a collaborative team effort to improve performance by focus on improving process output quality by identifying and removing the causes of defects (errors) and minimizing variability in (manufacturing and business) processes. This results in an error-free and high-quality process.[28,29] The cornerstone of "Lean Six Sigma" is *DMAIC*, an acronym for *Define, Measure, Analyze, Improve, and Control* which refers to a data-driven improvement cycle used for improving, optimizing, and stabilizing business processes and designs.[2,30,31]

Artificial intelligence (AI) is machine based intelligence which revolves around usage of algorithms and learning by feedback. Data intensive analysis with the help of AI can help to prognosticate outcomes. In the healthcare industry, this will lead to effective and economical delivery of high-quality medical care. The vast spectrum of AI will help to shorten the learning curve and detect "near misses" to help prevent complications. IBM Watson Oncology was built to guide decision making for oncologists and to keep up-to-date with current evidence.[32]

Involvement of AI in perioperative management includes formulating accurate risk predictions as part of the preoperative assessment. The available categorical risk scales or risk prediction models like the Lee Revised Cardiac Risk Index, Surgical Apgar Score, P-POSSUM Scoring system and the American College of Surgeons National Surgical Quality Improvement Program (ACS NSQIP) generic Surgical Risk Calculator have many fallacies and shortcomings.[33] Machine learning (ML) platforms can analyze vast databases of the variables available from the "Electronic Health Records (EHR)" of patients and the outcomes. These can then identify and accurately predict risk. The *MySurgeryRisk platform* used the EHR data of 285 patients' variables and has been shown to demonstrate more valid and precise perioperative risk and mortality prediction than clinical judgment.[34] ML has been shown to accurately predict sepsis, acute kidney injury, and mortality using intraoperative data.[35-39] The *Predictive OpTimization Trees in Emergency Surgery Risk* (POTTER) calculator is an ML platform based on the *American College of Surgeons National Surgical Quality Improvement Program* (ACS-NSQIP) database to calculate perioperative risk and mortality. POTTER is accurate, uncomplicated, and user-friendly. Integrated with EHR data, it can be useful in identifying and preventing risks like SSI, sepsis, pneumonia, urinary tract infection, cardiac complications, and prolonged intensive care unit (ICU) stay in postoperative patients.[40] Similarly, for the prevention of anesthesia-related complications, ML algorithms can interpret patient's risk factors and postoperative outcomes data from previous surgery to recommend the anesthetic drugs to be used.[35,37,39,41]

Machine learning can assist in monitoring the depth of anesthesia (DOA) and early detection of anesthesia and surgery related complications. AI can also be used in intubating and operating robots and automated drug infusions. Postoperatively, AI has shown a role in early detection of complications such as postoperative surgical site infections (SSI) and identifying anastomotic leaks. Intervention can be faster with better prognosis.[35,36]

Nociception level (NOL) index, a multiparameter AI-driven index designed to monitor nociception during surgery, was used to study postoperative abdominal surgery pain in 50 patients in a randomized controlled trial. No differences were found in the total perioperative opioid (fentanyl and morphine) consumption, but there was a 1.6-point improvement in postoperative pain scores in the NOL-guided group was seen.[42]

▍ELEMENTS OF PERIOPERATIVE SURGICAL HOME

In the PSH model, the surgical decision is not made only by the surgeon. The patient is actively involved in the shared-decision making. The strategic doctrine of the PSH as identified by the ASA is that it is patient-centric with an emphasis on an active patient engagement with shared decision-making. The individualized PSH model affects all stages of perioperative period. A fully developed PSH is more than just strict implementation of predefined ERAS protocol.[14,16,23,43] To order to ensure that consistent and standardized evidence-based practices are applied to every patient undergoing surgery, the model has two additional features:

1. Coordination of all aspects of perioperative care to ensure adherence to individualized care plans.
2. Adaptability to patient-specific requirements and local environment.

When best evidence/best practice does not exist or is not clear, the PSH team should develop a standardized appropriate practice based on local systems and policies that will be applied to all patients. At each step of this continuum, the patient is informed and involved in the decision making and treatment planning with cognizance given to their preferences and values in all healthcare decisions.[1,2,5,6]

Preoperative elements include expectation management, targeted prehabilitation programs (e.g., smoking cessation and exercise), standardized protocol-driven health and risk stratification, i.e., identifying those patients most likely to experience postoperative problems at risk-specific PACs. Preoperative care is essentially the same in the PSH as in traditional care delivery models, except that the PSH model aims to optimization underlying medical conditions by beginning much sooner before surgery. PSH also includes a centralized clinic for admission to hospital and development of individualized care plans. These plans encompass the complete perioperative period from the preoperative outpatient setting to the inpatient surgical setting and back to the postoperative outpatient setting.

Intraoperative standardized and evidence-based anesthetic/nursing/surgical protocols are all determined in advance through the PSH pathway. Algorithmic management strategies for all clinical intraoperative elements including potential situations and complication are laid out. Examples of PSH include intraoperative elements such as integrated operating room scheduling, techniques to reduce waiting periods and delays in surgical scheduling and maintenance of EHR bridging outpatient and inpatient care.

Similarly, *PSH postoperative elements* include continuation of initiatives and interventions started in pre- and intraoperative phases, monitoring, early mobilization, and incorporation of other ERAS recommendations. PSH pathway in the postoperative period consists of initiation of consistent postoperative patient follow-up beyond the postanesthesia care unit and includes a multimodal plan for postoperative analgesia, early ambulation, nutrition management, rescue from complications, and smooth transition of care to an appropriate discharge setting. There is emphasis on developing new clinical pathways, and creation of an accessible database to track outcomes. This also includes education protocols for patients and caregivers.[1,4-6,18,25-29,44-46] The differences between the traditional surgical care and the PSH is listed in **Table 1**.

PERIOPERATIVE SURGICAL HOME TEAM (FIG. 2)

The team is structured with various departmental experts such as, surgeons, specialist physicians as required, nursing staff, pharmacists, information technology experts, and case managers. By virtue of the

TABLE 1: Difference between the traditional surgical care and perioperative surgical home.

Phase	Decision to operate	Preoperative	Intraoperative	Postoperative	Postdischarge
Traditional surgical care	Variable preoperative assessment, testing and optimization	• Variable preoperative assessment, testing and optimization • Admission often day prior to surgery	• Anesthesia management as per providers preference • Lack of standardized protocols for all similar cases	• Postoperative management by surgeon • Few protocols	• Variable follow-up and postoperative support • Possible delay in return to work or normal activities
Perioperative surgical home	• Shared decision with outline of the best course of management • Patient information, education and expectation management • Discharge planning • Referral to specific consultations for optimal planning	• Early preoperative assessment and intervention • Shared decision making to outline best anesthesia plan, recovery and postoperative pain management • Tailored medical optimization • Patient education and expectation management • Preoperative prescriptions and instructions	• Standardized protocols for tailored anesthesia care • Standardized equipment and nursing protocols • Infection prevention strategies • Optimization of fluid management • Multimodal analgesia	• Targeted recovery plan • Early ambulation • Multimodal analgesia with minimal systemic analgesics/opioids • Early removal of drains and catheters • Nutritional; management • Early interventions protocols for deviation from expected timeline of recovery • Discharge readiness protocols	• Personal recovery plans • Early remote follow-up • Wound management • Physiotherapy • Early return to work or normal activities

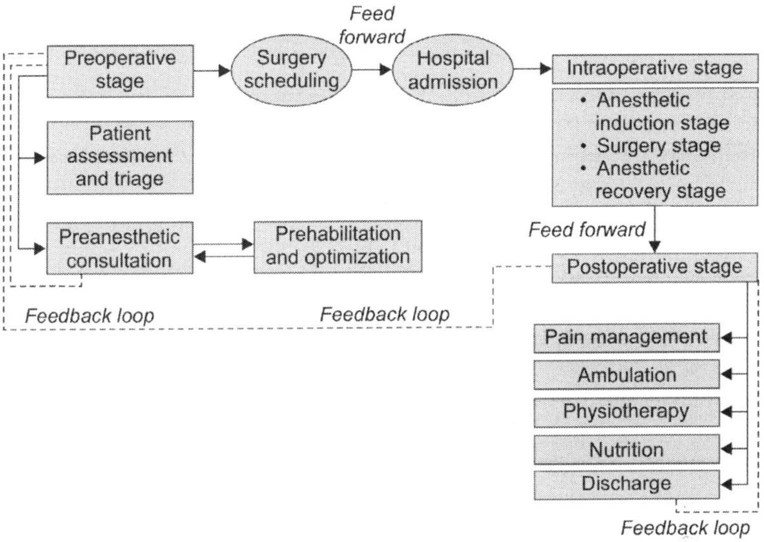

Fig. 2: Perioperative surgical team concept.

training, the anesthesiologist forms an integral and principal of the team. The team looks at all aspects of the perioperative period from the clinical, operations, information technology/finance, patient experience, and change management aspects. Apart from standardized care and goal-directed individual plans, extensive education for the medical staff is integrated in every step of the PSH protocol.[45-47]

The complete reach of perioperative care is not covered by any single specialty. By virtue of their training, surgeons are often not well conversant of the preoperative medical optimization and management of various anesthesia related intraoperative problems. In addition, physicians are also not very acquainted with the anesthetic or surgical procedures or possible complications as well as with acute pain management.

The anesthesiologist's involvement in PSH is to help lead the team to provide the best surgical care for the patient. Anesthesiologists undergo extensive specialized training to acquire core knowledge and disciplinary skills ranging from preoperative preparation, intraoperative anesthetic management, and postoperative management including that of both acute and subacute pain. They can superintend the entire range of age and various comorbidities. Anesthesiologists are typically "system-thinkers" as demonstrated by the improvement made in patient safety. In the past, the role of the anesthesiologist was limited to the preanesthetic examination just before surgery and the first 24 hours in the postoperative care unit with the surgical team providing most of the preoperative preparation and postoperative and postdischarge care of the patient. In recent decades, the role of anesthesiologists in perioperative care has been expanding.

The current interaction of the anesthesiologists with the patient before, during, and after the operation can positively influence the patient and PSH is seen as a natural extension of this trend.[1,5-7,18,25-27,29]

However, the current anesthesiology training is still lacking continuing training for patient recovery in the ward beyond the initial 24 hours postoperative. With additional training, anesthesiologist can expand into perioperative care as a constructive way to provide high-quality healthcare. However, anesthesiologists will not be abandoning the traditional role in the "Operation Theater". This will emerge as an expansion into a new area within a larger framework of anesthesiology. This expansion will be similar to existing subspecialties like critical care medicine and pain medicine. The intraoperative anesthetic role will continue to be intact and unique.[48]

From the standpoint of the surgeon, the PSH model has some ingenious value. It is a new model aimed to increase the competence of care throughout whole perioperative period. There is no displacement of the role of the surgeon in postoperative management.[49,50]

Surgeons and anesthesiologists have always been cooperative and synergistic. With the induction of the anesthesiologist in the perioperative care team a more advanced surgical patient care can be achieved. The knowledge of perioperative conditions can be augmented the care in the future.[5,6,14,28,29]

Hospital administrators by virtue of their pedagogy and lack of surgical experience lack the fundamental understanding of perioperative physiology and thus are not ideally positioned to deliver optimal postoperative care. They can be part of the PSH team but not as the team leaders.[5,6,50,51]

■ BENEFITS OF PERIOPERATIVE SURGICAL HOME

The PSH is designed to improve the experience of patients by uniting all aspects of their surgical journey. From the viewpoint of the patient, the PSH model is promising value and quality care. Patients these days have easy access to medical information and are aware of the various lacunae in healthcare systems. The trio of "underuse, misuse, and overuse" of resources is apparent to them. Team-based effective care is way forward in this new medical setting and this is the need rather than performance by individual physicians. Patients experience more seamless healthcare, with higher quality of care, shorter hospital stays, improved safety, improved effectiveness, more cohesive education, and equity in service availability and standards.[5,8,10,11,24,51]

Statistical analyses have shown that patient-centered integrated care models like PSH reduces the wastage of both tangible and intangible 3M of resources, i.e., man, material, and money and improves quality of life, patient satisfaction and clinical outcomes. This reflects as excellent healthcare at lower costs and is a good business model. The changes of remuneration paradigm such as value-based purchasing of healthcare, *"pay for performance"* or *"bundled payments"* are all potent incentives to improve the quality of perioperative surgical care.[2,4,24,25,26,29,45]

Benefits for the surgical teams are many since collaboration and communication is at the model's core. The streamlined patient journey creates opportunities to improve the workflow and job satisfaction of every member of the clinical team, resulting in improved efficiency, less unjustified variation, fewer redundant tests and laboratories, and decreased waste of resources, higher productivity, and individualized surgical plans. This will also boost the reputation of the hospital and the team.[24,25,51]

Health plan providers also see substantial benefits from the implementation of a PSH, including higher cost-effectiveness and improved reliability.

■ BARRIERS TO IMPLEMENTATION

Consistent evidence of effectiveness of PSH programs as a model of perioperative care delivery is still not available. This is because of the variability of content and implementation is lacking. A review was undertaken by Kash et al. to analyze the improvement, if any, in the cost and efficiency outcomes as well as the clinical outcomes when PSH was implemented. The authors found improvement in cost and efficiency outcomes in 75–88% of PSH studies. They also reported that clinical outcomes were significantly improved in 80–90% studies. But, significant heterogeneity was observed among the studies. Most of the included studies were observational in nature and thus are likely limited by publication bias.[52] Given these limitations, it was concluded that there is a paucity of strong evidence that suggested PSH implementation leads to improved patient care and healthcare system outcomes.[3,5,52-54]

Since there is intensive human resources and financial implications necessary for implementing PSH, a pragmatic trial design to evaluate the program *in toto* or partially. Designs such as a stepped-wedge cluster-randomized trial or hospital cluster-randomized trial along with implementation scientists will allow adequate evaluation of the PSH. Apart from a formal study of implementation, other outcomes can also be studied like patient-centered clinical outcomes and cost and efficiency outcomes. With this in mind, the ASA has committed financial support for a multihospital collaborative PSH implementation study.

One of the greatest challenges to the implementation of the PSH model is postoperative pain management. Currently, postoperative pain is managed by the "Acute Pain Team". However, with a substantial increase in patient volume, this model will not be sustainable. A dedicated anesthesiologist may be required to supervise dedicated nurse practitioners for coordination and adherence to protocols of these patients.[53]

The skills needed to build such a program need to be differentiated from the skills needed to maintain it. For the development phase, anesthesiologists need to be skilled in team-building, change management techniques, and streamlining protocols such as LEAN, and Six Sigma methodology. Once a PSH program is developed, skillsets in the postoperative management of complex surgical patients may be improved upon with more training in perioperative medicine with particular stress on postoperative care.

There is no provision to reimburse the "extra services" provided by team within the existing payment system. This financial constraint presents a major barrier to a PSH mode. In the future, medical payments may move from the existing fee-for-service system where the team members are paid, based on time units to a "bundle payment" system, where the team members will be compensated for their "overall value" to the surgical episode. This would offset the costs associated with the implementation and maintenance of a PSH. If PSH is as successful as the ERAS program, financial savings will be realized by hospitals which may be a strong motivator.[5,7,8,53]

CONCLUSION

The PSH is a novel perioperative care system developed as a team working under the supervision of an anesthesiologist. This aims to provide coordinated, consistent, and integrated care from the preoperative to the postdischarge phases. This model has now emerged as an organizing idea for ERAS pathways and perioperative medicine with a goal to improve the quality of perioperative care delivered, improve patient outcomes and satisfaction, decrease utilization of expensive tests and procedures, decrease postencounter discomfort, and reduce the cost of surgical care. The model will provide standardized, evidence-based perioperative strategies to improve outcome for each hospital. By this manner, patients can receive better medical care at a more reasonable cost. This new model will also be an attractive subspecialty for anesthesiologists. It has been heralded as a breakthrough in medical reality with optimal usage of all surgical personnel involved in perioperative care of patients.

REFERENCES

1. Cline KM, Clement V, Rock-Klotz J, Kash BA, Steel C, Miller TR. Improving the cost, quality, and safety of perioperative care: a systematic review of the literature on implementation of the perioperative surgical home. J Clin Anesth. 2020;63:109760.
2. Chopra SS, Schmidt SC, Fotopoulou C, Sehouli J, Schumacher G. Evidence-based perioperative management: strategic shifts in times of fast track surgery. Anticancer res. 2009;29(7):2799-802.

3. Paiste J, Simmons JW, Vetter TR. Enhanced recovery after surgery in the setting of the perioperative surgical home. Int Anesth Clin. 2017;55(4):135-47.
4. Desebbe O, Lanz T, Kain Z, Cannesson M. The perioperative surgical home: an innovative, patient-centred and cost-effective perioperative care model. Anaesth Crit Care Pain Med. 2016;35(1):59-66.
5. Vetter TR, Goeddel LA, Boudreaux AM, Hunt TR, Jones KA, Pittet JF. The perioperative surgical home: how can it make the case so everyone wins? BMC Anesthesiol. 2013;13(1):6.
6. Kain ZN, Vakharia S, Garson L, Engwall S, Schwarzkopf R, Gupta R, et al. The perioperative surgical home as a future perioperative practice model. Anesth Analg. 2014;118(5):1126-30.
7. Dexter F, Wachtel RE. Strategies for net cost reductions with the expanded role and expertise of anesthesiologists in the perioperative surgical home. Anesth Analg. 2014;118(5):1062-71.
8. Raphael DR, Cannesson M, Schwarzkopf R, Garson LM, Vakharia SB, Gupta R, Kain ZN. Total joint perioperative surgical home: an observational financial review. Perioper Med. 2014;3(1):1-7.
9. Schweitzer M, Fahy B, Leib M, Rosenquist R, Merrick S. The perioperative surgical home model. ASA Monitor. 2013;77(6):58-9.
10. Schonberger RB. Rebranding the perioperative surgical home: lessons from the duke experience. J Cardiothorac Vasc Anesth. 2016;30(4):1064-6.
11. Chimento GF, Thomas LC. The perioperative surgical home: improving the value and quality of care in total joint replacement. Curr Rev Musculoskelet Med. 2017;10(3):365-9.
12. Black N. Surgical waiting lists are inevitable: time to focus on work undertaken. J R Soc Med. 2004;97(4):159-60
13. Ray S, Kirtania J. Waiting time of inpatients before elective surgical procedures at a State Government Teaching Hospital in India. Indian J Public Health. 2017;61(4):284-9.
14. Segelman J, Nygren J. Evidence or eminence in abdominal surgery: recent improvements in perioperative care. World Journal of Gastroenterology: WJG. 2014;20(44):16615.
15. Udayasankar M, Udupi S, Shenoy A. Comparison of perioperative patient comfort with 'enhanced recovery after surgery (ERAS) approach' versus 'traditional approach' for elective laparoscopic cholecystectomy. Indian J Anaesth. 2020;64(4):316.
16. Li J, Li H, Xv ZK, Wang J, Yu QF, Chen G, et al. Enhanced recovery care versus traditional care following laminoplasty: a retrospective case-cohort study. Medicine. 2018;97(48):e13195.
17. Li ZE, Lu SB, Kong C, Sun WZ, Wang P, Zhang ST. Comparative short-term outcomes of enhanced recovery after surgery (ERAS) program and non-ERAS traditional care in elderly patients undergoing lumbar arthrodesis: a retrospective study. BMC Musculoskelet Disord. 2021;22(1):283.
18. Kwon MA. Perioperative surgical home: a new scope for future anesthesiology. Korean J Anesthesiol. 2018;71(3):175-81.
19. Kehlet H. Multimodal approach to control postoperative pathophysiology and rehabilitation. Br J Anaesth. 1997;78(5):606-17.

20. Kehlet H. Beneficial effects of stress response blockade on patients undergoing surgery. Host defense dysfunction in trauma, shock and sepsis. Berlin, Heidelberg: Springer; 1993. pp. 67-71.
21. Lewis KS, Whipple JK, Michael KA, Quebbeman EJ. Effect of analgesic treatment on the physiological consequences of acute pain. Am J Health Syst Pharm. 1994;51(12):1539-54.
22. Li C, Cheng Y, Li Z, Margaryan D, Perka C, Trampuz A. The pertinent literature of enhanced recovery after surgery programs: a bibliometric approach. Medicina. 2021;57(2):172.
23. Brindle M, Nelson G, Lobo DN, Ljungqvist O, Gustafsson UO. Recommendations from the ERAS® Society for standards for the development of enhanced recovery after surgery guidelines. BJS Open. 2020;4(1):157-63.
24. Maeng DD, Graf TR, Davis DE, Tomcavage J, Bloom Jr FJ. Can a patient-centered medical home lead to better patient outcomes? The quality implications of Geisinger's Proven Health Navigator. Am J Med Qual. 2012;27(3):210-6.
25. Fix GM, VanDeusen Lukas C, Bolton RE, Hill JN, Mueller N, LaVella SL, et al. Patient-centred care is a way of doing things: How healthcare employees conceptualize patient-centred care. Health Expect. 2018;21(1):300-7.
26. Vetter TR, Ivankova NV, Goeddel LA, McGwin Jr G, Pittet JF. UAB Perioperative Surgical Home Group. An analysis of methodologies that can be used to validate if a perioperative surgical home improves the patient-centeredness, evidence-based practice, quality, safety, and value of patient care. Anesthesiology. 2013;119(6):1261-74.
27. Grocott MP, Pearse RM. Perioperative medicine: the future of anaesthesia? Br J Anaesth. 2012;108:723-6.
28. Alem N, Rinehart J, Lee B, Merrill D, Sobhanie S, Ahn K, et al. A case management report: a collaborative perioperative surgical home paradigm and the reduction of total joint arthroplasty readmissions. Perioper Med (Lond). 2016;5:27. eCollection 2016.
29. Nicolescu TO. Perioperative Surgical Home. Meeting tomorrow's challenges. Rom J Anaesth Intensive Care. 2016;23(2):141-7.
30. Irizarry-Alvarado JM, Lundy M, McKinney B, Ray FA, Reynolds VE, Pai SL. Preoperative evaluation clinic redesign: an initiative to improve access, efficiency, and staff satisfaction. Am J Med Qual. 2019;34(4):348-53.
31. Latessa I, Picone I, Fiorillo A, Sorrentino A, Orabona GD, Valente AS. DMAIC Approach to Reduce LOS in Patients Undergoing Oral Cancer Surgery. In: Jarm T, Cvetkoska A, Mahnič-Kalamiza S, Miklavcic D (Eds). 8th European Medical and Biological Engineering Conference. EMBEC 2020. IFMBE Proceedings, vol 80. Cham: Springer; 2020. pp. 424-33.
32. Somashekhar S, Sepúlveda M, Norden AD, Rauthan A, Arun K, Patil P, et al. Early experience with IBM Watson for Oncology (WFO) cognitive computing system for lung and colorectal cancer treatment. J Clin Onco. 2017;35:8527.
33. Lee TH, Marcantonio ER, Mangione CM, Thomas EJ, Polanczyk CA, Cook EF, et al. Derivation and prospective validation of a simple index for prediction of cardiac risk of major noncardiac surgery. Circulation. 1999;100:1043-9.

34. Brennan M, Puri S, Ozrazgat-Baslanti T, Feng Z, Ruppert M, Hashemighouchani H, et al. Comparing clinical judgment with the MySurgeryRisk algorithm for preoperative risk assessment: A pilot usability study. Surgery. 2019; 165:1035-45.
35. Solanki SL, Pandrowala S, Nayak A, Bhandare M, Ambulkar RP, Shrikhande SV. Artificial intelligence in perioperative management of major gastrointestinal surgeries. World J Gastroenterol. 2021;27(21):2758-70.
36. Soguero-Ruiz C, Hindberg K, Rojo-Alvarez JL, Skrovseth SO, Godtliebsen F, Mortensen K, et al. Support Vector Feature Selection for Early Detection of Anastomosis Leakage From Bag-of-Words in Electronic Health Records. IEEE J Biomed Health Inform. 2016;20:1404-15.
37. Adhikari L, Ozrazgat-Baslanti T, Ruppert M, Madushani RWMA, Paliwal S, Hashemighouchani H, et al. Improved predictive models for acute kidney injury with IDEA: intraoperative data embedded analytics. PLoS One. 2019;14:e0214904.
38. Henry KE, Hager DN, Pronovost PJ, Saria S. A targeted real-time early warning score (TREWScore) for septic shock. SciTransl Med. 2015;7:299ra122.
39. Delahanty RJ, Kaufman D, Jones SS. Development and evaluation of an automated machine learning algorithm for in-hospital mortality risk adjustment among critical care patients. Crit Care Med. 2018;46:e481-8.
40. Bertsimas D, Dunn J, Velmahos GC, Kaafarani HMA. Surgical risk is not linear: derivation and validation of a Novel, User-friendly, and Machine-learning-based Predictive OpTimal Trees in Emergency Surgery Risk (POTTER) Calculator. Ann Surg. 2018;268:574-83.
41. Karpagavalli S, Jamuna KS, Vijaya MS. Machine learning approach for pre-operative anaesthetic risk prediction. Int J Rece Trends Engineering. 2009;1: 19-22.
42. Meijer F, Honing M, Roor T, Toet S, Calis P, Olofsen E, et al. Reduced postoperative pain using nociception level-guided fentanyl dosing during sevoflurane anaesthesia: a randomised controlled trial. Br J Anaesth. 2020;125:1070-8.
43. Harrison TG, Ronksley PE, James MT, Brindle ME, Ruzycki SM, Graham MM, et al. The perioperative surgical home, enhanced recovery after surgery and how integration of these models may improve care for medically complex patients. Canadian J Surg. 2021;64(4):E381.
44. Prielipp RC, Morell RC, Coursin DB, Brull SJ, Barker SJ, Rice MJ, et al. The future of anesthesiology: should the perioperative surgical home redefine us? Anesth Analges. 2015;120(5):1142-8.
45. Mariano ER, Vetter TR, Kain ZN. The perioperative surgical home is not just a name. Anesth Analges. 2017;125(5):1443-5.
46. Duncan MJ. Perioperative surgical home, fixing a fragmented process to improve quality of care. Missouri Med. 2019;116(1):53.
47. Cannesson M, Mahajan A. Vertical and horizontal pathways: intersection and integration of enhanced recovery after surgery and the perioperative surgical home. Anesth Analges. 2018;127(5):1275-7.
48. Zaccagnino MP, Bader AM, Sang CN, Correll DJ. The perioperative surgical home: a new role for the acute pain service. Anesth Analges. 2017;125(4):1394-402.

49. Powell AC, Thearle MS, Cusick M, Sanderson DJ, Van Lew H, Lee C, et al. Early results of a surgeon-led, perioperative surgical home. J Surg Res. 2017;211:154-62.
50. Butterworth IV JF, Green JA. The anesthesiologist-directed perioperative surgical home: a great idea that will succeed only if it is embraced by hospital administrators and surgeons. Anesth Analges. 2014;118(5):896-7.
51. Holt NF. Trends in healthcare and the role of the anesthesiologist in the perioperative surgical home: the US perspective. Curr Opin Anesthesiol. 2014;27(3):371-6.
52. Kash B, Cline K, Menser T, Zhang Y. (2014). The Perioperative Surgical Home (PSH): a comprehensive literature review for the American Society of Anesthesiologists. [online] Available from https://www.asahq.org/psh/~/media/sites/psh/files/pshlitreview.pdf [Last accessed October, 2022].
53. Kash BA, Zhang Y, Cline KM, Menser T, Miller TR. The perioperative surgical home (PSH): a comprehensive review of US and non-US studies shows predominantly positive quality and cost outcomes. Milbank Quarterly. 2014;92(4):796-821.
54. Vetter TR, Boudreaux AM, Jones KA, Hunter Jr JM, Pittet JF. The perioperative surgical home: how anesthesiology can collaboratively achieve and leverage the triple aim in health care. Anesth Analges. 2014;118(5):1131-6.

CHAPTER 21

Overview of Point-of-Care Ultrasound for the Anesthesiologist

C Adam Coridan, Sanjib Das Adhikary

ABSTRACT

Point-of-care ultrasound (POCUS) is the bedside use of ultrasound technology to aid clinicians with pathological diagnosis or procedural techniques. POCUS can be used to assess most areas of the body and can help in the diagnosis of a wide variety of pathologies. The benefits of POCUS lie in its relative safety, portability, quickness, and reliability. It has not been until recently that many anesthesiologists have begun to see POCUS as a valuable tool for the wider perioperative period, from preoperative assessment through a patient's stay in the postoperative care unit (PACU). Beyond the obvious benefit of cardiac and pulmonary POCUS use, it also has been shown to improve clinical decision-making related to a patient's airway, aspiration risk, and hemodynamic status, among others. Additionally, POCUS has been shown to help the anesthesiologist more successfully perform bedside procedures for regional anesthesia, neuraxial anesthesia, and vascular access. The purpose of this review is to provide anesthesiologists and trainees with an overview of the many uses and benefits of POCUS in the perioperative setting.

Keywords: Point-of-care-ultrasound; Gastric ultrasound; Focused cardiovascular ultrasound (FOCUS); Lung ultrasound; Focused assessment with sonography for trauma (FAST); Perioperative.

KEY POINTS

- The benefits of POCUS lie in its relative safety (i.e., lack of radiation), reproducibility, portability, quickness, and reliability.
- Point-of-care ultrasound use by anesthesiologists for regional anesthetic procedures has become so prevalent that it is considered the gold standard for care in this area.
- Beyond the obvious benefit of cardiac and pulmonary POCUS use, it also has been shown to improve assessment and outcomes related to a patient's airway, aspiration risk, and vascular access, among others.
- The use of airway POCUS is beneficial for preoperative identification of patients with potentially difficult laryngoscopy, confirmation of endotracheal tube placement, and assistance with cricothyrotomy procedures.

- Well-validated POCUS protocols exist to diagnose causes of respiratory failure and shock in trauma and critically ill patients [e.g., the bedside lung ultrasound in emergency (BLUE) and the failure and fluid administration limited by lung sonography (FALLS) protocols].
- In certain situations (e.g., pneumothorax, pleural effusion, and diaphragmatic dysfunction), lung POCUS has superior diagnostic accuracy (both sensitivity and specificity) over some of the more traditional pulmonary imaging modalities (e.g., chest X-ray).
- Focused cardiovascular ultrasound is a valuable perioperative tool for the anesthesiologist to quickly and reliably assess a patient's general cardiac function and hemodynamic status, as well as examine for ischemia, valvular pathologies, or pericardial effusion.
- Gastric POCUS is reliable in determining the fasting status when the status is unknown. Gastric POCUS provides a modality that allows anesthesiologists to visually assess the gastric contents in a patient's stomach before a procedure and make an informed decision about the proper anesthetic and airway plans given the qualitative and quantitative assessment of the gastric contents.
- The focused assessment with sonography for trauma and rapid ultrasound for shock and hypotension (RUSH) examinations are helpful for the anesthesiologist in the perioperative setting to assess for possible postoperative bleeding or undifferentiated shock.
- Point-of-care ultrasound use by anesthesiologists for regional anesthetic procedures has become so prevalent that it is considered the gold standard for care.
- Point-of-care ultrasound use for neuraxial procedures can identify a given lumbar intervertebral space more accurately when compared to landmark palpation while measuring depth to the epidural or intrathecal space and increasing success rates.

INTRODUCTION

Ultrasound technology in medicine traces its origins to the period following World War II.[1] Research supporting the use of ultrasound grew during the 1950s, and by the mid-1960s, commercially-available ultrasound machines allowed for wider use of the technology in hospitals and clinics. Since that time, the use of ultrasound has expanded to the point that it is now the most widely utilized imaging modality in clinical medicine.[2] With decreasing cost and increasing portability of ultrasound technology, its use as a bedside diagnostic tool has grown exponentially over the last 2 decades, allowing the physician to evaluate patients quickly and reliably.

Point-of-care ultrasound (POCUS) is the bedside use of ultrasound technology to aid clinicians with pathological diagnosis or procedural techniques. The benefits of POCUS lie in its relative safety (i.e., lack of radiation), reproducibility, portability, quickness, and reliability. POCUS can be used to assess most areas of the body and can help in the diagnosis of a wide variety of pathologies. A growing amount of research shows that POCUS has greater sensitivity and specificity to diagnose conditions (e.g., pneumothorax) in real-time compared to traditional imaging modalities. Additionally, POCUS can improve anatomic visualization, allowing a proceduralist to more safely complete bedside procedures [e.g., regional anesthesia or central venous catheter (CVC) placement] in less time and with fewer attempts.

Initially, POCUS was most widely implemented by emergency and critical care physicians because of POCUS ability to assess traumatically injured rapidly and also critically ill patients in shock. However, it has not been until more recently that many anesthesiologists have begun to see POCUS as a valuable tool for the wider perioperative period, from preoperative assessment through a patient's stay in the postoperative care unit (PACU). Beyond the obvious benefit of cardiac and pulmonary POCUS use, it also has been shown to improve assessment and outcomes related to a patient's airway, aspiration risk, and vascular access, among others. From the cardiac operating room to the ambulatory surgery center, new anesthesia-related applications for POCUS are constantly arising and becoming more readily utilized.

POINT-OF-CARE ULTRASOUND FOR DIAGNOSTIC EVALUATION

Ultrasound of the Lungs

Pulmonary ultrasound has great utility for preoperative evaluation and pathology diagnosis throughout the perioperative period. Well-validated protocols exist to diagnose causes of respiratory failure and shock in trauma and critically ill patients [e.g., the bedside lung ultrasound in emergency (BLUE) and the failure and fluid administration limited by lung sonography (FALLS) protocols]. Lung POCUS can help an anesthesiologist to assess patients with respiratory/ventilation difficulty or hemodynamic changes in real-time. In certain situations, lung POCUS has superior diagnostic accuracy (sensitivity and specificity) over some more traditional pulmonary imaging modalities (e.g., chest X-ray).

Pneumothorax is a rare but serious condition encountered by anesthesiologists, especially when dealing with patients with traumatic injuries. On pulmonary ultrasound, the presence of pneumothorax is usually noted by the absence of lung sliding on the affected side using the M-mode function.[3] The absence of lung sliding and "B lines" (a representation of the ratio of fluid-to-air content), along with the presence of a "lung point" (the transition

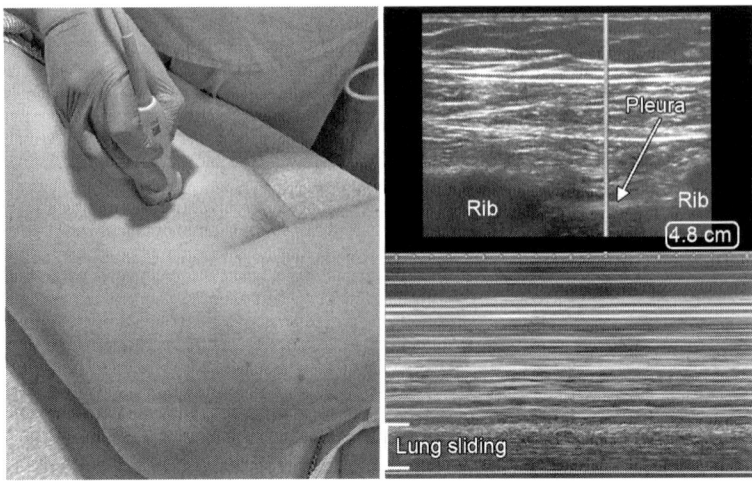

Fig. 1: Example of lung point-of-care ultrasound (POCUS) visualizing the left lung via the axilla utilizing M-mode. The pleura can be identified as the hyperechoic stripe between the two ribs. Lung sliding is the rough, granulated portion apparent in M-mode below the depth of the pleura. This is sometimes referred to as a "Seashore Sign" or "Sand on the Beach", indicating the physiologic motion of an inflated lung and excluding the presence of a pneumothorax.

between collapsed lung tissue and normal lung tissue) is characteristic of the finding of pneumothorax via ultrasound. Pulmonary ultrasound is more reliable than chest X-ray for the diagnosis of pneumothorax with accuracy approaching that of CT.[4] A 2020 Cochrane Review of studies that examined the use of lung ultrasound versus chest X-ray for the diagnosis of pneumothorax in trauma patients found the sensitivity and specificity of ultrasound to be 91% and 99%, respectively.[5] Comparatively, the sensitivity of chest X-ray was only found to be 47%.

The diagnosis of pulmonary edema, pneumonia, chronic obstructive pulmonary disease (COPD)/asthma, and pleural effusion with ultrasound depends largely on the interpretation of sonographic artifacts. The most common are the "A and B lines".[6] The lines are acoustic impedances between the pleura and the surrounding lung parenchyma, creating horizontal artifacts. Essentially, they represent air in the lung, whether it is normal or pathologic. B lines can be more pathognomonic for fluid in the lungs. They are described as three or more vertical hyperechoic reverberation artifacts (comet tails) that move synchronously with the lung. Pathologic B lines are commonly found in conditions like pulmonary edema, acute respiratory distress syndrome (ARDS), and pneumonia.

Ultrasound has been shown to have high accuracy in the diagnosis of pleural effusions, outperforming chest X-ray, auscultation, and other physical examination modalities (e.g., dullness to percussion or monitoring for the presence of asymmetric chest rise).[7,8] Similarly, lung POCUS is a beneficial tool for anesthesiologists in diagnosing pulmonary edema. Multiple meta-analyses have shown lung ultrasound to be 94–97% sensitive and 92–98% specific in diagnosing acute pulmonary edema.[9,10] When compared to chest X-ray, lung ultrasound was shown in a 2019 meta-analysis to be a more sensitive tool in the detection of pulmonary edema in patients with decompensated heart failure.[11]

Diaphragmatic paralysis is a possible complication associated with regional anesthesia of the brachial plexus secondary to blockade of the phrenic nerve. So, understanding how to evaluate diaphragmatic dysfunction with ultrasound can benefit anesthesiologists. Ultrasound M-mode can assess diaphragmatic displacement and contraction (thickening) at the zone of apposition via hepatic and splenic ultrasound windows. A thickening coefficient can be calculated to estimate the degree of paresis.[12] Diaphragmatic ultrasound has also been found to be beneficial for helping to determine readiness for tracheal extubation, especially in the critically ill population.[13]

Ultrasound of the Cardiovascular System

The use of cardiac POCUS often referred to as focused transthoracic echocardiographic examination has been well established for patients in the emergency department and intensive care unit for several decades. The focus assessed transthoracic echocardiography (FATE) protocol is the most well-known and validated example of cardiac POCUS.[14] Other protocols have been put forth since by anesthesiologists for cardiac evaluation in the perioperative period.[15] FOCUS is a valuable perioperative tool for the anesthesiologist to quickly and reliably assess a patient's general cardiac function and hemodynamic status, as well as examine for ischemia, valvular pathologies, or pericardial effusion. In the preoperative setting, assessing a patient with FOCUS provides vital information for the development of an anesthetic plan for a given surgery or for determining whether further workup would be beneficial before proceeding with surgery. Intraoperatively, FOCUS is a real-time tool to assess issues like extreme hypotension of unknown etiology or intraoperative myocardial ischemia. Postoperatively, FOCUS can allow for continued evaluation of volume status for patient-driven fluid resuscitation or quick evaluation in the postoperative care unit if acute ischemia or other cardiac pathology is suspected.

Ideally, FOCUS should be completed with a phased-array transducer. The basic views for FOCUS are the parasternal long axis, parasternal short axis, apical four-chamber, and subcostal four-chamber, with the addition of the subcostal caval view if evaluation of volume status is desired. When employed to answer a specific clinical question (e.g., is there significant ventricular dysfunction or severe valvular regurgitation?), using FOCUS in the perioperative period has been shown to cause a significant change in clinical care for up to 82% of patients.[16]

Ultrasound can provide an anesthesiologist with in-time feedback regarding a patient's volume status before, during, or after surgery. Evaluating fluid resuscitation status utilizing FOCUS relies on viewing the inferior vena cava (IVC) via the subcostal view and/or left ventricle via the parasternal short axis view. For the IVC, hypovolemia is indicated when its diameter will measure 1.5 cm or less with >50% collapse during inspiration.[17] For the left ventricle, hypovolemia with normal contractility will cause the ventricle to appear hyperdynamic with apparent underfilling and often ventricular wall touching at the end of systole. In the setting of hypervolemia, the IVC will appear dilated with minimal change in size with inspiration, and the right ventricle will appear abnormally large. A systematic literature review found that assessing IVC diameter and collapsibility with FOCUS, in conjunction with a passive leg raise to provide a fluid bolus, was an effective method for predicting fluid responsiveness.[18] Also, routine preoperative FOCUS examinations to assess volume status have been shown to reliably predict which patients will have hypotension after the induction of general anesthesia for elective surgery.[19]

Cardiac evaluation with POCUS can quickly assess for ischemia, ventricular dysfunction, and valvular abnormalities. The parasternal views are frequently used to assess for cardiac ischemia, presenting as wall akinesis or hypokinesis.[20] A recent meta-analysis found FOCUS to be highly sensitive but not highly specific for correct diagnosis of left ventricular dysfunction or valvular abnormalities versus clinical examination alone.[21] More specific to the anesthesiologist, using FOCUS can help to identify undiagnosed valvular dysfunction and characterize the severity of the pathology present during the perioperative period. One prospective study of hip fracture patients who lacked an audible murmur found that 31% of patients had notable aortic stenosis when examined with routine POCUS.[22] Awareness of previously unknown or worsened ventricular dysfunction or valvular pathology may alter the anesthetic technique employed.

Echocardiography is the gold standard for diagnosing pericardial effusion and cardiac tamponade. FOCUS has been shown to decrease the time to diagnosis of pericardial effusion significantly and therapeutic intervention with pericardiocentesis in symptomatic patients compared to diagnosing with clinical evaluation, ECG, and chest X-ray alone.[23] The subcostal four-chamber view provides the best view for the anterior pericardium, where effusions are most likely to occur.[20]

Cardiac arrest can occur anytime during the perioperative period. Cardiac POCUS can be used during resuscitation for cardiac arrest without

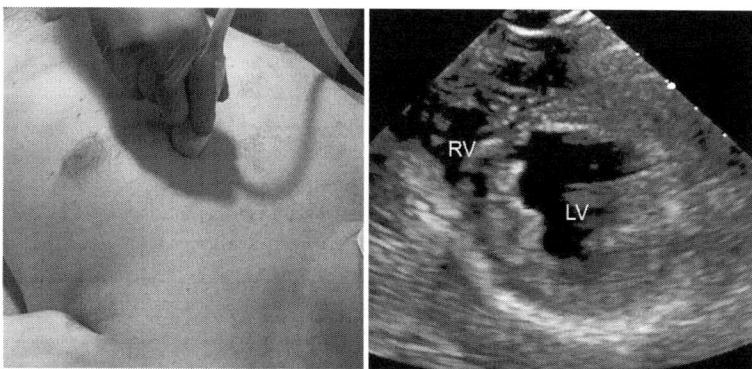

Fig. 2: Example of cardiovascular point-of-care ultrasound (POCUS) visualizing the left ventricle (LV) and right ventricle (RV) of the heart via a parasternal short-axis view.

interrupting chest compressions, utilizing the brief intermittent pause of compressions to assess cardiac rhythm and pulse activity.[24] One study that compared cardiac POCUS to doppler ultrasonography and manual palpation found that cardiac POCUS more quickly and accurately identified cardiac pulsatility than the other two techniques.[25]

Ultrasound of the Gastrointestinal System

Aspiration of gastric contents is a significant risk to patients undergoing a surgical procedure or anesthetic. Aspiration pneumonitis or pneumonia carries high morbidity and mortality for the patient.[26] Aspiration is a risk for all types of anesthetics, especially ones without a secure airway (e.g., endoscopic procedures). Fasting or nil per os (NPO) guidelines exist to help anesthesiologists to minimize the risk of aspiration when allowable. However, delayed gastric emptying can occur in patients with pathologies such as diabetes, chronic kidney disease, or neuromuscular diseases. Obesity, pregnancy, and certain medications (e.g., opioids) can cause delayed gastric emptying. The standard fasting guidelines may not hold for these patients, so using gastric ultrasound can be beneficial for guiding decision-making by the anesthesiologist.

Gastric POCUS provides a modality that allows anesthesiologists to visually assess the gastric contents in a patient's stomach before a procedure and make an informed decision about the proper anesthetic and airway plans given the qualitative and quantitative assessment of the gastric contents. Gastric ultrasound is done ideally in the supine and right lateral decubitus positions to allow for optimal visualization of gastric contents and measurement of gastric antral cross-sectional area.[27]

In average-sized adults, a curved (low-frequency) array transducer is utilized. A linear (high-frequency) probe can often be utilized for small adult or pediatric patients. To assess fasting status with gastric POCUS, any

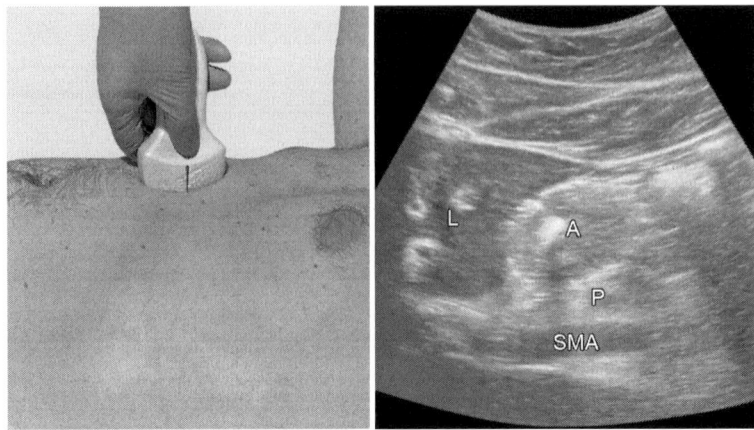

Fig. 3: Example of gastric point-of-care ultrasound (POCUS) visualizing the stomach antrum (A) with the patient in the right lateral decubitus position. Also visible are the liver (L), pancreas (P), and superior mesenteric artery (SMA). In this Figure, the antrum contains solid food.

amount of thick fluid or solid material should be considered a "full stomach" because of the dire pulmonary outcomes that could occur with the aspiration of solid particulates.[28] If only thin fluid is visualized, then determining the gastric volume is necessary. The cross-sectional area of the gastric antrum allows for an estimation of the gastric volume to be made. A volume of thin fluid <1.5 mL/kg can be considered appropriately fasted, while a volume of ≥1.5 mL/kg should be considered a "full stomach".[29]

Gastric POCUS is reliable in determining the fasting status when the status is unknown. A recent random control trial found that bedside gastric POCUS has a sensitivity of 1.0, a specificity of 0.975, a positive predictive value of 0.976, and a negative predictive value of 1.0 in ruling out a full stomach in patients with a pre-test probability of 50% for having a full stomach.[30] Though research has been promising regarding the use of gastric POCUS for determining fasting status, the use of gastric POCUS has not yet been adopted into societal fasting guidelines.

Ultrasound for Trauma Patients

The focused assessment with sonography for trauma (FAST) examination has become a standard examination of trauma patients over the last 3 decades when assessing for the presence of fluid in the pericardium, abdomen, or pelvis. The FAST examination is the most widely utilized and validated POCUS protocol, incorporated into the trauma algorithms at >96% of the US level 1 trauma centers.[31] The FAST examination components include scanning the right upper quadrant to visualize Morrison's Pouch, the left upper quadrant, subxiphoid region for pericardial assessment, and the suprapubic region.[32] The extended FAST (eFAST) protocol has recently replaced the traditional

FAST for many providers. In addition to the traditional FAST examination components, the eFAST examination looks at the bilateral thoracies for the presence of fluid, blood, or air.[33]

In the perioperative setting, the FAST examination can be used quickly to assess for intra-abdominal fluid collection postoperatively. A positive FAST examination in the PACU can help to expedite the decision to return to the operating room if postoperative intra-abdominal bleeding is suspected. The suprapubic portion of the FAST examination also can help to assess a patient's bladder for urine output measurement. Additionally, the FAST examination has been used to assess intra-abdominal fluid extravasation (IAFE) after hip arthroscopies, which in rare circumstances can lead to serious complications like abdominal compartment syndrome. A 2017 study used the FAST examination to show that the presence of IAFE after hip arthroscopies correlated with increased pain scores in the PACU.[34]

The rapid ultrasound for shock and hypotension (RUSH) examination may be of additional benefit to the anesthesiologist in the perioperative setting as it is designed to assess the patient with undifferentiated shock rather than specifically the trauma patient.[35] The RUSH examination includes a POCUS evaluation of the heart, IVC, abdomen, aorta, and thoracies to identify reversible causes of hypotension. While not as well-validated as the FAST examination, a 2019 meta-analysis found that the RUSH examination was beneficial in assessing shock, especially to rule in specific etiologies.[36]

While it is a generally beneficial tool for the anesthesiologist, the FAST examination has limitations that impact its applicability in the perioperative period. The accuracy of the FAST examination decreases as the amount of fluid present gets smaller, with more fluid needing to be detected by a low or moderately trained practitioner.[37] Visualizing retroperitoneal fluid collection is notably difficult with the FAST examination. Additionally, nonacute fluid collection (e.g., ascites or ventriculoperitoneal shunt outflow) may cause false positive FAST results. Lastly, significant fluid shifts from the intravascular to the intraperitoneal space due to large-scale volume resuscitation have the potential to cause a false positive FAST result.[33]

■ POINT-OF-CARE ULTRASOUND FOR PROCEDURES
Ultrasound of the Airway

Expertise in airway management, especially the ability to handle complex and difficult intubations, is a staple of the anesthesiologist's toolbox. Failed or prolonged intubation can increase the risk of serious complications (e.g., severe hypoxia or pulmonary aspiration of gastric contents). The use of airway POCUS is beneficial for preoperative identification of patients with potentially difficult laryngoscopy,[38] confirmation of endotracheal tube placement, and identification of anatomical structures to assist with cricothyrotomy procedures.

While visualization of an endotracheal tube passing through the vocal cords and adequate end-tidal carbon dioxide levels on capnography are often adequate confirmation to the anesthesiologist of successful endotracheal tube placement, there are situations where visualization of the glottic opening is obscured or capnography is not reliable (e.g., cardiac arrest). Airway ultrasound can be a useful tool in these difficult situations. With successful tracheal intubation, a single air-mucosal interface with posterior shadowing will be visualized, along with bilateral lung sliding. Esophageal intubation will have the absence of bilateral lung sliding and has a "double-tract sign" appearance, which is a hyperechoic structure with posterolateral shadowing to the trachea.[39] Two meta-analyses showed transtracheal ultrasonography was at least 98% sensitive and 97% specific in confirming endotracheal intubation.[40,41] Ultrasound confirmation took only an average of 13 seconds across the studies analyzed by Gottlieb et al. Additionally, a double-blinded, randomized study comparing the use of ultrasound to auscultation found that ultrasound had a sensitivity of 93% and a specificity of 96% for differentiating tracheal versus endobronchial intubation.[42] Auscultation's sensitivity and specificity were only 66% and 59%, respectively. The reliability of auscultation is likely worse in obese patients.

All major guidelines for difficult airway management recommend placement of an emergency surgical airway when the airway cannot be managed successfully with tracheal intubation, mask ventilation, or supraglottic device. Traditional visual and palpatory techniques used by trained physicians to identify the cricothyroid membrane during emergency cricothyrotomy are relatively inaccurate.[43,44] Utilization of POCUS for visualizing the cricothyroid membrane is superior to palpatory techniques, especially for obese patients or those with poorly defined or difficult anatomy.[45] Using ultrasound for cricothyrotomy has the potential to have higher success rates and less tracheal damage from misguided attempts.

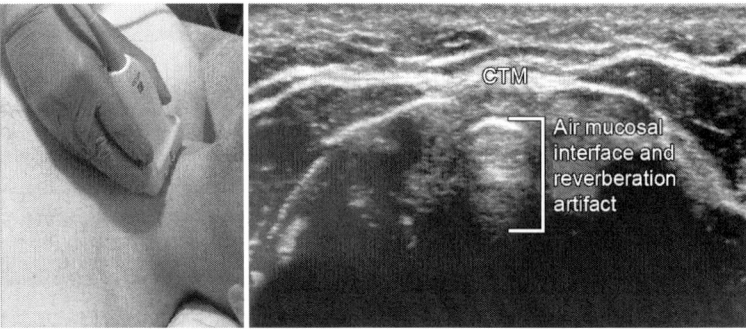

Fig. 4: Example of airway point-of-care ultrasound (POCUS) visualizing the cricothyroid membrane (CTM).

Ultrasound for Regional and Neuraxial Anesthesia

Historically, regional anesthesia injections were completed via landmark- and palpatory-based methods. Nerve stimulation techniques then appeared for regional anesthesia due to the perceived benefits of improvement in block accuracy and visual feedback from the elicited motor response. However, ultrasound for regional anesthesia allows for actual visualization of the local anatomy for a given nerve block, allowing for real-time monitoring of injectate to assure desired distribution. Ultrasound also helps to avoid unwanted trauma to structures like blood vessels or nerves. Two meta-analyses showed that ultrasound-guided peripheral nerve blocks were more successfully placed and had greater efficacy while also reducing the risk of vascular injury when compared to landmark- and nerve-stimulator-guided approaches.[46,47] The anatomic visualization that ultrasound technology permits have led to an explosion of new peripheral nerve block variants (e.g., fascial plane blocks) and the enhancement of techniques employed for more traditional blocks. POCUS use by anesthesiologists for regional anesthesia procedures has become so prevalent that it is considered the gold standard for care in this area.[48]

Unlike regional anesthesia, most anesthesiologists still rely on landmark- and palpatory-based techniques for spinal and epidural procedures, even for patients with clearly difficult anatomy on surface visualization or prior imaging. While difficult to use in a real-time manner, POCUS can be used to visualize spinal anatomy, identify the ideal location for needle insertion, and estimate the depth of the epidural or intrathecal space. A 2016 systematic review and meta-analysis found significant evidence supporting the use of POCUS for neuraxial anesthesia.[49] The analysis showed that POCUS use for neuraxial procedures identified a given lumbar intervertebral space more accurately when compared to landmark palpation, precisely measured the depth from the skin to the epidural or intrathecal space, and increased procedural success rates. The analysis found that using POCUS decreased the risk of traumatic procedures. Still, the evidence was not strong enough to indicate a truly significant improvement in safety using POCUS. Additionally, when considering patients with known spinal anatomical abnormalities or difficult surface landmarks, preprocedural ultrasound evaluation for lumbar spinal anesthetic techniques has improved first-pass success rates without extending the procedural duration.[50,51] These findings also hold for obese patients with BMIs >35.

Ultrasound for Vascular Access

Central venous catheterization is frequently performed by anesthesiologists in the operating room and the intensive care unit for volume resuscitation, vasopressor administration, central venous pressure (CVP) monitoring,

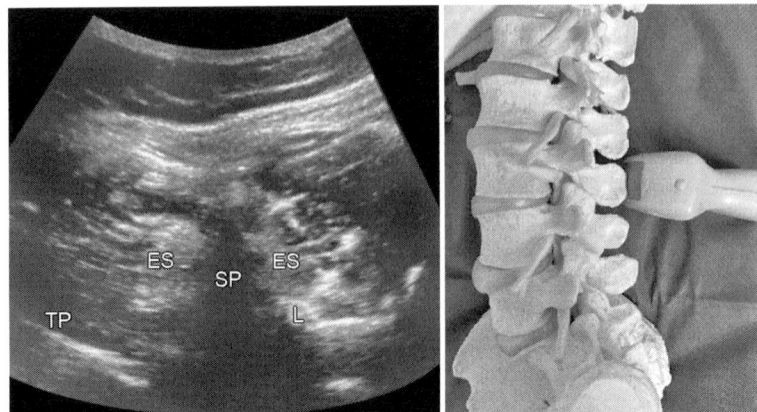

Fig. 5: Example of neuraxial point-of-care ultrasound (POCUS) visualizing lumbar vertebrae in the transverse plane at the level of a spinous process (SP). Also visible is the lamina (L), transverse process (TP), and erector spinae muscles (ES).

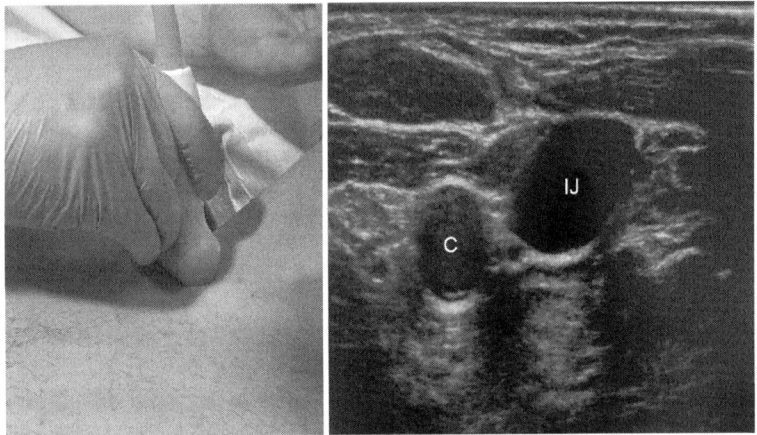

Fig. 6: Example of vascular point-of-care ultrasound (POCUS) visualizing the right internal jugular (IJ) vein and common carotid artery (C).

or renal replacement therapy. Ultrasound use has largely replaced the landmark-based approach due to several benefits. Many studies, including meta-analyses, have been performed since the 1980s comparing the landmark-based technique versus the ultrasound-guided technique. These studies showed that ultrasound for CVC placement corresponded to fewer failures and attempts than the traditional, landmark-based technique while reducing the instances of pneumothorax and inadvertent arterial puncture.[52]

The placement of peripheral intravenous (PIV) catheters is a very common procedure performed by anesthesiologists. An increasing number of patients have conditions (e.g., obesity) associated with difficult PIV access. One meta-analysis comparing ultrasound-guided PIV placement to traditional PIV techniques in patients with difficult peripheral venous access found that while ultrasound did not necessarily reduce the time to successful cannulation or the number of puncture attempts, the use of ultrasound did increase the overall success rate of PIV catheter placement.[53] Increasing the success rate for PIV catheter placement in patients with difficult peripheral access reduces the need for CVC placement by up to 80%. It reduces the risk of serious complications that accompany CVC placement.[54]

While the use of ultrasound for CVC placement has become more commonplace, the use of ultrasound for arterial line placement has lagged. While the femoral, brachial, and dorsalis pedis arteries can be used for arterial catheterization, the radial artery is the most common site accessed. Most studies investigating the efficacy of ultrasound guidance and arterial catheterization versus palpatory techniques involve radial artery canalization. Much like with CVC placement, research, including two recent meta-analyses, shows that the use of ultrasound-guided techniques for arterial catheterization improves first-attempt success rates and requires fewer overall attempts when compared to palpatory techniques.[55,56]

■ CONCLUSION

The application of POCUS has more recently gained significant interest from anesthesiologists. While this article has highlighted the numerous benefits of POCUS use perioperatively, limitations of this modality exist and merit mentioning. POCUS is limited in scope, only helping answer a focused clinical question (e.g., does the patient have a pneumothorax?). Additionally, though the technology is becoming more portable and affordable, the cost is still prohibitive for hospitals and clinics in a large portion of the world. The benefit of POCUS is most appreciably limited by the user's training and experience. There has been a strong push by several national and international organizations to increase POCUS training for anesthesiologists across the globe.[57,58] However, the scope and quality of training programs vary greatly. POCUS protocols help to overcome the variance of competence across practitioners. However, they are largely limited in their scope to a specific patient population or organ system. Other generalizable POCUS frameworks, like the Indication, Acquisition, Interpretation, and Medical management (I-AIM) model, describe a broader stepwise approach to POCUS examinations that can be applied to any situation or patient population to improve examination reliability and performance.[59]

Point-of-care ultrasound is a valuable bedside diagnostic tool for the expedient diagnosis of various acute conditions in the perioperative period in an easy and cost-effective manner. It is gaining a base of evidence to support its validity as an aide to traditional procedural and diagnostic techniques in the perioperative setting. POCUS cannot supplant all aspects of physical examination. However, it can enhance physical examination findings. As discussed in this article, applying POCUS by anesthesiologists can enhance clinician decision-making for various organ systems from the preoperative period through a patient's stay in the PACU. POCUS also has shown great value for the anesthesiologist performing bedside procedures. As technology becomes more portable and affordable, POCUS will become more widely available for anesthesiologists to utilize during the perioperative period.

REFERENCES

1. British Medical Ultrasound Society. The history of ultrasound. [online] Available from https://www.bmus.org/for-patients/ history-of-ultrasound/. [Last accessed October, 2022].
2. Klibanov AL, Hossack JA. Ultrasound in radiology: from anatomic, functional, molecular imaging to drug delivery and image-guided therapy. Invest Radiol. 2015;50(9):657-70.
3. Zhang G, Huang XY, Zhang L. Ultrasound guiding the rapid diagnosis and treatment of perioperative pneumothorax: a case report. World J Clin Cases. 2021;9(35):11043-9.
4. Abu Arab W, Abdulhaleem M, Eltahan S, Elhamami M. Comparative study between bedside chest ultrasound and chest CT scan in the diagnosis of traumatic pneumothorax. Cardiothorac Surg. 2021;29:15.
5. Chan KK, Joo DA, McRae AD, Takwoingi Y, Premji ZA, Lang E, et al. Chest ultrasonography versus supine chest radiography for diagnosis of pneumothorax in trauma patients in the emergency department. Cochrane Database Syst Rev. 2020;7:CD013031.
6. Kruisselbrink R, Chan V, Cibinel GA, Abrahamson S, Goffi A. I-AIM (Indication, acquisition, interpretation, medical decision-making) framework for point-of-care lung ultrasound. Anesthesiology. 2017;127(3):568-82.
7. Tasci O, Hatipoglu ON, Cagli B, Ermis V. Sonography of the chest using linear-array versus sector transducers: correlation with auscultation, chest radiography, and computed tomography. J Clin Ultrasound. 2016;44(6):83-9.
8. Walsh MH, Zhang KX, Cox EJ, Chen JM, Cowley NG, Oleynick CJ, et al. Comparing accuracy of bedside ultrasound examination with physical examination for detection of pleural effusion. Ultrasound J. 2021;13(1):40.
9. Wang Y, Shen Z, Lu X, Zhen Y, Li H. Sensitivity and specificity of ultrasound for the diagnosis of acute pulmonary edema: a systematic review and meta-analysis. Med Ultrason. 2018;1(1):32-6.
10. Al Deeb M, Barbic S, Featherstone R, Dankoff J, Barbic D. Point-of-care ultrasonography for the diagnosis of acute cardiogenic pulmonary edema in patients presenting with acute dyspnea: a systematic review and meta-analysis. Acad Emerg Med. 2014;21(8):843-52.
11. Maw AM, Hassanin A, Ho PM, McInnes MDF, Moss A, Juarez-Colunga E, et al. Diagnostic accuracy of point-of-care lung ultrasonography and chest radiography in adults with symptoms suggestive of acute decompensated heart failure: a systematic review and meta-analysis. JAMA Netw Open. 2019;2(3):e190703.

12. Boussuges A, Rives S, Finance J, Brégeon F. Assessment of diaphragmatic function by ultrasonography: current approach and perspectives. World J Clin Cases. 2020;8(12):2408-24.
13. Zambon M, Greco M, Bocchino S, Cabrini L, Beccaria PF, Zangrillo A. Assessment of diaphragmatic dysfunction in the critically ill patient with ultrasound: a systematic review. Intensive Care Med. 2017;43(1):29-38.
14. Jensen MB, Sloth E, Larsen KM, Schmidt MB. Transthoracic echocardiography for cardiopulmonary monitoring in intensive care. Eur J Anaesthesiol. 2004;21:700-7.
15. Zimmerman JM, Coker BJ. The nuts and bolts of performing focused cardiovascular ultrasound (FOCUS). Anesth Analges. 2017;124:753-60.
16. Cowie B. Three years' experience of focused cardiovascular ultrasound in the peri-operative period. Anaesthesia. 2011;66(4):268-73.
17. Haskins SC, Tanaka CY, Boublik J, Wu CL, Sloth E. Focused cardiac ultrasound for the regional anesthesiologist and pain specialist. Reg Anesth Pain Med. 2017;42(5):632-44.
18. Ansari BM, Zochios V, Falter F, Klein AA. Physiological controversies and methods used to determine fluid responsiveness: a qualitative systematic review. Anaesthesia. 2016;71(1):94-105.
19. Zhang J, Critchley LA. Inferior Vena Cava Ultrasonography before general anesthesia can predict hypotension after induction. Anesthesiology. 2016; 124(3):580-9.
20. Li L, Yong RJ, Kaye AD, Urman RD. Perioperative point-of-care ultrasound (POCUS) for anesthesiologists: an overview. Curr Pain Headache Rep. 2020; 24(5):20.
21. Marbach JA, Almufleh A, Di Santo P, Jung R, Simard T, McInnes M, et al. Comparative accuracy of focused cardiac ultrasonography and clinical examination for left ventricular dysfunction and valvular heart disease: a systematic review and meta-analysis. Ann Intern Med. 2019;171(4):264-72.
22. Loxdale SJ, Sneyd JR, Donovan A, Werrett G, Viira DJ. The role of routine pre-operative bedside echocardiography in detecting aortic stenosis in patients with a hip fracture. Anaesthesia. 2012;67(1):51-4.
23. Hanson MG, Chan B. The role of point-of-care ultrasound in the diagnosis of pericardial effusion: a single academic center retrospective study. Ultrasound J. 2021;13(1):2.
24. Kedan I, Ciozda W, Palatinus JA, Palatinus HN, Kimchi A. Prognostic value of point-of-care ultrasound during cardiac arrest: a systematic review. Cardiovasc Ultrasound. 2020;18(1):1.
25. Zengin S, Gümüşboğa H, Sabak M, Eren ŞH, Altunbas G, Al B. Comparison of manual pulse palpation, cardiac ultrasonography and Doppler ultrasonography to check the pulse in cardiopulmonary arrest patients. Resuscitation. 2018;133:59-64.
26. Komiya K, Rubin BK, Kadota JI, Mukae H, Akaba T, Moro H, et al. Prognostic implications of aspiration pneumonia in patients with community acquired pneumonia: a systematic review with meta-analysis. Sci Rep. 2016;6:38097.
27. Kruisselbrink R, Gharapetian A, Chaparro LE, Ami N, Richler D, Chan VWS, Perlas A. Diagnostic accuracy of point-of-care gastric ultrasound. Anesth Analg. 2019;128(1):89-95.
28. Perlas A, Arzola C, Van de Putte P. Point-of-care gastric ultrasound and aspiration risk assessment: a narrative review. Can J Anaesth. 2018;65(4):437-48.

29. Perlas A, Van de Putte P, Van Houwe P, Chan VW. I-AIM framework for point-of-care gastric ultrasound. Br J Anaesth. 2016;116(1):7-11.
30. Kruisselbrink R, Gharapetian A, Chaparro LE, Ami N, Richler D, Chan VWS, et al. Diagnostic accuracy of point-of-care gastric ultrasound. Anesth Analg. 2019;128(1):89-95.
31. Richards JR, McGahan JP. Focused assessment with sonography in trauma (FAST) in 2017: what radiologists can learn. Radiology. 2017;283(1):30-48.
32. Manson WC, Kirksey M, Boublik J, Wu CL, Haskins SC. Focused assessment with sonography in trauma (FAST) for the regional anesthesiologist and pain specialist. Reg Anesth Pain Med. 2019;44(5):540-8.
33. Desai N, Harris T. Extended focused assessment with sonography in trauma. BJA Educ. 2018;18(2):57-62.
34. Haskins SC, Desai NA, Fields KG, Nejim JA, Cheng S, Coleman SH, et al. Diagnosis of intraabdominal fluid extravasation after hip arthroscopy with point-of-care ultrasonography can identify patients at an increased risk for postoperative pain. Anesth Analg. 2017;124(3):791-9.
35. Shokoohi H, Boniface KS, Pourmand A, Liu YT, Davison DL, Hawkins KD, et al. Bedside ultrasound reduces diagnostic uncertainty and guides resuscitation in patients with undifferentiated hypotension. Crit Care Med. 2015;43(12):2562-9.
36. Stickles SP, Carpenter CR, Gekle R, Kraus CK, Scoville C, Theodoro D, et al. The diagnostic accuracy of a point-of-care ultrasound protocol for shock etiology: a systematic review and meta-analysis. CJEM. 2019;21(3):406-17.
37. Richards JR, McGahan JP. Focused assessment with sonography in trauma (FAST) in 2017: what radiologists can learn. Radiology. 2017;283(1):30-48.
38. Koundal V, Rana S, Thakur R, Chauhan V, Ekke S, Kumar M. The usefulness of point of care ultrasound (POCUS) in preanaesthetic airway assessment. Indian J Anaesth 2019;63:1022-8.
39. Kristensen MS, Teoh WH. Ultrasound in confirming endotracheal intubation. In: Rosenblatt WH, Popescu WM (Eds). Master techniques in upper and lower airway management. Philadelphia: Wolters Kluwer Health; 2015. pp. 28-9.
40. Das SK, Choupoo NS, Haldar R, Lahkar A. Transtracheal ultrasound for verification of endotracheal tube placement: a systematic review and meta-analysis. Can J Anaesth. 2015;62:413-23.
41. Gottlieb M, Holladay D, Peksa GD. Ultrasonography for the confirmation of endotracheal tube intubation: a systematic review and meta-analysis. Ann Emerg Med. 2018;72:627-36.
42. Ramsingh D, Frank E, Haughton R, Schilling J, Gimenez KM, Banh E, et al. Auscultation versus point-of-care ultrasound to determine endotracheal versus bronchial intubation: a diagnostic accuracy study. Anesthesiology. 2016;124(5):1012-20.
43. Campbell M, Shanahan H, Ash S, Royds J, Husarova V, McCaul C. The accuracy of locating the cricothyroid membrane by palpation: an intergender study. BMC Anesthesiol. 2014;14:108.
44. Lamb A, Zhang J, Hung O, Flemming B, Mullen T, Bissell MB, et al. Accuracy of identifying the cricothyroid membrane by anesthesia trainees and staff in a Canadian institution. Can J Anaesth. 2015;62(5):495-503.
45. Siddiqui N, Yu E, Boulis S, You-Ten KE. Ultrasound is superior to palpation in identifying the cricothyroid membrane in subjects with poorly defined neck landmarks: a randomized clinical trial. Anesthesiology. 2018;129(6):1132-9.

46. Abrahams MS, Aziz MF, Fu RF, Horn JL. Ultrasound guidance compared with electrical neurostimulation for peripheral nerve block: a systematic review and meta-analysis of randomized controlled trials. Br J Anaesth. 2009;102(3):408-17.
47. Gelfand HJ, Ouanes JP, Lesley MR, Ko PS, Murphy JD, Sumida SM, et al. Analgesic efficacy of ultrasound-guided regional anesthesia: a meta-analysis. J Clin Anesth. 2011;23(2):90-6.
48. Boselli E, Hopkins P, Lamperti M, Estèbe JP, Fuzier R, Biasucci DG, et al. European Society of Anaesthesiology and Intensive Care Guidelines on peri-operative use of ultrasound for regional anaesthesia (PERSEUS regional anesthesia): Peripheral nerves blocks and neuraxial anaesthesia. Eur J Anaesthesiol. 2021;38(3):219-50.
49. Perlas A, Chaparro LE, Chin KJ. Lumbar neuraxial ultrasound for spinal and epidural anesthesia: a systematic review and meta-analysis. Reg Anesth Pain Med. 2016;41(2):251-60.
50. Chin KJ, Perlas A, Chan V, Brown-Shreves D, Koshkin A, Vaishnav V. Ultrasound imaging facilitates spinal anesthesia in adults with difficult surface anatomic landmarks. Anesthesiology. 2011;115:94-101.
51. Park SK, Bae J, Yoo S, Kim WH, Lim YJ, Bahk JH, et al. Ultrasound-assisted versus landmark-guided spinal anesthesia in patients with abnormal spinal anatomy: a randomized controlled trial. Anesth Analg. 2020;130(3):787-95.
52. Srinivasan S, Govil D, Gupta S, Patel S, Jagadeesh KN, Tomar DS. Incidence of posterior wall penetration during internal jugular vein cannulation: a comparison of two techniques using real-time ultrasound. Indian J Anaesth. 2017;61(3):240-4.
53. Stolz LA, Stolz U, Howe C, Farrell IJ, Adhikari S. Ultrasound-guided peripheral venous access: a meta-analysis and systematic review. J Vasc Access. 2015;16(4):321-6.
54. Shokoohi H, Boniface K, McCarthy M, Khedir Al-tiae T, Sattarian M, Ding R, et al. Ultrasound-guided peripheral intravenous access program is associated with a marked reduction in central venous catheter use in noncritically ill emergency department patients. Ann Emerg Med. 2013;61(2):198-203.
55. Bhattacharjee S, Maitra S, Baidya DK. Comparison between ultrasound guided technique and digital palpation technique for radial artery cannulation in adult patients: an updated meta-analysis of randomized controlled trials. J Clin Anesth. 2018;47:54-9.
56. Zhao W, Peng H, Li H, Yi Y, Ma Y, He Y, et al. Effects of ultrasound-guided techniques for radial arterial catheterization: a meta-analysis of randomized controlled trials. Am J Emerg Med. 2021;46:1-9.
57. ACGME. (2020). ACGME program requirements for graduate medical education in anesthesiology. [online] Available from https://www.acgme.org/Portals/0/PFAssets/ProgramRequirements/040_Anesthesiology_2020.pdf. [Last accessed October, 2022].
58. Volpicelli G, Lamorte A, Tullio M, Cardinale L, Giraudo M, Stefanone V, et al. Point-of-care multiorgan ultrasonography for the evaluation of undifferentiated hypotension in the emergency department. Intensive Care Med. 2013;39(7):1290-8.
59. Bahner DP, Hughes D, Royall NA. I-AIM: a novel model for teaching and performing focused sonography. J Ultrasound Med. 2012;31(2):295-300.

CHAPTER

22

Artificial Intelligence in Anesthesia

Shaloo Garg

▓ ABSTRACT

Artificial intelligence (AI) plays a crucial role in various fields of application. In one way or the other, it influences our everyday lives. AI is being rapidly developed in the field of medicine. As advancements are happening in medicine, AI researchers are keeping pace with practical applications for most disciplines of medicine. Anesthesia has found various applications of AI, which help in many ways in the perioperative period and are being tested in clinical settings. With the need for anesthetics widening and the global pandemic not showing any signs of abatement, anesthesiologists need to exploit the advantages of AI to become more efficient and innovative.

Keywords: Artificial Intelligence; Anesthesia; Perioperative care; Predictive therapy; Postoperative analgesia; Ultrasound, and operating room logistics.

▓ KEY POINTS

- AI is being rapidly developed in the field of medicine.
- AI is useful in perioperative care, critical care, pain management, and drug delivery.
- AI can play a role in the preanesthetic evaluation of the airway, risk stratification, planning of anesthesia, monitoring depth of anesthesia, hemodynamic monitoring, and prediction of hypotension.
- Automated closed-loop anesthesia delivery (CLAD) systems use hemodynamics and bispectral index (BIS) monitoring to forecast and deliver drugs for anesthesia.
- AI helps start pre-emptive therapy, effective use of resources and predict long-term outcomes in critical care.
- Wireless intelligent patient-controlled analgesia (PCA) and AI-controlled analgesia by remote monitoring, intelligent alarms, and analysis can be used to treat acute and chronic pain.
- Ultrasound in regional blocks and for epidural placement helps identify critical anatomical structures.

- AI can be used for operating room (OR) logistics, i.e., scheduling OR time, tracking movements and actions of anesthesiologists, staffing/limiting wastage of resources, OR use per procedure, and staff coordination.
- 5G can be used to reach out to a larger base of patients by creating more operation theatre (OT) hubs within the premises or at different off-campus locations.

INTRODUCTION

Humans have been dreaming about the possibilities of artificial intelligence (AI) for a long time. It was almost a century ago when AI first appeared in a German movie titled *Metropolis*, and technology has become more prevalent since then.

Artificial intelligence is often referred to synonymously with computers and robots. However, we can trace the roots across multiple fields such as philosophy, psychology, linguistics, and statistics. Many visionaries helped in providing the foundation for the modern elements of artificial intelligence across those fields. Charles Babbage, Alan Turing, Claude Shannon, Richard Bellman, and Marvin Minsky helped in cutting-edge innovation and sophisticated analytics. Furthermore, significant advances in computer science such as hardware-based improvements in processing and storage, have enabled the base technologies required for the advent of artificial intelligence.

Our healthcare system faces the challenges of an increasing amount of patient data, subsets of diseases, diagnostic tools, monitoring, and treatment modalities. The big data, AI, and development of machine learning (ML) algorithms offer massive relief to physicians from the information overload concerning the complexity of health care, predicting clinical events, improving diagnostic accuracy, and providing targeted treatments.

Almost all specialties of medicine are using AI, ranging from primarily diagnostic applications in radiology and pathology to more therapeutic and interventional applications in cardiology, critical care, and surgery.[1] With the developing applications of AI in medicine, clinicians in every field need to understand what these technologies are and how they can help deliver safer, more efficient, and more cost-effective care.

The anesthesiology practice has the potential to benefit from AI in multiple areas. By applying AI to perioperative care, critical care, pain management, and drug delivery, anesthesiologists can try to be ahead of their patient's condition by the monitoring and predictive functions of AI. Surgeons, not to be left behind, are applying AI to sit in a different room or a city and operate upon a patient with the da Vinci robotic system. With the advent of 5G systems, Internet of Medical Things (IoMT)/smart healthcare, shorter latency, and enhanced throughput, anesthesia can easily be replicated at a remote OT, with real-time monitoring from a distant OT hub.[2]

ARTIFICIAL INTELLIGENCE

What is artificial intelligence?

Artificial intelligence has been defined in numerous manners by various scientists. John McCarthy described AI as "the science and engineering of making intelligent machines". AI is the ability of a *digital computer* or *computer-controlled robot* to perform tasks commonly associated with the intellectual process characteristics of humans. It is essentially the algorithms that help the machines to reason, discover meaning, solve problems, recognize features, make decisions, and learn from experience. This is made possible due to large datasets, rapid processing hardware, AI architecture, and algorithms.[3]

Artificial intelligence came into being as an academic discipline in 1956. In the subsequent years, AI has ridden waves of optimism, disappointment, and loss of funding known as an "AI winter", followed by new approaches, success, and renewed funding. AI researchers have attempted to simulate the brain, model human problem-solving and formal logic, and imitate animal behavior.[4]

Three factors that form the backbone of AI and have contributed to its rapid development are as follows:
1. Large datasets.
2. Improved hardware that can simultaneously perform large processing tasks.
3. A new wave of AI architectures and algorithms.

Machine Learning

Machine learning is one of the major subfields of AI. With the onset of the 21st century, *machine learning* has dominated the field with a highly mathematical statistical model. Machine learning is training a *computer* to learn from its inputs and react to data (numerical, images, text, sound, etc.) without explicit programming.

There are different learning algorithms with various techniques used to solve a problem—supervised learning, unsupervised learning, and reinforcement learning.

- *Supervised learning:* Supervised learning is a task-driven process by which an algorithm(s) is trained to predict a prespecified output. It requires both the training and test datasets. The training dataset allows the machine to analyze and learn the associations between input and desired output. In contrast, the test dataset allows for the assessment of the performance of the algorithm on new data.

    Kendale et al., conducted a study on electronic health record data to identify patients who experienced postinduction hypotension [mean arterial pressure (MAP) <55 mm Hg). The training dataset included 70% of the patients and variables such as the American Society of Anesthesiologists (ASA) physical status, age, body mass index, comorbidities, medications, and the blood pressure of the patients. The various algorithms used by Kendale et al., could then analyze the training dataset to learn which variables were predictive of postinduction hypotension. The test dataset was then analyzed to assess how accurately the algorithm could predict postinduction hypotension in the remaining 30% of patients.[5]

- *Unsupervised learning:* In unsupervised learning, algorithms identify patterns or structures within a dataset. It can be used to identify patients who could most benefit from certain drugs such as asthmatics, who would benefit most from glucocorticoid therapy, based on genomic analysis.[6]
- *Reinforcement learning:* Reinforcement learning refers to the process by which an algorithm is asked to attempt a specific task, e.g., deliver inhalational anesthesia to a patient.[7] Padmanabhan et al., used reinforcement learning to develop an anesthesia controller that used feedback from a patient's bispectral index (BIS) and MAP to control the infusion rates of propofol (in a simulated patient model). In this scenario, achieving BIS and MAP values within a set range result in a reward for the algorithm. In contrast, values outside the range result in errors that prompt the algorithm to perform further fine-tuning.[8]
- *Fuzzy logic:* Often uses rule-based systems where precise mathematical functions do not accurately model phenomena.[9] A monitor was developed to detect hypovolemia using fuzzy logic. It classified hypovolemia into mild, moderate, and severe based on normalized values of heart rate (HR), blood pressure, and pulse volume that was further divided into categories of mild, moderate, and severe. Using fuzzy logic, "if electrocardiogram-HR and blood pressure are mild and pulse volume is severe, hypovolemia is moderate". Progress in AI research has focused on using more data-driven techniques in machine learning to achieve goals first explored by researchers working with fuzzy logic.[10]
- *Classical machine learning:* Uses features, or properties within the data, to perform the tasks. Hu et al., used decision trees to predict total patient-controlled analgesia (PCA) consumption from patient demographics, vital signs, and aspects of their medical history, surgery type, and PCA doses delivered, with the promise of using such approaches to optimize PCA dosing regimens.[11]
- *Convoluted neural networks and deep learning:* These are one of the most popular methods today for performing work in machine learning. These networks are inspired by biological nervous systems and process signals in layers of computational units (neurons).[12,13] Each network comprises an input layer of neurons comprised of features that describe the data, at least one hidden layer of neurons that conduct different mathematical transformations on the input features, and an output layer that yields a result as depicted in **Figure 1**.[14] Within the field of anesthesia, multiple examples of the applications of neural networks exist, including depth of anesthesia monitoring and control of anesthesia delivery.

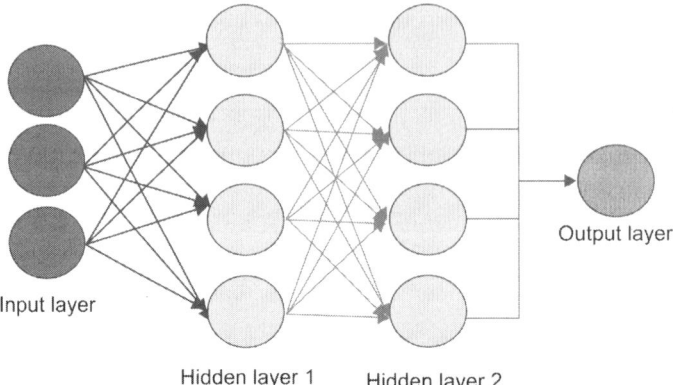

Fig. 1: Convolutional neural network—a representation.

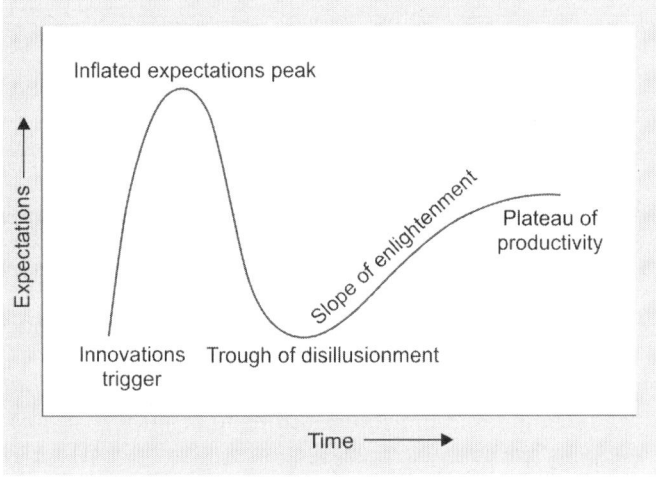

Fig. 2: Gartner hype cycle.[15]

Gartner Hype Cycle

How does one discern the hype from commercial viability in AI? Whenever new technologies make bold promises, do the claims payoff? If yes, how long does it take? Gartner hype cycles **(Fig. 2)** is a graphic representation of the maturity and adoption of technologies and their relevance to solving real problems and exploiting new opportunities.[15]

Each technological advancement has five key phases in its life cycle:
1. *Innovation trigger:* A technology breakthrough leads to proof-of-concept stories often, there is no usable product, and commercial viability is unproven.
2. *The peak of inflated expectations:* Early publicity produces a number of success stories and failures. Anesthesiology is currently in this phase where plenty of experimental robots and models are being tested.

3. *Trough of disillusionment:* Interest wanes as experiments and implementations fail to deliver.
4. *The slope of enlightenment:* The benefits of technology become better understood, and products appear from technology providers.
5. *Plateau of productivity:* Mainstream adoption starts to take off, and applicability and relevance of technology become apparent.

How can AI be used in healthcare?
The CEO of DataRobot, Jeremy Achin, while addressing a crowd at the Japan AI experience in 2017, said, "AI is a computer system able to perform tasks that ordinarily require human intelligence. Many of these artificial intelligence systems are powered by machine learning, some of them are powered by deep learning, and some of them are powered by very boring things like rules".

Artificial intelligence has made inroads into different medical fields, from diagnostics to therapy. AI can assist in situations where health professionals disagree in their diagnosis, and for this, developers at Elinext have devised a tool that analyzes lung X-ray images to identify signs of pneumonia or tuberculosis.[16]

United States Food and Drug Administration approved the first software in 2018, which uses AI to diagnose diabetic retinopathy. Several studies have shown that AI can outdo dermatologists in classifying suspicious skin lesions. Artificial intelligence has been used widely in mental health interventions and pain management. It has significantly contributed to the research and evaluation of new medications, which would otherwise take years to process, given the overwhelming number of existing drugs.

Anesthesiology touches on multiple elements of clinical care, including perioperative and intensive care, pain management, drug delivery, and discovery. A review of the literature for artificial intelligence and anesthesia research identified and summarized six themes of applications of artificial intelligence in anesthesiology: (1) depth of anesthesia monitoring, (2) control of anesthesia, (3) event and risk prediction, (4) ultrasound guidance, (5) pain management, and (6) operating room logistics. The advances in AI are potentially beneficial to the specialty and would also allow anesthesiologists to be more efficient and innovative.[17]

■ APPLICATIONS OF ARTIFICIAL INTELLIGENCE

Artificial Intelligence and Preanesthetic Evaluation

The most critical area in anesthesia is the management of the airway. AI, through a convoluted neural network, uses attention-based multiple instance learning and predicts airway as easy or difficult on an image directly by learning "features" on the image. This is similar to how the visual cortex in the human brain processes images. Deep learning through the neural network has been giving encouraging results in airway assessment.[18]

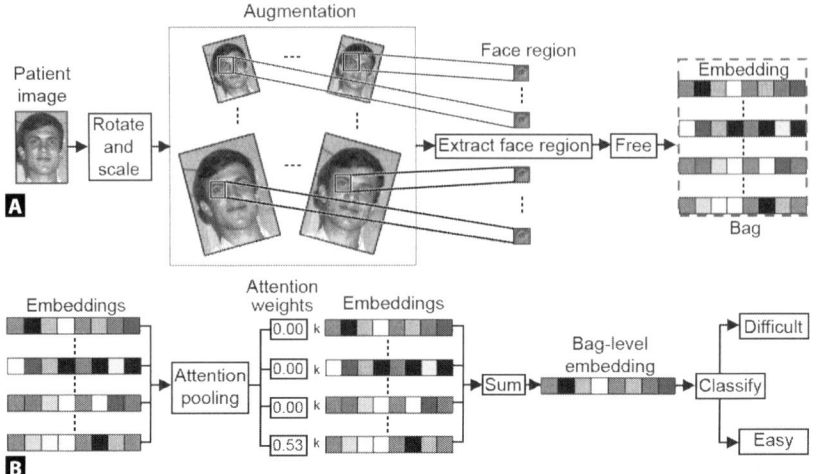

Fig. 3: Attention-based multiple instance learning composition and aggregation. (A) Patient image features are extracted by random forests and recursive feature elimination (FRFE) models; (B) Attention pooling computes a weighted sum of embeddings and classifies them as difficult or easy to intubate.

As can be seen in **Figure 3**, AI rotates, scales, augments, and extracts data from the facial features. With serial embeddings, attention pooling of the data and sum augmentation can predict the difficulty of the airway.

Machine learning can be used for risk stratification based on the analysis of millions of perioperative data and intervention-based outcomes extracted from the electronic health record (EHR) of multiple centers. This helps in preoperative counseling, optimization, and planning anesthetic management of individual cases with rare comorbidities. Preoperative checklists have contributed to increased surgical safety. A clinical decision support system (CDSS) has been developed and widely tested in multicenter trials.[19]

A model provides automated physician order decision support suggestions for inpatient care regarding antibiotics and other drugs through a feed-forward neural network. This is based on the patient's current status data mined from EHR and the deep learning that the model has acquired.

Artificial Intelligence and Monitoring

Alarm fatigue is a significant factor responsible for oversight or error. During delivery of anesthesia for long-duration cases, automated monitoring, response to hemodynamic changes, and support in clinical decision helps prevent errors. Analysis of multiple parameters such as heart rate, blood pressure, Train of Four (TOF), BIS, etc., can be integrated into the alarm system with the help of AI using cognitive robots. This prevents alarm fatigue and reduces the incidence of false alarms, and also prevents miscommunication between various teams.[20,21]

The depth of anesthesia has been a problem during surgery where the need is to avoid excessive depth and the light plane of anesthesia. AI-based models predict the depth of anesthesia with fair accuracy by monitoring BIS, electroencephalography (EEG), or midlatency auditory evoked potential (AEP). The accuracy is BIS 84.2%, EEG 88.4%, and mid latency AEP 86%. This can obviate the risk of awareness under anesthesia and postoperative cognitive dysfunction. It helps reduce hospital stays, new complications, and higher medical expenses.

Mirsadeghi et al., studied 25 patients and compared the accuracy of their machine learning method of analyzing the BIS index with the direct features from EEG signals [e.g., power in different bands (delta, theta, alpha, beta, and gamma), total power, spindle score, entropy, etc.] in identifying awake versus anesthetized patients.[22]

Zhang et al., recorded midlatency AEP from patients. They used neural networks to assess the accuracy of these signals in determining when patients were awake (96.8% accuracy), receiving adequate anesthesia (86% accuracy), and emerging from general anesthesia (86.6% accuracy). In addition, clinical variables such as heart rate variability have been investigated to approximate sedation levels typically measured by the Richmond Agitation Sedation Scale.[23] The neural network and deep learning engage in self-learning of the features in the dataset, and select features that will best predict a target value (e.g., awareness) rather than being fed the features thought to be the most predictive by a human expert.[24]

Artificial Intelligence and Anesthesia Delivery

Control of anesthesia delivery is possible by AI, where model parameters are learned from data by learning algorithms. As depicted in **Figure 4**, Wang et al., described the drug/procedure inputs to outcomes in surgery

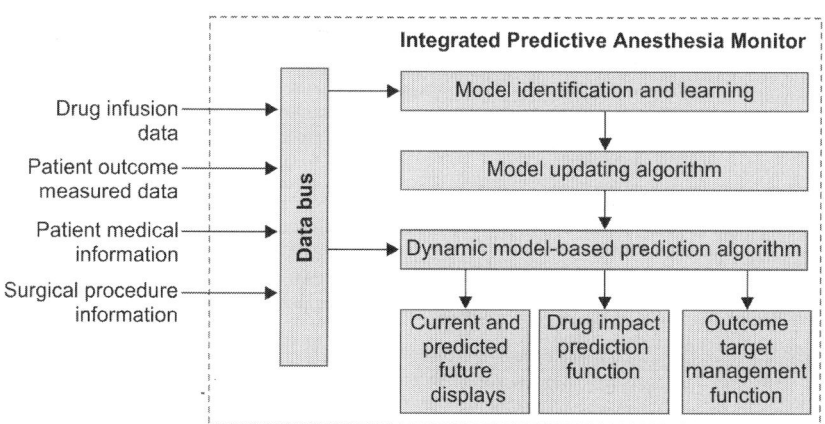

Fig. 4: Automated closed loop anesthesia delivery system.

or procedure and that the model must be tunable to fit specific patient parameters into a range of surgical procedures.[25]

Automated closed-loop anesthesia delivery (CLAD) has been designed to take the inputs of all patient parameters, run it through an ML system of data analysis and predict outcomes and help in target management through predictive anesthesia monitor. This has been used for propofol infusion, opioids, and muscle relaxants. Hemodynamic feedback mechanisms, noninvasive cardiac output monitoring, cerebral oximetry, EEG processing, and nociception assessment form the basis of predictive monitoring, drug impact, and outcome target management.

Monitoring parameters related to sympathetic and/or parasympathetic systems and various pain scores such as nociception level index, analgesia-nociception index, surgical plethysmographic index, pupillometry, and pupillary pain index help in fine-tuning the opioid infusion for pain relief.[26,27]

Artificial Intelligence and Event Prediction

Anesthesiologists can harness AI and ML optimally for event prediction under anesthesia, thus also alleviating the shortage of anesthesiologists. During actual surgeries, data is collected using machine learning models. This is then analyzed and helps predict events like return of consciousness and rate of neuromuscular blockade (NMB) recovery. The hypotension prediction index is also made easy with AI. Real-time monitoring and hospital records of patients undergoing complex surgical procedures were studied. This helped predict the onset of myocardial perfusion compromise like a fall in ejection fraction. Thus armed with this information, the clinician can do early intervention, reducing the incidence of perioperative morbidity and mortality. This can be followed up with confirmatory tests such as echocardiography and biomarker assay and further definitive management.[27]

The process of manifold learning is a subtype of AI. The prediction of long-term outcomes for early pre-emptive intervention will optimally utilize resources. The concept of "artificial intelligence clinician" has been studied and validated in critical care for lowering mortality rates in sepsis.[28] 3D ECG imaging and arterial waveform analysis can diagnose coronary insufficiency early and help in definitive intervention.[29,30]

Artificial Intelligence and Postoperative Pain

Postoperative pain is a major patient concern, and achieving optimum analgesia is an eternal pursuit for anesthesiologists. Wireless intelligent PCA and AI-controlled analgesia are the way forward through remote monitoring, intelligent alarm and analysis, assessment, and automatic recording. Machine learning can help in predicting opioid dosing, individual opioid requirements, and the need for preoperative acute pain counseling.

Many studies have successfully used remotely controlled pumps, without physical intervention by nurses or physicians, for postoperative analgesia.[31] One study used a system with telemonitoring of patients for pain, which could control the patient's infusion pump remotely, without the need to visit him personally. The advent of 5G technology will help to safeguard health systems and restrict hacking/intrusion.

Gram et al., used machine learning to analyze EEG signals from 81 patients. The results had a 65% predictive value in identifying patients who would respond to opioid therapy for acute pain.[32]

Artificial Intelligence and Ultrasound Guidance

Many articles have been identified that describe the use of AI techniques to assist in performing ultrasound-based procedures. The neural networks help classify ultrasound images with an average accuracy of 94.5% ± 2.9%.[33] Smistad et al., used ultrasound images of the groin from 15 patients to train a convolutional neural network to identify the femoral artery or vein while distinguishing it from other potentially similar appearing ultrasound images such as muscle, bone, or even acoustic shadow.

Neural networks are also valuable for the identification of the vertebral level and other anatomical landmarks for epidural placement and identifying the anterior base of the vertebral lamina, Hetherington et al., used convolutional neural networks with up to 95% accuracy to identify the sacrum and the L1–L5 vertebrae and vertebral spaces from ultrasound images in real-time.[34]

Artificial Intelligence and Operative Room Logistics

Operative room logistics is an area where AI can play a big role in optimizing resources by precisely scheduling operating room time, tracking movements and actions of anesthesiologists, staffing/limiting wastage of resources, OR use per procedure and staff, coordinating multiple spaces simultaneously such as postanesthesia care unit (PACU) and OR. Cancellation has an important economic repercussion, and identifying surgeries with high risks of cancellation and pre-empting it can prevent wastefulness.

Combes et al., used a hospital database containing extensive information on staffing, operating room use per procedure and staff, and postanesthesia care unit use with the electronic health record to train a neural network to predict the duration of an operation based on the team, type of operation and a patient's relevant medical history; however, the prediction accuracy of their models never exceeded 60%.[35]

Houliston et al., analyzed radio frequency identification tags to determine the location, orientation, and stance of anesthesiologists in the operating room. The study was limited to simulated operating rooms with mannequins. Still, the authors proposed the use of this application of ML with actual patients to understand better potential impacts on patient safety based on the interaction of anesthesiologists with the various equipment in the room.[36]

Artificial Intelligence and Robots in Anesthesia

- *Mechanical robots:* Kepler intubation system[37] depicted in **Figures 5A and B**, Mc Sleepy, the anesthesia robot, and iControl RP anesthesia robot are a few robots making a foray into the anesthesiologists' workplace.
- *Pharmacological robots:* AI-assisted closed-loop titration of drugs may lessen workload and free a solitary anesthesiologist to initiate and monitor multiple anesthetics simultaneously from a control booth via multiple video screens and interface displays, maintain a stable anesthetic and detect if the patient has begun to drift outside the control parameters. AI has the potential to impact the clinical practice of anesthesia for perioperative support, critical care delivery, and outpatient pain management.

Handling all tasks by an automated robotic device is still the stuff of science fiction. AI-based machines are fast, more accurate, and consistently rational. They are, however, not intuitive, emotional, or culturally sensitive. These deficiencies make humans more effective.

An early role for the robot and AI, where an anesthesiologist is unavailable, could be in war zones, remote areas, outer space, and the current severe acute respiratory syndrome (SARS) COVID-19 pandemic for anesthesia delivery and critical care. One could conjecture that a closed-loop anesthesia system may be used to facilitate surgery in outer space as well.

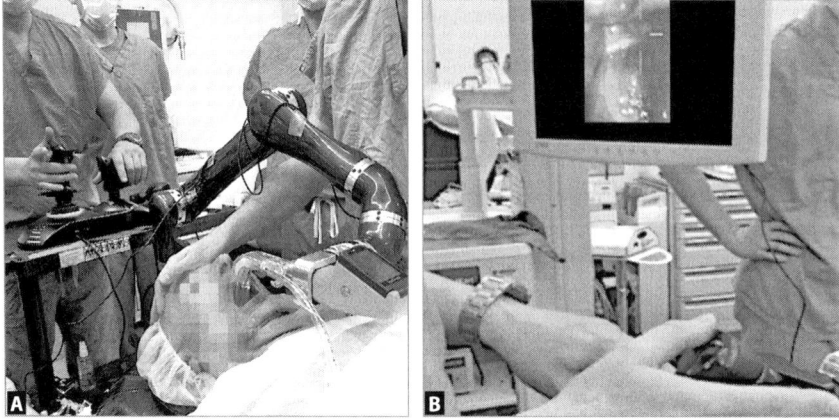

Figs. 5A and B: Video laryngoscopy and a robotic arm to introduce an endotracheal tube.

■ LIMITATIONS AND ETHICS

A critical realization is that anesthetizing patients requires far more skill than merely titrating two drug levels. Every patient requires preoperative assessment, including history, physical exam, and laboratory evaluation, so the anesthesiologist can plan and prescribe the appropriate type of anesthesia.

Placement of an intravenous line, mask ventilation followed by the placement of an airway to control the ventilation, and removal of the airway on completion of the surgery, are all human interventions, which will be difficult to replace by the robots.

Observation of all vital monitors during surgery to determine the diagnosis and treatment of any complication that occurs perioperatively due to anesthesia or the surgical procedure will also require human intervention.

The possibilities of AI are limited and will not always result in classifications or predictions superior to traditional methods. A machine would not be able to replace the warmth, reassurance, and allaying of an anxious patient's fears.

Artificial intelligence methods often lack transparency, wherein an algorithm can make a prediction but cannot explain why such a prediction was made. Similarly, AI methods demonstrate correlations and identify patterns easily but cannot yet determine causal relationships. Clinicians and researchers expect more transparency, and the "correlation does not mean causation" rule is applicable to AI as well.

Artificial intelligence algorithms are prone to biases, just like the humans. The healthcare system is full of implicit and explicit biases which can impact the big data implementation and affect the types of predictions that AI makes based on this data.[38]

In medical practice, patient data and sound ethical practices are the strong pillars of patient care and research. AI thus has a big role to play keeping in mind patient privacy. A strong regulatory body is the need of the hour to protect patient rights, ethical practices, humane approach and privacy before the medical records are outsourced to researchers or companies for developing newer interventions.[39]

■ FUTURE OF ARTIFICIAL INTELLIGENCE

Artificial intelligence algorithms have not yet surpassed human performance. Greater productivity, the automation of cognitively routine work, ability to quickly and accurately sift through large stores of data and uncover correlations and patterns that are imperceptible to human cognition will make it a valuable tool for clinicians.

Artificial intelligence can contribute to monitoring the depth of anesthesia, maintaining drug infusions, and predicting hypotension. Creating inclusive teams by aligning man and machine will allow practicing anesthesiologists to be more effective and efficient in the care they provide. The teams should compose of humans and nonhumans working to integrate the new technologies ambitiously and strategically.

Anesthesiology is both a science and art, and at its core, it is still a uniquely human endeavor. Algorithms may exceed human capabilities in integrating complex, gigantic, and structured datasets. Still, much data is obtained from the clinician-patient relationship established when patients bestow trust in their doctor.

For humans to align the strengths and weaknesses of man and machine, they will need to be educated about how AI works. Integration and data analysis by models do not mean the models understand the implications of that data for specific patients.[40,41] Thus, anesthesiologists using their judgment abilities, can optimally use AI to foster performance serving human interests and continue innovations in the delivery of safe anesthesia care.

ARTIFICIAL INTELLIGENCE, 5G, AND ANESTHESIA

5G has the advantage of lowest communication latency, highest speed, enhanced throughput, minimum end-to-end (E2E) delay, and minimizing packet loss has made it a potent tool for use in the field of the IoMT/smart healthcare.[2] Recent studies indicate that 5G can accommodate a much higher number of devices than 4G, making network security much more robust, which can now be used without worrying about information leakage.

Studies have shown successful use of remote control pumps for postoperative analgesia without physical intervention by the nurse or the physician.[42] Another study suggests a system that could combine telemonitoring of patients with the ability to remote control the patient's infusion pump from afar for pain management without the need to visit him personally.[43] Another study concludes that a remote-controlled system is feasible for propofol infusion in patients undergoing magnetic resonance imaging (MRI) with the recommendation that the syringe adaptor needs improvements.[44]

Hence a study to simulate the OT environments of anesthesia and life support mechanisms is the need of the hour, which could be useful in scenarios when operating in remote areas or with constrained resources. With the advances in remote surgery protocols developing day by day, this remote anesthesia component could further refine the compositeness of distance OT management. Hospitals can take advantage of new connectivity capabilities provisioned through 5G to reach out to a more extensive base of patients by creating more OT hubs within the premises or at different off-campus locations. Care should be taken in the security and safety of the teletherapy system to eliminate harm to the patient caused at any stage by benign and malignant intrusions.[45] The overall benefits would include an increase in productivity and a care support system where an adequate number of trained medical practitioners are a challenge. This will also allow ubiquitous healthcare philosophy for a welfare state.

■ CONCLUSION

Will we ever know how to handle AI? Will it evolve into something genocidal like Terminator's Skynet, or will helpful robots like WALL-E and Jarvis harmlessly improve the quality of our lives? Only the future can bring the answers to these questions, but the way we envision this future in our media has consistently given us a glimpse at what could be.

Artificial intelligence has come a long way from the initial Turing test to its current *avatar*. As we enter the "roaring twenties", we are at the dawn of a new medical era when AI begins immersion into daily clinical practice. The potential applications for the role of AI in anesthesia currently have no boundaries.

Many AI applications for anesthesiology are now being tested in clinical settings. We are yet to find more about how they work and which limitations and benefits they have. Just as the AI technologies, we too, will learn more as more data becomes available. AI has the potential to impact the clinical practice of anesthesia for perioperative support, critical care delivery, and outpatient pain management.

There are challenges to adopting AI in healthcare, including having to meet regulatory requirements and overcoming trust issues with machine learning results. Despite these challenges, bringing AI and machine learning to the healthcare industry has brought numerous benefits to healthcare organizations by streamlining workflows, leading to better experiences for patients, members, citizens, and consumers.

■ REFERENCES

1. Mayo RC, Leung J. Artificial intelligence and deep learning-radiology's next frontier? Clin Imaging. 2018;49:87-8.
2. Mishra L, Vikash, Varma S. Seamless health monitoring using 5G NR for internet of medical things. Wireless pers commun. 2021;120(3):2259-89.
3. Amisha, Malik P, Pathania M, Rathaur VK. Overview of artificial intelligence in medicine. J Family Med Prim Care. 2019;8(7):2328-31.
4. Crevier D. The Tumultuous History of the Search for Artificial Intelligence. New York, NY: Basic Books; 1993.
5. Kendale S, Kulkarni P, Rosenberg AD, Wang J. Supervised machine-learning predictive analytics for prediction of postinduction hypotension. Anesthesiology. 2018;129(4):675-88.

6. Hakonarson H, Bjornsdottir US, Halapi E, Bradfield J, Zing F, Mouy M, et al. Profiling of genes expressed in peripheral blood mononuclear cells predicts glucocorticoid sensitivity asthma patients. Proc Natl Acad Sci USA. 2005;102(41):14789-94.
7. Sutton RS, Barto AG. Reinforcement Learning: An Introduction. Massachusetts: The MIT Press; 1998.
8. Padmanabhan R, Meskin N, Haddad WM. Closed-loop control of anesthesia and mean arterial pressure using reinforcement learning. Biomed Signal Process Control. 2015;22:54-64.
9. Zadeh LA. Fuzzy sets. Inf Control. 1965;8:338-53.
10. Baig MM, Gholamhosseini H, Kouzani A, Harrison MJ. Anaesthesia monitoring using fuzzy logic. J Clin Monit Comput. 2011;25(5):339-47.
11. Hu YJ, Ku TH, Jan RH, Wang K, Tseng YC, Yang SF. Decision tree-based learning to predict patient controlled analgesia consumption and readjustment. BMC Med Inform Decis Mak. 2012;12:131.
12. McCulloch WS, Pitts W. A logical calculus of the ideas immanent in nervous activity. Bull Math Biophys. 1943;5:115-33.
13. LeCun Y, Bengio Y, Hinton G. Deep learning. Nature. 2015;521(7553):436-44.
14. LISA lab. (2014). Convolutional Neural Networks (LeNet). [online] Available from https://www.cs.virginia.edu/yanjun/teach/2014f/lecture/L20-handout-deeplearningTutorial.pdf [Last accessed October, 2022].
15. Gartner, Inc. Gartner hype cycle. [online] Available from https://www.gartner.com/en/research/methodologies/gartner-hype-cycle [Last accessed October 2022].
16. Elinext. Pneumonia diagnostic tool. [online] Available from https://www.elinext.com/case-study/web/pneumonia-diagnosis-tool/. [Last accessed October 2022].
17. Singh M, Nath G. Artificial intelligence and anesthesia: a narrative review. Saudi J Anaesth. 2022;16(1):86-93.
18. Connor CW, Segal S. Accurate classification of difficult intubation by computerized facial analysis. Anesth Analg. 2011;112(1):84-93.
19. Wang JX, Sullivan DK, Wells AJ, Wells AC, Chen JH. Neural Networks for Clinical Order Decision Support. AMIA Jt Summits Transl Sci Proc. 2019;2019:315-24.
20. Freundlich RE, Grondin L, Tremper KK, Saran KA, Kheterpal S. Automated electronic reminders to prevent miscommunication among primary medical, surgical and anesthesia providers: a root cause analysis. BMJ Qual Saf. 2012;21:850-4.
21. Edworthy J, Hellier E. Alarms and human behaviour: implications for medical alarms. Br J Anaesth. 2006;97(1):12-7.
22. Mirsadeghi M, Behnam H, Shalbaf R, Moghadam JH: Characterizing awake and anesthetized states using a dimensionality reduction method. J Med Syst. 2016;40(1):13.
23. Nagaraj SB, Biswal S, Boyle EJ, Zhou DW, McClain LM, Bajwa EK, et al. Patient-specific classification of ICU sedation levels from heart rate variability. Crit Care Med. 2017;45(7):e683-90.
24. Ranta SO, Hynynen M, Räsänen J. Application of artificial neural networks as an indicator of awareness with recall during general anaesthesia. J Clin Monit Comput. 2002;17(1):53-60.

25. Wang LY, McKelvey GM, Wang H. Multi-outcome predictive modelling of anesthesia patients. J Biomed Res. 2019;33(6):430-34.
26. Upton HD, Ludbrook GL, Wing A, Sleigh JW. Intraoperative "analgesia nociception index"-guided fentanyl administration during sevoflurane anesthesia in lumbar discectomy and laminectomy: A randomized clinical trial. Anesth Analg. 2017;125(1):81-90.
27. Funcke S, Pinnschmidt HO, Wesseler S, Brinkmann C, Beyer B, Jazbutyte V, et al. Guiding opioid administration by 3 different analgesia nociception monitoring indices during general anesthesia alters intraoperative sufentanil consumption and stress hormone release: a randomized controlled pilot study. Anesth Analg. 2020;130(5):1264-73.
28. Komorowski M, Celi LA, Badawi O, Gordon AC, Faisal AA. The artificial intelligence clinician learns optimal treatment strategies for sepsis in intensive care. Nat Med. 2018;24(11):1716-20.
29. Wang SC, Wu HT, Huang PH, Chang CH, Ting CK, Lin YT. Novel imaging revealing inner dynamics for cardiovascular waveform analysis via unsupervised manifold learning. Anesth Analg. 2020;130(5):1244-54.
30. Mathis MR, Engoren MC, Joo H, Maile MD, Aaronson KD, Burns ML, et al. Early detection of heart failure with reduced ejection fraction using perioperative data among noncardiac surgical patients: a machine-learning approach. Anesth Analg. 2020;130(5):1188-200.
31. Grossmann U, Schiessl C, Jatobá L, Ottenbacher J, Stork W, Mueller-Glaser KD. Securely control Infusion Pumps via Internet for efficient Remote Therapy of Pain. In: Magjarevic R, Nagel JH (Eds.). World Congress on Medical Physics and Biomedical Engineering, 6th edition. Heidelberg: IFMBE Proceedings Beitrag; 2006.
32. Gram M, Erlenwein J, Petzke F, Falla D, Przemeck M, Emons MI, et al. Prediction of postoperative opioid analgesia using clinical-experimental parameters and electroencephalography. Eur J Pain. 2017;21(2):264-77.
33. Smistad E, Løvstakken L. Vessel Detection in Ultrasound Images Using Deep Convolutional Neural Networks. In: Deep Learning and Data Labeling for Medical Applications. Springer: Lecture Notes in Computer Science; 2016.
34. Hetherington J, Lessoway V, Gunka V, Abolmaesumi P, Rohling R. SLIDE: Automatic spine level identification system using a deep convolutional neural network. Int J Comput Assist Radiol Surg. 2017;12(7):1189-98.
35. Combes C, Meskens N, Rivat C, Vandamme JP. Using a KDD process to forecast the duration of surgery. Int J Prod Econ. 2008;112(1):279-93.
36. Houliston BR, Parry DT, Merry AF. TADAA: Towards automated detection of anaesthetic activity. Methods Inf Med. 2011;50(5):464-71.
37. Hemmerling TM, Wehbe M, Zaouter C, Taddei R, Morse J. The Kepler intubation system. Anesth Analg. 2012;114(3):590-4.
38. Hashimoto DA, Witkowski E, Gao L, Meireles O, Rosman G. Artificial Intelligence in Anesthesiology: Current Techniques, Clinical Applications, and Limitations. *Anesthesiology*. 2020;32(2):379-94.
39. Keyes KM, Westreich D. UK Biobank, big data, and the consequences of non-representativeness. Lancet. 2019;393(10178):1297.

40. Weber GM, Mandl KD, Kohane IS. Finding the missing link for big biomedical data. JAMA. 2014;311(24):2479-80.
41. Cremer DD, Kasparov G. (2021). AI Should Augment Human Intelligence, Not Replace It. [online] Available from https://hbr.org/2021/03/ai-should-augment-human-intelligence-not-replace-it [Last accessed October, 2022].
42. Macaire P, Nadhari M, Greiss H, Godwin A, Elhanfi O, Sainudeen S, et al. Internet remote control of pump settings for postoperative continuous peripheral nerve blocks: a feasibility study in 59 patients. Ann Fr Anesth Reanim. 2014;33(1):e1-7.
43. Masterflex. Remote Peristaltic Pump Monitoring. [online] Available from https://www.masterflex.com/tech-article/remote-peristaltic-pump-monitoring-reduces-costs. [Last accessed October, 2022].
44. Sesay M, Tauzin-Fin P, Verdonck O, Dousset V, Maurette P. A wireless remote controlled infusion pump for anaesthesia during magnetic resonance imaging. Br J Anaesth. 2008;100(6):862-3.
45. TechCrunch. (2019). A widely used infusion pump can be remotely hijacked, say researchers. [online] Available from https://techcrunch.com/2019/06/13/alaris-infusion-pump-security-flaws/ [Last accessed October, 2022].

CHAPTER

23

Technologies Likely to Impact Cardiopulmonary Resuscitation in the Near Future

Tommaso Scquizzato, Federico Semeraro

ABSTRACT

Technology is present in every link of the chain of cardiac arrest survival, from prediction, prevention, and rapid recognition to early cardiopulmonary resuscitation, defibrillation, and advanced life support. Smartphones are used in numerous countries to notify citizen first responders of nearby out-of-hospital cardiac arrest, improving bystanders' interventions and outcomes. Drones delivering defibrillators and artificial intelligence to support the dispatcher in recognizing cardiac arrest are already being used in real-life out-of-hospital cardiac arrest. Wearables, smart speakers, surveillance cameras, and artificial intelligence technologies are being developed and studied to prevent and recognize out-of-hospital and in-hospital cardiac arrest. Percutaneous and extracorporeal circulatory supports and technologies for real-time rhythm analysis without interrupting chest compressions are becoming common in managing cardiac arrest. Further research is needed to understand the best role of different technologies in the chain of survival and how these may ultimately improve outcomes.

Keywords: Cardiopulmonary resuscitation; Out-of-hospital cardiac arrest; Technology; Smartphones; Applications; Artificial intelligence; Drones and Basic life support.

KEY POINTS

- Technology will help every link of the survival chain, from prediction, prevention, and rapid recognition of cardiac arrest to systems to increase basic and advanced life support and defibrillation.
- The intersection of different disciplines is at the base of the innovation to increase survival from cardiac arrest. Therefore, it is fundamental that the integration of technology follows a "system approach" based on a solid collaboration between communities and institutions.
- High-quality research is needed to determine the effectiveness of current or future technologies in improving the chain of survival and patient-oriented outcomes.

INTRODUCTION

Technology has revolutionized our lives in the past decade, and nowadays, it has numerous applications also in healthcare.[1] Smartphones, wearables, unmanned aerial systems (also known as drones), and machine learning and artificial intelligence (AI) are being increasingly adopted in the prevention and treatment of out-of-hospital cardiac arrest (OHCA) and in-hospital cardiac arrest (IHCA).[2,3]

Technology is already used successfully in several countries to activate citizen first responders in the case of OHCA,[4-6] leading to higher rates of bystander-initiated cardiopulmonary resuscitation (CPR), use of defibrillators and improved survival.[7-9] While many technologies are still in the early phases of the development, unmanned aerial systems (drones) used to deliver automated external defibrillators (AEDs) and AI to support dispatchers in increasing rates of cardiac arrest recognized during the emergency call are already implemented in the treatment of real-life OHCAs.[10-12]

On the contrary, the use of smartwatches, smart speakers, surveillance cameras, and wearables to anticipate and recognize OHCA are still being investigated and developed.[13] Moving to the hospital setting, AI and machine learning algorithms are being developed and studied to early identify deterioration and risk factors[14] to prevent cardiac arrest through early detection.[15]

Percutaneous and extracorporeal circulatory supports such as extracorporeal CPR and more recently, resuscitative endovascular balloon occlusion of the aorta (REBOA) are becoming common in the management of refractory OHCA. Novel techniques like real-time rhythm analysis without interrupting chest compressions are being developed and investigated to improve resuscitation quality.

In this chapter, we discuss how current and emerging technologies are likely to improve each link of the survival chain and patient outcomes after cardiac arrest and CPR.

PREVENTING CARDIAC ARREST

Out-of-hospital cardiac arrest is frequently preceded by chest pain, dyspnea, and syncope in approximately half of the cases,[16,17] and patients may present signs of clinical and physiological deterioration immediately before a cardiac arrest occurs. When not ignored, warning symptoms allow a more rapid activation of emergency medical service (EMS) and a seven-fold increase in survival.[18] Therefore, the prediction and prevention of cardiac arrest before its onset constitute an important area of research.[19] Thanks to recent technological advances, wearable devices can be embedded within clothes, watches, or accessories[20] that could potentially allow monitoring patients outside the hospital continuously. In the future, biometrics signals[21] may alert patients days, hours, or minutes before a life-threatening major cardiovascular event. Furthermore, AI, particularly machine learning, can potentially improve cardiac arrest prediction by integrating and analyzing different parameters from multiple sources. This will lead to faster recognition and alert to patients at risk of cardiac arrest and timely activation of EMS to prevent cardiac arrest, anticipate treatments, reduce delays, and improve outcomes.

In the hospital, systems for identifying deteriorating patients, such as early warning systems, are crucial to prevent cardiac arrest. Patients admitted to the hospital have their vital signs continuously assessed or monitored (i.e., telemetry). Clinicians and researchers are using AI and machine learning (i.e., analysis of vital parameters, prediction models, risk stratification of patients) to improve the early detection of deterioration to prevent cardiac arrest. In the following years, AI could play a significant role.[14,15]

TECHNOLOGIES FOR RECOGNIZING CARDIAC ARREST
During Emergency Phone Calls

Early bystanders' interventions followed by a rapid EMS arrival are essential for patients to survive an OHCA. One crucial element of the chain of survival is prompt recognition by EMS dispatchers. However, EMS dispatchers may fail to recognize OHCA during the phone call[22] leading to delayed EMS response, reduced rates of dispatcher-assisted CPR provided,[23] and worse outcomes.

Artificial intelligence is an encouraging technology to improve recognition of OHCA by providing real-time support to EMS dispatchers on the phone.[11,24,25] AI listens to the emergency call live and estimates the probability of facing cardiac arrest based on the words spoken. Such systems were retrospectively studied in observational studies suggesting a similar specificity, but a higher sensitivity of AI compared to dispatchers.[24,25] In a randomized trial, dispatchers' ability to recognize OHCA was not significantly improved by AI, even though AI did surpass human recognition.[11] AI could play a key role in helping dispatchers in handling complex calls like OHCA, in particular in EMS systems with suboptimal rates of OHCA recognition during the phone call. However, future developments are still needed to improve specificity, relevance of alerts, and interaction between the dispatcher and the computer.

Unwitnessed Cardiac Arrests

About half of OHCA occur unwitnessed,[26] and these patients usually die because the chain of survival is not timely activated and CPR is not promptly initiated. In this situation, smartphones, AI, and wearables could recognize a cardiac arrest occurring unwitnessed outside the hospital and facilitate rapid response of bystanders and EMS.

First, wearables (e.g., wrist-worn wearables including smartwatches, smart bands, and others) measure and monitor vitals (i.e., heart rate) or detect falls[27,28] and could alert emergency numbers automatically in case of a suspected out-of-hospital cardiac arrest (OHCA) (a motionless patients as detected by technology implemented in wearable devices) unless the smartwatch wearer manually stops the process within 5–10 seconds.

Second, OHCA recognition is often delayed in uncrowded or remote places, such as during off-peak hours in parking lots and some streets. The high number of installed closed-circuit surveillance cameras can be leveraged to automatically identify someone collapsing, like in OHCA.[29,30] Video analysis combined with AI can detect a collapse and absence of movement, suggesting a cardiac arrest, and trigger an alert.

Finally, agonal breathing is often present immediately after cardiac arrest.[31] Smartphones and smart speakers are progressively present at home and represent an innovative approach to identify cardiac arrest thanks to passive and contactless detection of abnormal or absent breathing.[32]

TECHNOLOGIES FOR CPR AND DEFIBRILLATION

Video Call

Dispatcher-assisted CPR improves rates of CPR initiated before EMS arrival and improves outcomes.[33-36] Dispatchers must still first recognize cardiac arrest, often a challenging task when only information communicated over the phone are available. Moreover, dispatchers have no real-time, direct feedback about bystander CPR quality. Technological improvements of smartphones have made video calls more efficient and therefore widespread, allowing to live stream the scene of a cardiac arrest to dispatchers through smartphones. Simulation studies showed that providing dispatcher-assisted CPR instructed through video calls was feasible and improved bystander CPR quality.[37,38] Therefore, the implementation of live video streaming could help improve both OHCA recognition and CPR quality.

In real-life OHCAs, video calls showed to be feasible, and the EMS dispatcher could successfully instruct bystanders in performing CPR that was improved in quality thanks to video calls.[37-39] Nonrandomized studies showed that video-instructed dispatcher-assisted CPR was associated with increased survival and neurological outcomes.[40,41]

Smartphone-Activated Citizen First Responders

Nowadays, smartphone technology allows to alert citizens willing to intervene in case an OHCA strikes in their vicinity.[4,42] They are called citizen first responders and, in Europe, they are available in more than half of the countries.[43,44] In countries where these systems are active, EMS dispatchers alert citizen first responders localized within a variable distance from the OHCA, usually from 150 m to 5 km or in the same neighborhood. Text messages or application notifications are used to notify citizen first responders simultaneously to ambulance dispatch. In most cases, volunteers are requested to be trained in basic life support (BLS).

Early studies showed that alerting citizen first responders was feasible and helpful.[45] Cardiopulmonary resuscitation and defibrillation were performed in more cases and with less delays before EMS arrival.[45-47] When investigated in a randomized clinical trial, the rate of CPR performed before EMS arrival proved to increase.[8] Moreover, recent studies and meta-analyses[4,7,9] demonstrated increased bystander CPR, AED use, and survival. In addition, regions that implemented a first responder system had higher rates of return of spontaneous circulation (ROSC) and survival compared to regions without such systems.[48]

Locating the Nearest Automated External Defibrillators

The likelihood of survival following OHCA is increased by early defibrillation. However, obtaining an AED can be difficult because citizens must be aware of its location. Despite major efforts, the accessibility and use of public AEDs are still quite low globally.[49] Numerous websites and smartphone applications have been created in the last 10 years to map and find AEDs, available in 78% of European countries.[43] Applications can determine the user's location in real-time and provide nearby AEDs with directions to the closest one thanks to smartphone geolocation technologies.

Additionally, these systems allow community members to add new AEDs or update the information on those that already exist. This raises community awareness and aids in the creation and upkeep of an updated AED registry. The efficacy of these systems is higher when integrated with citizen first responders and EMS dispatch centers.

Drone-Delivered Automated External Defibrillators

Despite the rise in AED installations, defibrillators are still infrequently present at OHCA sites. For improving survival after an OHCA, expanding access to AEDs and cutting down on the time it takes to shock a patient are essential.[50,51] For this reason, drones were suggested as a quick way to get an AED to the scene of an OHCA, in particular for mountain and rural areas.[52]

Drone-delivered AEDs was the subject of several simulation experiments, with promising findings that an AED might safely arrive by drone before an ambulance.[53-55] AEDs were properly delivered by drones in 92% of real-life OHCAs, and 64% of them arrived about a minute before EMS.[10] It was reported for the first time that a drone-delivered AED assisted in saving a 71-year-old patient in Sweden who was experiencing an OHCA.[56]

■ TECHNOLOGIES IN ADVANCED LIFE SUPPORT

Percutaneous and extracorporeal circulatory supports are becoming common in managing cardiac arrest. Extracorporeal CPR, the application of venoarterial extracorporeal membrane oxygenation (ECMO) during ongoing CPR, is a recent innovative technique increasingly being applied to treat refractory cardiac arrests in cardiac arrest centers with a high level of expertise. Observational and randomized studies showed the benefits of the extracorporeal CPR.[57,58] Further development of extracorporeal technology in the future will allow having smaller devices, possibly increasing and facilitating ECMO application also in the prehospital setting.[59] Resuscitative Endovascular Balloon Occlusion of the Aorta (REBOA), a percutaneous technique originally developed for the treatment of trauma patients with active bleeding,[60] has been introduced in the pre-hospital treatment of refractory OHCA.[61,62] The rationale behind the application of REBOA during ongoing CPR is that aortic occlusion can raise cerebral and coronary perfusion pressure by increasing left ventricular afterload leading to higher chances of ROSC and reducing brain hypoperfusion. Moreover, REBOA is applied percutaneously via a femoral artery, and the presence of a catheter could allow more precise hemodynamic monitoring during CPR and a faster transition to extracorporeal cardiopulmonary resuscitation (E-CPR) after hospital arrival.

Resuscitation guidelines require cyclical interruptions of chest compressions for the analysis of the rhythm and shock delivery (if needed) every two minutes. Ineffective defibrillations or underlying nonshockable rhythm cause unnecessary interruptions of chest compressions, reducing myocardial perfusion and the chance of successful defibrillation.[63] Real-time analysis of ECG implementing adaptive filters to suppress artifacts from the ECG derived from chest compressions is an effective technique to identify the rhythm during CPR and reduce hands-off time before a shock.[64] The employment of AI could further improve the distinction between shockable and no-shockable rhythms during CPR. Similarly, amplitude spectrum area (AMSA), the ventricular fibrillation waveform analysis, allows for reserve defibrillation when there is an elevated chance of successful defibrillation and postpone when termination of ventricular fibrillation is dubious.[65] Moreover, AMSA is being investigated for the early detection of myocardial infarction during ventricular fibrillation.[66]

■ CONCLUSION

Technology is completely revolutionizing the chain of survival, from methods to forecast, prevent, and quickly identify cardiac arrest to technologies to enhance and strengthen basic and advanced life support and defibrillation. Citizen first responders alerting of nearby OHCA have been implemented in numerous countries with improvement in bystanders' interventions and patient outcomes. In real-life OHCA, drones delivering AEDs and AI to help the dispatcher recognize cardiac arrest are already in use. Future technologies such as wearables, security cameras, and smart speakers will detect and prevent OHCA. Through early risk factor and deterioration detection and identification, AI will be able to prevent an impeding cardiac arrest. More research is required to determine the appropriate place for various technologies in the chain of survival and how they might finally improve outcomes.

■ CONFLICTS OF INTEREST

Tommaso Scquizzato is the Social Media Editor of Resuscitation and Resuscitation Plus and a member of the BLS Science and Education Committee of the European Resuscitation Council. Federico Semeraro is the Chair-Elect of the European Resuscitation Council, ILCOR Chair of Social Media Working Group, and ILCOR BLS Task Force member.

■ REFERENCES

1. Sim I. Mobile devices and health. N Engl J Med. 2019;381(10):956-68.
2. Myat A, Song K-J, Rea T. Out-of-hospital cardiac arrest: current concepts. Lancet. 2018;391(10124):970-9.
3. Andersen LW, Holmberg MJ, Berg KM, Donnino MW, Granfeldt A. In-hospital cardiac arrest: A review. JAMA. 2019;321(12):1200-10.
4. Scquizzato T, Pallanch O, Belletti A, Frontera A, Cabrini L, Zangrillo A, et al. Enhancing citizens response to out-of-hospital cardiac arrest: a systematic review of mobile-phone systems to alert citizens as first responders. Resuscitation. 2020;152:16-25.
5. Valeriano A, Van Heer S, de Champlain F, C Brooks S. Crowdsourcing to save lives: a scoping review of bystander alert technologies for out-of-hospital cardiac arrest. Resuscitation. 2021;158:94-121.
6. Semeraro F, Greif R, Böttiger BW, Burkart R, Cimpoesu D, Georgiou M, et al. European Resuscitation Council Guidelines 2021: Systems saving lives. Resuscitation. 2021;161:80-97.
7. Scquizzato T, Belloni O, Semeraro F, Greif R, Metelmann C, Landoni G, et al. Dispatching citizens as first responders to out-of-hospital cardiac arrests: A systematic review and meta-analysis. Eur J Emerg Med. 2022;29(3):163-72.
8. Ringh M, Rosenqvist M, Hollenberg J, Jonsson M, Fredman D, Nordberg P, et al. Mobile-phone dispatch of laypersons for CPR in out-of-hospital cardiac arrest. N Engl J Med. 2015;372(24):2316-25.
9. Andelius L, Hansen CM, Lippert FK, Karlsson L, Torp-Pedersen C, Ersbøll KA, et al. Smartphone Activation of Citizen Responders to Facilitate Defibrillation in Out-of-Hospital Cardiac Arrest. J Am Coll Cardiol. 2020;76(1):43-53.
10. Schierbeck S, Hollenberg J, Nord A, Svensson ·L, Nordberg P, Ringh M, et al. Automated external defibrillators delivered by drones to patients with suspected out-of-hospital cardiac arrest. Eur Heart J. 2021;43(15):1478-87.

11. Blomberg SN, Christensen HC, Lippert F, Ersbøll AK, Torp-Petersen C, Sayre MR, et al. Effect of Machine Learning on Dispatcher Recognition of Out-of-Hospital Cardiac Arrest During Calls to Emergency Medical Services: A Randomized Clinical Trial. JAMA Netw Open. 2021;4(1):e2032320.
12. Olasveengen TM, Semeraro F, Ristagno G, Castren M, Handley A, Kuzovlev A, et al. European Resuscitation Council Guidelines 2021: Basic Life Support. Resuscitation. 2021;161:98-114.
13. Scquizzato T, Semeraro F. No more unwitnessed out-of-hospital cardiac arrests in the future thanks to technology. Resuscitation. 2022;170:79-81.
14. JayaSree M, Koteswara Rao L. (2020). Survey on - Identification of Coronary Artery Disease using Deep Learning. [online] Available from: https://www.sciencedirect.com/science/article/pii/S2214785320372424 [Last accessed October, 2022].
15. Kumari CU, Murthy ASD, Prasanna BL, Reddy MPP, Panigrahy AK. An automated detection of heart arrhythmias using machine learning technique: SVM. Mater Today Prac. 2021;45:1393-8.
16. Nehme Z, Bernard S, Andrew E, Cameron P, Bray JE, Smith K. Warning symptoms preceding out-of-hospital cardiac arrest: Do patient delays matter? Resuscitation. 2018;123:65-70.
17. Nishiyama C, Iwami T, Kawamura T, Kitamura T, Tanigawa K, Sakai T, et al. Prodromal symptoms of out-of-hospital cardiac arrests: a report from a large-scale population-based cohort study. Resuscitation. 2013;84(5):558-63.
18. Marijon E, Uy-Evanado A, Dumas F, Karam N, Reinier K, Teodorescu C, et al. Warning symptoms are associated with survival from sudden cardiac arrest. Ann Intern Med. 2016;164(1):23-9.
19. Mann KD, Good NM, Fatehi F, Khanna S, Campbell V, Conway R, et al. Predicting patient deterioration: A review of tools in the digital hospital setting. J Med Internet Res. 2021;23(9):e28209.
20. Khundaqji H, Hing W, Furness J, Climstein M. Smart shirts for monitoring physiological parameters: Scoping review. JMIR Mhealth Uhealth. 2020;8(5):e18092.
21. Krittanawong C, Rogers AJ, Johnson KW, Wang Z, Turakhia MP, Halperin JL, et al. Integration of novel monitoring devices with machine learning technology for scalable cardiovascular management. Nat Rev Cardiol. 2021;18(2):75-91.
22. Vaillancourt C, Charette ML, Bohm K, Dunford J, Castrén M. In out-of-hospital cardiac arrest patients, does the description of any specific symptoms to the emergency medical dispatcher improve the accuracy of the diagnosis of cardiac arrest: a systematic review of the literature. Resuscitation. 2011;82(12):1483-9.
23. Fukushima H, Imanishi M, Iwami T, Seki T, Kawai Y, Norimoto K, et al. Abnormal breathing of sudden cardiac arrest victims described by laypersons and its association with emergency medical service dispatcher-assisted cardiopulmonary resuscitation instruction. Emerg Med J. 2015;32(4):314-7.
24. Blomberg SN, Folke F, Ersbøll AK, Christensen HC, Torp-Pedersen C, Sayre MR, et al. Machine learning as a supportive tool to recognize cardiac arrest in emergency calls. Resuscitation. 2019;138:322-9.
25. Byrsell F, Claesson A, Ringh M, Svensson L, Jonsson M, Nordberg P, et al. Machine learning can support dispatchers to better and faster recognize out-of-hospital

cardiac arrest during emergency calls: A retrospective study. Resuscitation. 2021;162:218-26.
26. Fukuda T, Matsubara T, Doi K, Fukuda-Ohashi N, Yahagi N. Predictors of favorable and poor prognosis in unwitnessed out-of-hospital cardiac arrest with a non-shockable initial rhythm. Int J Cardiol. 2014;176(3):910-5.
27. Perez MV, Mahaffey KW, Hedlin H, Rumsfeld JS, Garcia A, Ferris T, et al. Large-scale assessment of a smartwatch to identify atrial fibrillation. N Engl J Med. 2019;381(20):1909-17.
28. Apple Inc. (2022). Use fall detection with Apple Watch. [online] Available from: https://support.apple.com/en-us/HT208944 [Last accessed October, 2022].
29. Scquizzato T. Cardiac arrest detection through artificial intelligence-based surveillance camera: A working prototype. Resuscitation. 2018;130:e114.
30. Douma MJ. Automated video surveillance and machine learning: Leveraging existing infrastructure for cardiac arrest detection and emergency response activation. Resuscitation. 2018;126:e3.
31. Bobrow BJ, Zuercher M, Ewy GA, Clark L, Chikani V, Donahue D, et al. Gasping during cardiac arrest in humans is frequent and associated with improved survival. Circulation. 2008;118(24):2550-4.
32. Chan J, Rea T, Gollakota S, Sunshine JE. Contactless cardiac arrest detection using smart devices. NPJ Digit Med. 2019;2:52.
33. Song KJ, Shin SD, Park CB, Kim JY, Kim DK, Kim CH, et al. Dispatcher-assisted bystander cardiopulmonary resuscitation in a metropolitan city: a before-after population-based study. Resuscitation. 2014;85(1):34-41.
34. Wu Z, Panczyk M, Spaite DW, Hu C, Fukushima H, Langlais B, et al. Telephone cardiopulmonary resuscitation is independently associated with improved survival and improved functional outcome after out-of-hospital cardiac arrest. Resuscitation. 2018;122:135-40.
35. Rajan S, Wissenberg M, Folke F, Hansen SM, Gerds TA, Kragholm K, et al. Association of bystander cardiopulmonary resuscitation and survival according to ambulance response times after out-of-hospital cardiac arrest. Circulation. 2016;134(25):2095-104.
36. Eberhard KE, Linderoth G, Gregers MCT, Lippert F, Folke F. Impact of dispatcher-assisted cardiopulmonary resuscitation on neurologically intact survival in out-of-hospital cardiac arrest: a systematic review. Scand J Trauma Resusc Emerg Med. 2021;29(1):70.
37. Lin Y-Y, Chiang W-C, Hsieh M-J, Sun J-T, Chang Y-C, Ma MH-M. Quality of audio-assisted versus video-assisted dispatcher-instructed bystander cardiopulmonary resuscitation: A systematic review and meta-analysis. Resuscitation. 2018;123:77-85.
38. Lee SGW, Kim TH, Lee HS, Shin SD, Song KJ, Hong KJ, et al. Efficacy of a new dispatcher-assisted cardiopulmonary resuscitation protocol with audio call-to-video call transition. Am J Emerg Med. 2021;44:26–32.
39. Linderoth G, Rosenkrantz O, Lippert F, Østergaard D, Ersbøll AK, Meyhoff CS, et al. Live video from bystanders' smartphones to improve cardiopulmonary resuscitation. Resuscitation. 2021;168:35-43.
40. Lee SY, Song KJ, Shin SD, Hong KJ, Kim TH. Comparison of the effects of audio-instructed and video-instructed dispatcher-assisted cardiopulmonary resuscitation on resuscitation outcomes after out-of-hospital cardiac arrest. Resuscitation. 2020;147:12-20.

41. Lee HS, You K, Jeon JP, Kim C, Kim S. The effect of video-instructed versus audio-instructed dispatcher-assisted cardiopulmonary resuscitation on patient outcomes following out of hospital cardiac arrest in Seoul. Sci Rep. 2021;11(1):15555.
42. Folke F, Andelius L, Gregers MT, Hansen CM. Activation of citizen responders to out-of-hospital cardiac arrest. Curr Opin Crit Care. 2021;27(3):209-15.
43. Scquizzato T, Burkart R, Greif R, Monsieurs KG, Ristagno G, Scapigliati A, et al. Mobile phone systems to alert citizens as first responders and to locate automated external defibrillators: A European survey. Resuscitation. 2020;151:39-42.
44. Oving I, Masterson S, Tjelmeland IBM, Jonsson M, Semeraro F, Ringh M, et al. First-response treatment after out-of-hospital cardiac arrest: a survey of current practices across 29 countries in Europe. Scand J Trauma Resusc Emerg Med. 2019;27(1):112.
45. Ringh M, Fredman D, Nordberg P, Stark T, Hollenberg J. Mobile phone technology identifies and recruits trained citizens to perform CPR on out-of-hospital cardiac arrest victims prior to ambulance arrival. Resuscitation. 2011;82(12):1514-8.
46. Zijlstra JA, Stieglis R, Riedijk F, Smeekes M, van der Worp WE, Koster RW. Local lay rescuers with AEDs, alerted by text messages, contribute to early defibrillation in a Dutch out-of-hospital cardiac arrest dispatch system. Resuscitation. 2014;85(11):1444-9.
47. Scholten AC, van Manen JG, van der Worp WE, Ijzerman MJ, Doggen CJM. Early cardiopulmonary resuscitation and use of Automated External Defibrillators by laypersons in out-of-hospital cardiac arrest using an SMS alert service. Resuscitation. 2011;82(10):1273-8.
48. Oving I, de Graaf C, Masterson S, Koster RW, Zwinderman AH, Stieglis R, et al. European first responder systems and differences in return of spontaneous circulation and survival after out-of-hospital cardiac arrest: A study of registry cohorts. Lancet Reg Health Eur. 2020;1:100004.
49. Bækgaard JS, Viereck S, Møller TP, Ersbøll AK, Lippert F, Folke F. The Effects of Public Access Defibrillation on Survival After Out-of-Hospital Cardiac Arrest: A Systematic Review of Observational Studies. Circulation. 2017;136(10):954-65.
50. Hasselqvist-Ax I, Riva G, Herlitz J, Rosenqvist M, Hollenberg J, Nordberg P, et al. Early cardiopulmonary resuscitation in out-of-hospital cardiac arrest. N Engl J Med. 2015;372(24):2307-15.
51. Kitamura T, Kiyohara K, Sakai T, Matsuyama T, Hatakeyama T, Shimamoto T, et al. Public-access defibrillation and out-of-hospital cardiac arrest in Japan. N Engl J Med. 2016;375(17):1649-59.
52. Vögele A, Ströhle M, Paal P, Rauch S, Brugger H. Can drones improve survival rates in mountain areas, providing automated external defibrillators? Resuscitation. 2020;146:277-8.
53. Claesson A, Bäckman A, Ringh M, Svensson L, Nordberg P, Djärv T, et al. Time to delivery of an automated external defibrillator using a drone for simulated out-of-hospital cardiac arrests vs emergency medical services. JAMA. 2017;317(22):2332-4.
54. Boutilier JJ, Brooks SC, Janmohamed A, Byers A, Buick JE, Zhan C, et al. Optimizing a drone network to deliver automated external defibrillators. Circulation. 2017;135(25):2454-65.

55. Sanfridsson J, Sparrevik J, Hollenberg J, Nordberg P, Djärv T, Ringh M, et al. Drone delivery of an automated external defibrillator — a mixed method simulation study of bystander experience. Scand J Trauma Resusc Emerg Med. 2019;27(1):40.
56. Schierbeck S, Svensson L, Claesson A. Use of a Drone-Delivered Automated External Defibrillator in an Out-of-Hospital Cardiac Arrest. N Engl J Med. 2022;386(20):1953-4.
57. Holmberg MJ, Geri G, Wiberg S, Guerguerian A-M, Donnino MW, Nolan JP, et al. Extracorporeal cardiopulmonary resuscitation for cardiac arrest: A systematic review. Resuscitation. 2018;131:91-100.
58. Scquizzato T, Bonaccorso A, Consonni M, Scandroglio AM, Swol J, Landoni G, et al. Extracorporeal cardiopulmonary resuscitation for out-of-hospital cardiac arrest: A systematic review and meta-analysis of randomized and propensity score-matched studies. Artif Organs. 2022;46(5):755-62.
59. Singer B, Reynolds JC, Lockey DJ, O'Brien B. Pre-hospital extra-corporeal cardiopulmonary resuscitation. Scand J Trauma Resusc Emerg Med. 2018;26(1). Available from: http://dx.doi.org/10.1186/s13049-018-0489-y
60. Petrone P, Pérez-Jiménez A, Rodríguez-Perdomo M, Brathwaite CEM, Joseph DK. Resuscitative endovascular balloon occlusion of the aorta (REBOA) in the management of trauma patients: a systematic literature review. Am Surg. 2019;85(6):654-62.
61. Gamberini L, Coniglio C, Lupi C, Tartaglione M, Mazzoli CA, Baldazzi M, et al. Resuscitative endovascular occlusion of the aorta (REBOA) for refractory out of hospital cardiac arrest. An Utstein-based case series. Resuscitation. 2021;165:161-9.
62. Mazzoli CA, Chiarini V, Coniglio C, Lupi C, Tartaglione M, Gamberini L, et al. Resuscitative endovascular balloon occlusion of the aorta (REBOA) in non-traumatic cardiac arrest: A narrative review of known and potential physiological effects. J Clin Med. 2022;11(3):742.
63. Babini G, Ruggeri L, Ristagno G. Optimizing defibrillation during cardiac arrest. Curr Opin Crit Care. 2021;27(3):246-54.
64. Affatato R, Li Y, Ristagno G. See through ECG technology during cardiopulmonary resuscitation to analyze rhythm and predict defibrillation outcome. Curr Opin Crit Care. 2016;22(3):199-205.
65. Ristagno G, Mauri T, Cesana G, Li Y, Finzi A, Fumagalli F, et al. Amplitude spectrum area to guide defibrillation: a validation on 1617 patients with ventricular fibrillation. Circulation. 2015;131(5):478-87.
66. Nas J, van Dongen LH, Thannhauser J, Hulleman M, van Royen N, Tan HL, et al. The effect of the localisation of an underlying ST-elevation myocardial infarction on the VF-waveform: a multi-centre cardiac arrest study. Resuscitation. 2021;168:11-8.

CHAPTER

24

Comprehensive Care at the End-of-Life

Rakesh Garg, Ruparna Khurana

ABSTRACT

A good quality of life should also culminate in "good death". The disease conditions, including advanced cancer and organ failures, lead to a stage wherein comfort care is more desirable than longevity. However, attempts must be made to smoothen the transition and help patients achieve this important milestone with grace and dignity. The aim of end-of-life care (EOLC) is a good death. The death that is free of pain and suffering, with a sense of accomplishment and achievement. Recognition of symptoms and signs of dying is the first step toward initiating EOLC. A physician should be able to predict impending death to initiate the processes of EOLC, like communication with the family, and alleviate physical and psychological symptoms. The understanding of these symptoms and appropriate management remains important for its optimal delivery. This chapter describes various aspects of comprehensive care at the end-of-life in patients with advanced diseases.

Keywords: End-of-life care; Palliative care; Advanced diseases; Palliative sedation; Comfort care.

KEY POINTS

- The aim of EOLC is a good death.
- Recognition of symptoms and signs of dying is the first step toward initiating EOLC.
- Based on the underlying disease and its trajectory, symptom burden may vary at the end-of-life, and thus individualized goals of care need to be set for the patients.
- Understanding these symptoms and initiation for various management strategies, including drugs, counseling, and other aspects of comfort care, is the key to good EOLC.

CASE VIGNETTE

A 72-year-old diabetic, hypertensive male with a history of coronary artery disease with chronic liver disease, portal hypertension, hepatitis C associated hepatocellular carcinoma with periportal lymphadenopathy with portal vein thrombosis, post-targeted cancer therapy presents to the palliative care outpatient clinic with complaints of extreme weakness, bedridden status, decreased oral intake, restlessness, irrational and incoherent talk, muffled speech and coated tongue, decreased urine output of 5 days duration, hematemesis, and melena of 3 days duration, hallucinations of 1 day duration. Her investigations revealed blood urea: 138 mg/dL, serum creatinine: 2.6 mg/dL, and bilirubin: 12.6 mg/dL.

Caregivers are anxious and worried, they had taken the patient to a local hospital where he was evaluated and admitted to the critical care unit, but the patient was too uncomfortable and felt so suffocated that he begged the family to take him; he wanted to die at home.

They know somehow that the end is near. They need validation from a medical professional that the decision to bring him home is right. They fear unforeseen circumstances where they would not know what to do, what to expect, how much time they have, whether there will be more suffering, whether they can hasten his death, or can they sedate him so that he does not feel the pain.

■ INTRODUCTION

Death is the overwhelming reality of human existence. The medical fraternity, with its myriad feats, may have accomplished cures to deadly ailments, but death cannot be conquered. However, attempts must be made to smoothen the transition and help patients achieve this important milestone with grace and dignity. The aim of end-of-life care (EOLC) is a good death. The death that is free of pain and suffering, with a sense of accomplishment and achievement. The end-of-life is generally associated with losing control, a desperate search for meaning, and making sense of what is happening.[1]

Patients and caregivers want to know what is happening, what is expected to happen shortly or in distant future, what options are available, what they should do if troublesome symptoms arise, should they rush to the hospital, should they get intravenous medications or hydration, how will they know it is the very last moment, there were some unresolved issues in the family, and some ongoing family feud.

Recognition of symptoms and signs of dying is the first step toward initiating EOLC. A physician should be able to predict impending death to initiate the processes of EOLC, such as communication with the family and alleviate physical and psychological symptoms. This should be followed by establishing consensus amongst all the treating teams and stakeholders and communication to the patient and family unit.[2]

The EOLC is applicable for three groups of patients, that includes[3]:
1. Patients who have advanced, progressive, and incurable conditions like malignancy.

2. Those who are generally frail with underlying morbidity.
3. Patients with chronic medical conditions make them susceptible to acute events that can be life-threatening.

In all these three groups, the expected patient survival is <12 months.

DEFINITIONS AND IMPLICATIONS OF OPERATIONAL TERMS

End-of-life care: EOLC is an "approach for a terminally ill patient that shifts the focus of care to symptom control, comfort, dignity, quality of life and quality of dying rather than treatments aimed at cure or prolongation of life".[4] The General Medical Council UK defines EOLC as "approaching the end-of-life when a patient is expected to live <12 months due to any of the following causes including but not limited to a terminal, progressive, incurable illness, fragility or sudden catastrophic event or patients in a persistent vegetative state who are likely to die if treatment and care are withdrawn".[4] This term may also be applied to extremely premature infants who are not expected to survive long.

End-of-life care is an integral component of palliative care, but is not the same as palliative care. Palliative care has a broad spectrum including the care of the patient and their families that begins with the diagnosis of a life-limiting, incurable illness along with other curative modalities, with the progressive increase in the palliative care, needs as the disease and simultaneously the symptom burden increases, ultimately with the exhaustion of curative options, the role of palliative care intensifies with aggressive symptom management and psychosocial support which finally give way to end-of-life care in the last few months or days of life, which is followed by bereavement care for the family and caregivers after the death of the patient **(Fig. 1)**.[5]

Terminal illness: It has been described as "An incurable and irreversible condition caused by injury, disease, or illness that would cause death within a reasonable period by accepted medical standards, and where the application of life-sustaining treatment would serve only to prolong the process of dying".[6]

Actively dying: This is described as "the hours or days preceding imminent death during which time the patient's physiological functions wane".[6] It is important to recognize the actively dying patient by various signs and symptoms, including decreased oral intake, dysphagia, dyspnea, delirium, death rattle, anxiety, and fatigue.[6]

Death: It is described as "irreversible cessation of the heart and circulatory function, or neurological function of the brain including the brain stem."[7] The confirmation of death is usually done by observing the irreversible nature of cardiopulmonary arrest for a minimum duration of 5 minutes, which can be done by palpation of central pulse and auscultation of heart

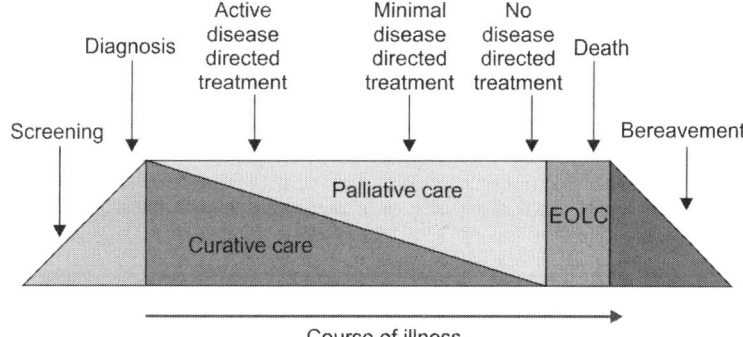

Fig. 1: Continuum of palliative care and end-of-life care (EOLC) in an illness trajectory.
Source: Myatra SN, Salins N, Iyer S, Macaden SC, Divatia JV, Muckaden M, et al. End-of-life care policy: an integrated care plan for the dying: A Joint Position Statement of the Indian Society of Critical Care Medicine (ISCCM) and the Indian Association of Palliative Care (IAPC). Indian J Crit Care Med. 2014;18(9):615-35.

sounds. Other modalities used for confirmation at a hospital setup include asystole on a continuous electrocardiographic (ECG) display, absence of pulsatile flow using direct intra-arterial pressure monitoring, or absence of contractile activity using echocardiography. If the cardiac or respiratory activity spontaneously returns during the observation period, a further 5 minute observation should be done. Cardiorespiratory arrest, followed by confirmation of the absence of pupillary responses to light, corneal reflexes, and motor response to supraorbital pressure, is confirmatory. The time of death is recorded as the time these criteria are fulfilled.[7]

■ END-OF-LIFE CARE: RECOGNITION AND MANAGEMENT

Based on the underlying disease and its trajectory, symptom burden may vary at the end-of-life. The end-of-life generally refers to patients approaching the last few months of life, and symptoms and signs also vary depending on how near to the end the patient is. There are characteristic physiological changes in the neurocognitive, neuromuscular, respiratory, and cardiovascular systems as a patient approaches death. The symptoms can be divided into physical, psychological, spiritual, and social.

Early signs >1 week from death may include decreased consciousness level, bedridden status, decreased or no oral intake, including dysphagia for liquids, and being completely dependent. Late signs <3 days of life include the inability to close eyelids, pulselessness of the radial artery, urine output <100 mL over 12 hours, nonreactive pupils, vocal fold grunting, and irregular breathing. A prognostic model suggests that poor performance status combined with drooping of nasolabial folds implies a 94% chance of mortality within 3 days.

Symptom constellation in the last few hours of life includes skin mottling and cool extremities, mouth breathing with hyperextended neck, changes in respiratory pattern, erratic breathing or Cheyne–Stokes breathing, calling out names of demised family members and friends, hallucinations, talking about packing bags or taking a trip, going for a car ride, and episodes of deep slumber. Although these factors predict mortality, their absence does not rule out the chances of impending death. Certain laboratory parameters such as elevated C reactive protein, reduced albumin levels, and leukocytosis suggest a poor prognosis.[8]

Various clinical tools and prognostic scales have been developed to predict mortality with a reasonable limit of certainty; these include Gold Standards Framework, the AMBER care bundle, the supportive and palliative care indicators tool (SPICT), palliative prognostic Score, the palliative prognostic index, and the Glasgow prognostic score.

Components of End-of-Life Care

End-of-life care comprises various components for its optimal delivery. These include:
- Timely and adequate symptom management.
- Effective communication and shared decision making.
- Expert, respectful, and compassionate care–formulation of a customized and pragmatic care plan for the patient by the patient's sociocultural values and beliefs.
- Aligning patients' goals of care with that of the healthcare team.
- Facilitating smooth transitions in care settings.
- Establishing a need for the surrogate decision-maker.
- Planning for a good death
- Advanced directives and care planning.
- Grief and bereavement care.

These components can be delivered effectively following the stepwise approach **(Table 1; Fig. 2)**.

Symptom Assessment and Management

Adequate symptom management is the cornerstone of providing quality EOLC. Qualitative research in EOLC revealed that adequate symptom control and relief of suffering were ranked as the topmost priority, followed by timely and honest dissemination of information by patients and their caregivers.[9] Most commonly reported symptoms at the end-of-life include fatigue, anorexia, xerostomia, pain, agitation, dyspnea, dysphagia, constipation, nausea, anxiety, myoclonus, death rattle, incontinence, restlessness, impaired cognition, confusion, drowsiness, dysphoria, delirium, noisy and moist breathing.[6] The management of these symptoms will be discussed

TABLE 1: Six-step approach in end-of-life care.

Steps	Description
Identify	Identify the target patient population eligible for end-of-life care (EOLC)
Assess	Assess for the need of EOLC–physical, psychosocial, spiritual symptoms and need for information regarding the disease, prognosis, what to expect and when
Plan	Formulation of a pragmatic care plan after consensus from all stakeholders, respecting patient and family wishes, and sociocultural beliefs
Provide	Adequate symptom management, support staff, medications, and after-hours care
Reassess	Ongoing assessment of pain and other symptom control. Documenting of variance and initiation of prompt action
Reflect	Constantly review and reflect on ongoing practice and identify key areas for the scope of improvement

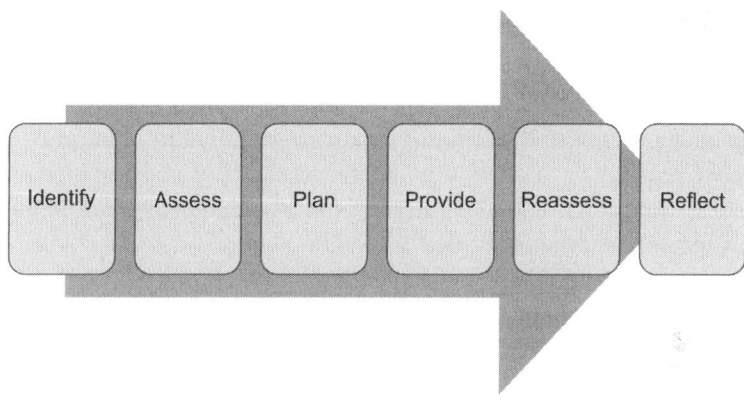

Fig. 2: Flow of steps to end-of-life care.

in a subsequent section of this chapter. These symptoms just need to be individually managed, but also emphasis is on managing the patient as a whole along with family. A comprehensive approach is required to provide comfort care and thus improve quality of life and death.

■ DEATH RATTLE

The death rattle is a characteristic sound produced at the time of breathing by patients in the last few days of life, in around 12–80% of cases.[10] It is more commonly reported in females and patients with advanced malignancies with pulmonary and cerebral metastases. It is caused by an ineffective clearance of the oropharyngeal and tracheobronchial secretions that tend to accumulate and produce a distinctive sound at each breath. Ineffective swallow and cough reflexes result in poor clearance.[11]

It is not painful for the patient, but may be distressing for the loved ones, so it is important to counsel and educate the caregivers about this expected symptom and its cause and reassure them. Decreasing overfeeding and properly positioning the patient's head down or lateral positions may reduce noisy breathing. Oral or nasal suctioning or routine use of anticholinergic is not recommended for its treatment.

PAIN

Pain is another common symptom at the end-of-life seen in 30–75% of patients. A proper assessment and reassessment of pain is an essential component of EOLC. This should include intensity, quality, aggravating, and relieving factors. Other important assessment components include efficacy and tolerability of analgesics, accompanying symptoms, associated psychological and spiritual distress, and its impact on daily functioning. Visual analog scale (VAS), verbal rating scale (VRS), numerical rating scale (NRS), and observational scales are available for intensity assessment.[12]

World Health Organization (WHO) analgesic leader remains the mainstay guide for pain management. Opioids remain the mainstay of treatment for moderate to severe pain at the end-of-life. Intravenous or subcutaneous routes may be preferred in case of a pain crisis. There is a lack of concrete evidence to suggest that opioids hasten death and shorten survival, so decisions should be made keeping in mind the clinical situation, goals of care, and risk versus benefit ratio.[13] Various analgesic drugs and adjuvants are used based on severity and type of pain **(Table 2)**.

There is insufficient evidence to support the use of nonsteroidal anti-inflammatory drugs (NSAIDs) or other adjuvants such as gabapentin, pregabalin, or serotonin-norepinephrine reuptake inhibitors in the last weeks of life, hence should be withdrawn timely.[14]

TABLE 2: Adjuvant analgesia at the end-of-life.[15]

Type of pain at end-of-life care (EOLC)	Analgesics and adjuvant medications
Musculoskeletal	• Paracetamol per-rectal suppository • Indomethacin per-rectal suppository • Dexamethasone subcutaneous
Neuropathic	• Dexamethasone subcutaneous • Clonazepam sublingual drops
Solid visceral	• Paracetamol per-rectal suppository • Indomethacin per-rectal suppository • Dexamethasone subcutaneous
Hollow visceral	• Hyoscine butylbromide subcutaneous • Ranitidine subcutaneous

■ NAUSEA AND VOMITING

Nausea and vomiting are troublesome and distressing symptoms at the end-of-life. Etiological factors include mechanical obstruction like gastric outlet obstruction or subacute intestinal obstruction or stasis, medications (e.g., opioids, chemotherapeutic agents), metabolic abnormalities such as hypercalcemia, hyponatremia, uremia, raised creatinine, mood-related causes (anxiety, fear), meningeal irritation due to brain or meningeal metastases increased intracranial pressure, vestibular dysfunction, excessive cough and ascites.[16]

The reversible causes, including optimal hydration and maintenance of electrolytes levels, remain paramount in these patients. Metoclopramide is the drug of choice for the management of nausea and vomiting. Other important drugs include haloperidol, levomepromazine, and olanzapine. The Multinational Association of Supportive Care in Cancer (MASCC) and European Society for Medical Oncology (ESMO) consensus recommendations of 2016 opined that antidopaminergic and 5-HT3 receptor antagonists are effective in opioid-induced emesis. Cannabinoids are not recommended in view of poor-quality evidence. Octreotide is the drug of choice in malignant bowel obstruction.

■ BREATHLESSNESS

Breathlessness is a very distressing symptom commonly encountered in the last few weeks and months of life. Estimates suggest its incidence is around 20-70% at the end-of-life and is a harbinger of a poor prognosis.[17] The intensity of dyspnea is assessed by patients' self-reported values of the sensation of dyspnea at rest and at moving, which may be expressed as a number from 1 to 10 (NRS) or its functional impact on walking or standing (modified Medical Research Council (march) breathlessness scale. The assessment aims at establishing the reversible causes and their correction. ESMO guidelines recommend oral or parenteral low-dose opioids, which have been shown to reduce the intensity of dyspnea by 20%.[16] The strategies of management of breathlessness depends on patient assessment and remains multipronged **(Fig. 3)**.

In patients already consuming opioids for other indications like pain, the dosage of opioids may have to be increased by 25-50%. Other nonopioid medications that have been reported in the literature to be of benefit in dyspnea include citalopram, sertraline, and mirtazapine.[18] Palliative sedation with midazolam infusion may be used in refractory cases.[19] Supplemental oxygen is not recommended routinely and may be reserved for patients with chronic severe hypoxemia, where the saturation falls below 90%.

■ DELIRIUM

Delirium is a common presentation in the last few weeks to days of life, with an estimated incidence of 90%. It is defined as a diminished cerebral

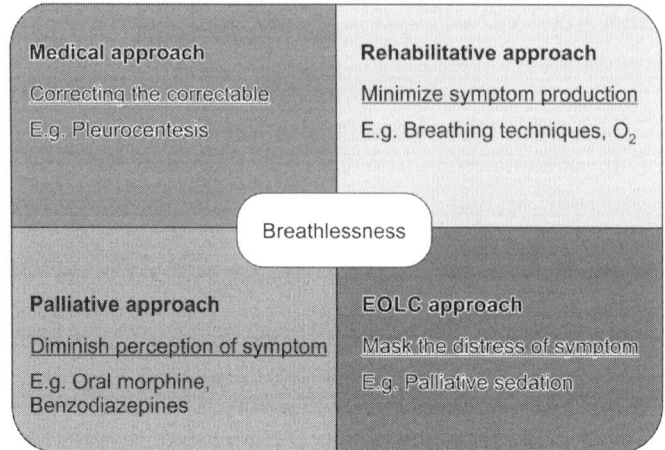

Fig. 3: Management strategies for breathlessness. (EOLC: End-of-life care)

function with associated disturbances in consciousness, thinking, attention, perception, behavior, memory, emotion, and sleep-wake cycle. It adversely affects the function and physical condition of the patient and their loved ones. Generally, it is an acute onset, and the course may fluctuate over the duration of the day. Common reversible causes of delirium include severe uncontrolled pain, medications, metabolic/electrolyte imbalance, urinary retention, constipation, and infections.

Patients suffering from delirium benefit from sunlight exposure and the comforting presence of family members, who can allay symptoms of fear, confusion, and anxiety.[20] Important drugs for managing delirium include haloperidol and risperidone. Benzodiazepines are not preferred as they can exacerbate the symptoms, but they can be used in case of increased anxiety and agitation as they have a sedative action. Palliative sedation may be required in case of distressing and refractory delirium.[21]

■ MASSIVE HEMORRHAGE

A massive hemorrhage, including carotid blowout, massive hematemesis, or oral bleed, maybe a terminal event in patients with head neck or gastric malignancy. The sudden and catastrophic nature of the bleed may leave the patient and caregiver in a state of panic and anxiety. Anticipatory counseling and prognostication in expected cases may prepare the family for such an event. They may be forewarned that such an event can occur, and they may use a dark-colored cloth to apply pressure over the affected area in case the bleeding is exogenous and try to calm the patient and not panic.

■ PSYCHOLOGICAL ISSUES

Important psychological issues at the end-of-life include depression, anxiety, emotional distress, and disturbed mood, and their incidence can be as high as 40% at the end-of-life. Patients may be screened for underlying psychiatric disorders as they are associated with an increased risk of psychological distress at the end-of-life and may warrant a specialist intervention. Nonpharmacological interventions such as life review and relaxation therapies have no role at the end-of-life as they are time and energy-consuming, and patients may lack the cognitive ability to comprehend such therapies. Antidepressant medications are the drugs of choice for anxiety. Benzodiazepines are used for insomnia, terminal sedation, and restlessness.[22]

SPIRITUAL DISTRESS

Spiritual distress is a significant factor at the end-of-life, and it must be assessed in totality. Active and compassionate listening skills should be used to reassure the patient and be present for them in time of need. Referral to spiritual care professional like a Chaplin may be required in certain cases. Other interventions such as mindfulness, art, narrative and music therapy, meaning-oriented therapy, and dignity therapy may be helpful.

GOOD DEATH

Good quality of life remains paramount. but equally important is to understand and provide good death as well. The principles of a good death are:
- Patients should be mentally prepared for death in terms of timeline and expectations.
- Patients should feel in control of what all is happening.
- Patient's dignity and privacy should be preserved.
- Pain and symptom control.
- Patients' choices about the place of death and who should be present at the time of death should be respected.
- Timely and honest communication and dissemination of information.
- Spiritual and emotional support.
- Access to hospice care.
- A facility for advance directives must be provided to the patient.
- To be able to bid final goodbyes.
- Patient should not undergo futile and invasive procedures to prolong life pointlessly.

These principles need to be followed while delivery various interventions for achieving the concept of good death **(Table 3)**.

ADVANCE DIRECTIVES AND ADVANCE CARE PLANNING

The National Hospice and Palliative Care Organization defines advance care planning as "making decisions about the care patients would like to receive if they become unable to speak for themselves." These decisions are made by patients irrespective of what care they choose for their future, based on their

TABLE 3: Concept of good death.

Themes	Description
Pain and symptom management	Effective symptom management and reassurance regarding relief of suffering–physical, psychological, and spiritual
Clear decision making	Timely and honest communication and keeping the patient and family wishes central in decision making
Preparation for death	Patients should be kept informed about the expected events around their death, probable timelines, and should be encouraged to plan ahead about their last wishes or things they would want after their death
Completion	• Sense of life well-lived, dreams fulfilled, resolution of conflicts, and making sense of it all • Saying final goodbyes • Existential and spiritual distress should be addressed
Contributing to others	Facilitating patients to contribute to others in one way or the other like donations or sharing knowledge and experience
Affirmation of the whole person	Affirmation of the patient as a whole, as a unique person with their set of likes, dislikes, preferences and choices, and not just a diagnoses or disease process

set of personal preferences, values, and beliefs after discussing with their loved ones. Advance care planning should include:

1. Equipping oneself with information regarding the different types of life-sustaining treatments available
2. Decisions regarding the types of care they would want at the end-of-life faced with adverse circumstances.
3. Making their loved ones aware of their choices and preferences
4. Advance directives should be put down in written format.

End-of-life care decision-making is a matter of personal choice and values. Discussions should be encouraged from broad perspectives to understand patients' preferences, what they consider fine and would rather not be subjected to.[23]

DO NOT INTUBATE/DO NOT ATTEMPT RESUSCITATION (DNI/DNAR)

Sometimes, medical fraternity needs to give in to the idea that death is not our ultimate enemy, but suffering is. Defeating death is not the blind aim of all our accumulated medical and technological feats. An objective assessment of the clinical situation, chances of meaningful survival postresuscitation, and risk versus benefit are essential to all medical decisions. Do not attempt resuscitation: the Indian Council of Medical Research published consensus guidelines on DNAR in April 2020, advocating that the option of DNAR be offered to all patients who are not likely to be benefitted from cardiopulmonary resuscitation in the event of a cardiopulmonary arrest. This includes patients with advanced, incurable, terminal illness or an advance disease with advanced age with fragility, where a successful resuscitation would not translate into a meaningful improvement in quality of life and may further the suffering. These conditions include advanced irreversible respiratory, cardiovascular, or neurological diseases, multiorgan failure, and advanced metastatic malignancy.[24]

■ EUTHANASIA AND PHYSICIAN-ASSISTED SUICIDE

Euthanasia is the performance of a deliberate act by the physician with an intent to end patients suffering and living with medical assistance. Euthanasia may be categorized as active or passive based on the mode of terminating a patient's life, inactive euthanasia. A deliberate act is performed, e.g., a lethal injection. In contrast, passive euthanasia patients' life is terminated by withholding or withdrawing life-sustaining therapy. Euthanasia is legal in Belgium and the Netherlands.

The Netherlands was the first country to legalize euthanasia, based on the act called "The Termination of Life on Request and Assisted Suicide Act" in 2002. According to this act, euthanasia and physician-assisted suicide are not liable to punishment under the following circumstances. The criteria include that the request for ending one's life must be made by a mentally competent patient suffering from unbearable and hopeless suffering. This is followed by a retrospective analysis by a regulatory commission to ascertain compliance with legal provisions.[25]

Physician-assisted suicide is providing medical help by a physician to enable terminally ill patients to terminate their life. Here the patient's autonomy and self-direction are important tenets as the patient actively decides and requests assistance and may self-administer the lethal agent to end their life. However, in euthanasia, it is the doctor's discretion and single-handedly decided and executed by him/her only.

The Death with Dignity Act of 1997 in the USA has led to the legalization of physician-assisted suicide in many states in the USA. It essentially means that if a set criterion is met, it is legal for a physician to aid a patient in fulfilling their expressed wish to end their sufferings. The criteria include:
1. Two doctors should confirm the patient's life expectancy to be 6 months or less.
2. The patient should be mentally competent and should make three requests in all that includes one oral and two in written format. The requests should be made at 15 days from each other.
3. The doctors must rule out any underlying psychiatric disorders.

However, the debate is still ongoing with the opponents dreading the potential misuse and abuse of these entities.[26]

■ PALLIATIVE SEDATION

Palliative sedation is a deliberate attempt to reduce the consciousness level of the patient to a level that they may not feel distressed anymore. It is the last resort treatment for refractory end-of-life symptoms that do not respond to standard therapies. Symptoms are termed refractory under the following circumstances:

i. Standard treatment options are ineffective in bringing about adequate symptom relief
ii. Relief of symptoms is not received in the stipulated time frame, or
iii. Intolerant side effects preclude the use of standard treatment options.

Severe pain, psychological distress, delirium, and dyspnea are the most compelling indications for trying palliative sedation. Other important scenarios are massive hemorrhage from any sire or status epilepticus. Before considering palliative sedation, patients and all the stakeholders must be included in detailed discussions about the procedure, alternatives, prognosis, and expected outcomes, and written informed consent must be taken. Palliative sedation is different from physician-assisted suicide and euthanasia in the intent. Here, the intent is only decreased consciousness and not death.

Contrary to popular belief, palliative sedation has not been shown to reduce survival in palliative care settings. Palliative sedation is controversial in cases of spiritual or existential distress, or the expected prognosis is >2 weeks. It can emotionally charge the caregivers so they may be reassured and checked upon regularly during the process. Before the sedation is started family should be allowed to communicate and engage with the patient as the patient may not be able to say their final goodbye once the process is initiated. Each center must establish its practice protocols based on its experience and expertise and devise a strategy best suited to its sociocultural environment. Respite sedation is another alternative that may be tried for transient sedation and then revival.[27]

The drugs which are commonly used for providing palliative sedation include benzodiazepines (midazolam, lorazepam) (first-line drug for palliative sedation), antipsychotics (levomepromazine, chlorpromazine), barbiturates (phenobarbitone) and less commonly certain anesthetic agents (propofol).[28]

■ ARTIFICIAL HYDRATION AND NUTRITION

The natural dying process is associated with decreased hunger and decreased eating ability. A physiological decline also reduces the body's nutritional requirement, this is associated with dysphagia, delirium, and anorexia cachexia leads to decreased feeding. The family must be counseled about this and reassured that is patient is not suffering because of decreased oral intake. Forcefully feeding the patients or subjecting them to parenteral and enteral nutritional supplementation is not recommended. It is not shown to improve quality of life or survival in patients with a poor prognosis of less than a few months. Artificial hydration may worsen edema, ascites, and respiratory secretions.[16]

Counseling regarding feeding, like encouraging liquid foods by mouth, small-quantity of meals, frequent meals instead of a few large meals, and other options is to feed the patient only when they demand instead of force-feeding or round-the-clock feeding is an important part in alleviating the family's worries regarding hastening of death due to starvation. Referral to a specialist dietician may be considered. The aim of feeding should be the alleviation of thirst. Decisions need to be individualized and tailored according to the clinical and ethical considerations after discussions with the patient and the caregivers. Pharmaceutical appetite-stimulating agents are not recommended at the end-of-life because of obscure evidence and efficacy. Short-term institution of corticosteroids or progesterone analogs may be considered under special circumstances.

■ WHERE DO WE STAND TODAY?

India was at the bottom of the 40 country list in 2010 for the quality of death index. Despite the improvement to reach 59 out of 81 recently, India still lies at grade D on the index, which is considered a "failing grade". In the last decade, much work has been done in India by the champions of palliative medicine, including EOLC in the undergraduate medical education curriculum recently, and the inclusion of palliative care in the 2017 National Health Policy. A lot needs to be done. Policy advocacy and ground-level work require to be done for further improvement. All stakeholders and palliative care champions should come together and make "good death" a priority in the coming time.[29,30]

■ REFERENCES

1. Meier EA, Gallegos JV, Montross-Thomas LP, Depp CA, Irwin SA, Jeste DV. Defining a Good Death (Successful Dying): Literature Review and a Call for Research and Public Dialogue. Am J Geriatr Psychiatry. 2016;24(4):261-71.
2. Macaden SC, Salins N, Muckaden M, Kulkarni P, Joad A, Nirabhawane V, et al. End-of-Life Care Policy for the Dying: Consensus Position Statement of Indian Association of Palliative Care. Indian J Palliat Care. 2014;20(3):171-81.
3. NICE. (2019). End of life care for adults: service delivery. [online] Available from https://www.nice.org.uk/guidance/ng142/chapter/recommendations [Last accessed October, 2022].

4. Salins N, Gursahani R, Mathur R, Iyer S, Macaden S, Simha N, et al. Definition of terms used in limitation of treatment and providing palliative care at the end of life: The Indian Council of Medical Research Commission Report. Indian J Crit Care Med. 2018;22(4):249-62.
5. Myatra SN, Salins N, Iyer S, Macaden SC, Divatia JV, Muckaden M, et al. End-of-life care policy: an integrated care plan for the dying: A Joint Position Statement of the Indian Society of Critical Care Medicine (ISCCM) and the Indian Association of Palliative Care (IAPC). Indian J Crit Care Med. 2014;18(9):615-35.
6. Hui D, Dev R, Bruera E. The Last Days of Life: Symptom Burden and Impact on Nutrition and Hydration in Cancer Patients. Curr Opin Support Palliat Care. 2015;9(4):346-54.
7. Gardiner D, Shemie S, Manara A, Opdam H. International perspective on the diagnosis of death. Br J Anaesth. 2012;108(suppl_1):i14-28.
8. Hui D, Dos Santos R, Chisholm G, Bansal S, Crovador CS, Bruera E. Bedside clinical signs associated with impending death in patients with advanced cancer: Preliminary findings of a prospective longitudinal cohort study. Cancer. 2015;121(6):960-7.
9. Lai XB, Wong FKY, Ching SSY. The experience of caring for patients at the end-of-life stage in non-palliative care settings: a qualitative study. BMC Palliat Care. 2018;17(1):116.
10. van Esch HJ, van Zuylen L, Geijteman ECT, Oomen-de Hoop E, Huisman BAA, Noordzij-Nooteboom HS, et al. Effect of prophylactic subcutaneous scopolamine butylbromide on death rattle in patients at the end-of-life: The SILENCE Randomized Clinical Trial. JAMA. 2021;326(13):1268-76.
11. Kompanje EJO. "The death rattle" in the intensive care unit after withdrawal of mechanical ventilation in neurological patients. Neurocrit Care. 2005;3(2):107-10.
12. Hagarty AM, Bush SH, Talarico R, Lapenskie J, Tanuseputro P. Severe pain at the end of life: a population-level observational study. BMC Palliat Care. 2020;19(1):60.
13. Nersesyan H, Slavin KV. The current approach to cancer pain management: Availability and implications of different treatment options. Ther Clin Risk Manag. 2007;3(3):381-400.
14. Lynch ME, Watson CPN. The pharmacotherapy of chronic pain: A review. Pain Res Manag. 2006;11(1):11-38.
15. Groninger H, Vijayan J. Pharmacologic management of pain at the end-of-life. Am Fam Physician. 2014;90(1):26-32.
16. Crawford GB, Dzierżanowski T, Hauser K, Larkin P, Luque-Blanco AI, Murphy I, et al. Care of the adult cancer patient at the end of life: ESMO Clinical Practice Guidelines. ESMO Open. 2021;6(4):100225.
17. Crisafulli E, Clini EM. Measures of dyspnea in pulmonary rehabilitation. Multidiscip Respir Med. 2010;5(3):202-10.
18. Hui D, Maddocks M, Johnson MJ, Ekström M, Simon ST, Ogliari AC, et al. Management of breathlessness in patients with cancer: ESMO Clinical Practice Guidelines. ESMO Open. 2020;5(6):e001038.
19. Prommer E. Midazolam: an essential palliative care drug. Palliat Care Soc Pract. 2020;14:2632352419895527.
20. Keeley PW. Delirium at the end of life. BMJ Clin Evid 2009;2009:2405.

21. Devlin JW, Skrobik Y. Antipsychotics for the prevention and treatment of delirium in the intensive care unit: what is their role? Harv Rev Psychiatry. 2011;19(2):59-67.
22. Block SD. Psychological issues in end-of-life care. J Palliat Med. 2006;9(3):751-72.
23. Fischhoff B, Barnato AE. Value Awareness: A new goal for end-of-life decision making. MDM Policy Pract. 2019;4(1):2381468318817523.
24. Mathur R. ICMR Consensus Guidelines on "Do Not Attempt Resuscitation". Indian J Med Res. 2020;151(4):303-10.
25. Banović B, Turanjanin V. Euthanasia: murder or not: a comparative approach. Iran J Public Health. 2014;43(10):1316-23.
26. Pereira J. Legalizing euthanasia or assisted suicide: the illusion of safeguards and controls. Curr Oncol. 2011;18(2):e38-45.
27. Kremling A, Schildmann J. What do you mean by "palliative sedation"? BMC Palliat Care. 2020;19:147.
28. Jadad AR, Browman GP. The WHO analgesic ladder for cancer pain management: Stepping up the quality of its evaluation. JAMA. 1995;274(23):1870-3.
29. Clark D, Baur N, Clelland D, Garralda E, López-Fidalgo J, Connor S, et al. Mapping levels of palliative care development in 198 countries: The situation in 2017. J Pain Symptom Manage. 2020;59(4):794-807.
30. Finkelstein EA, Bhadelia A, Goh C, Baid D, Singh R, Bhatnagar S, et al. Cross country comparison of expert assessments of the quality of death and dying 2021. J Pain Symptom Manage. 2022;63(4):e419-29.

Index

Page numbers followed by *b* refer to box, *f* refer to figure, *fc* refer to flowchart, and *t* refer to table.

A

Activated clotting time 123, 130
Active heated humidifier 26
Acute myocardial infarction 103
Acute respiratory distress syndrome 13, 19, 23, 312
Acute respiratory failure 1, 18, 20, 25
  causes 1
  diagnosis 1
  pathophysiology of 1, 13
Adenotonsillectomy 63
Adequate monitoring 127
Adjuvant analgesia 360*t*
Adjuvant drugs 89*t*
Adjuvant medication 360
Adult respiratory distress syndrome 11, 12
Advance care planning 276, 363
Advanced diseases 354
Advanced life support, technologies in 348
Adverse drug effects, opioid-related 251*b*
Air 26
  conditioning 263, 265
Airway 218
  exchange catheter 192*f*, 193
  management 161, 172, 190, 245
    progressive 245*b*
    strategies 191, 224
  obstruction 12
  occlusion pressure, measurement of 15
  point-of-care ultrasound 318*f*
  protection 127
  topicalization 171, 174
    different techniques of 174
  ultrasound of 317
Alpha 2 agonists 92
Alveolar concentration, minimum 162
Alveolar recruitment
  maneuver 34, 36, 42
  method for 43*f*
Alveolar-capillary interface, fracture of 37
Alveoli, higher compliance of 6*f*
Alzheimer's disease 149
American Heart Association 80, 109
American Society for Gastrointestinal Endoscopy 220
American Society of Anesthesiologists 191, 220, 296

Amyotrophic lateral sclerosis 12
Analgesia
  monitors 247
  nurse-controlled 167
  patient-controlled 167, 329
  postoperative 55, 87, 326
Analgesics medication 360
Anemia management 279
Anesthesia 114, 127, 206, 218, 326, 338
  agents, inhaled 261
  and intensive care 265*t*
  care, monitored 128
  concerns 151, 159
  delivery 333
  depth of 298
  emergence from 45
  environmental of 257
  induction of 44, 53
    general 160
  inhalation 53
  maintenance of 44, 53, 162
  management 114, 116, 122, 133
  monitoring ventilation during 44
  occupational considerations of 257
  robots in 336
  slow emergence from 120
  stages of general 44
  technique 116, 123, 129, 131
  types of 117
Anesthetic agents 12
  warming and inhalation 261
Anesthetic considerations 66, 128, 213
Anesthetic evaluation, preoperative 133
Anesthetic implications 218
Anesthetic management 197
Anesthetic pharmacology 69
Anesthetic techniques 140, 145
Aneurysm clipping, craniotomy for 133
Angiotensin receptor blockers 102, 108
  agents 159
Angiotensin-converting enzyme inhibitors 102, 108, 159
Anterograde guided retrograde intubation 179
Antithrombotic therapy 110
Antithymocyte 56
Anxiolysis 159

Index

Aortic aneurysm, abdominal 38
Arnold-Chiari malformation 153
Arrhythmias 59
Arterial blood gas 164
Arterial hypercapnia 11
Arterial hypoxemia 10, 12
    pathophysiologic mechanisms of 11
Arterial O_2 content, decreased 11
Arterial occlusion, temporary 136
Arterial partial pressure of oxygen 19
Arteriovenous malformation 127, 152
Artificial hydration 366
Artificial intelligence 297, 326, 328, 331, 333-336, 338, 343
    and monitoring 332
    applications of 331
    future of 337
Artificial nutrition 366
Aspiration 233
    risk
        assessment of 233
        considerations of 233
Assessing functional capacity 78
Asthma 11, 12, 312
    acute exacerbation of 23
Atelectasis 1
    role of 36
Atrial fibrillation, prevention of perioperative 111
Atrial septal defect 153
Auditory evoked potential 333
Automated closed-loop anesthesia delivery 326, 334
Automated external defibrillators 344, 347
Auto-positive end-expiratory pressure 196
Awake intubation rescue, failed 180
Awake tracheal intubation 171, 172, 181
    components of 174
Awake video laryngoscopy 177

B

Bain circuit assembly 227*f*
Basic life support 347
Bedside lung ultrasound in emergency 310, 311
Benzodiazepines 12
Bilevel positive airway pressure 20
Bispectral index 163, 241, 326
Blind nasal intubation 180
Blood
    lactate accumulation 83
    pressure monitoring, continuous intraoperative 109
    transfusion strategy 164

Body mass index 38, 210
Bore venous access, large 52
Borg dyspnea scale, modified 81, 81*b*
Borg scale 81
Bradycardia 120
Brain
    natriuretic peptide 107
    protection 131, 136
    relaxation 135
Brainstem
    compression 12
    infarction 12
Breath, shortness of 186
Breathing, increased work of 12
Breathlessness 361
    management strategies for 362*f*
British Society of Gastroenterology 220
Bronchoalveolar lavage 59
Bronchoscopy 59, 187
    preoperative 188
Buprenorphine 91
Burnout syndrome 268

C

Calcineurin inhibitors 56
Canadian Cardiovascular Society 109
Cancer 274
    care, enhanced recovery of 275*f*
    prehabilitation 278
Capnography monitoring 232
Carbon dioxide 187, 259*f*
    equivalency 260
    production 83
Carbon monoxide, diffusion capacity of 188
Cardiac arrest
    preventing 344
    unwitnessed 345
Cardiac output
    and partial pressure, effect of 4*f*
    decreased 11
Cardiac risk index 297
    revised 106
Cardiogenic pulmonary edema, acute 18, 20, 21
Cardiopulmonary
    bypass 54, 191
    disease 66
    exercise testing 78, 82, 83, 279
    interaction 14
    resuscitation 343
Cardiovascular and respiratory responses 12

Index

Cardiovascular assessment 117
Cardiovascular monitoring 120
Cardiovascular stability 127
Cardiovascular system 160
    ultrasound of 313
Carinal lesion 198, 199f
Carotid artery stenting 114, 121-123
    procedure 122
Carotid endarterectomy 114, 115, 118, 120, 124
    and stenting 114
Carotid vessels, atherosclerosis of 114, 115
Cavernous malformations 157
Central nervous system 102, 153
Central neuraxial blockades 90
Central venous
    catheter 311
    pressure 319
Cerebral aneurysm 127, 132
    endovascular coiling of 136
    intravascular treatment of 127
Cerebral artery, middle 119
Cerebral blood flow 132
Cerebral compromise 128
Cerebral hyperperfusion 124
    syndrome 121
Cerebral ischemia 134
Cerebrospinal fluid 153, 155
    drainage 131
Cerebrovascular accident 208, 210
Cervical
    approach 193
    epidural anesthesia 118
    incision, lower 193f
    meningomyelocele 154f
    plexus block 116
        superficial 118
Chest
    wall 12
    X-ray 58
Chiari malformation 155
Chronic obstructive pulmonary disease 11, 12, 18, 38, 52, 312
    acute exacerbation of 18, 20
Classical machine learning 329
Climate chemistry 261
Clinical decision support system 332
Clinical pulmonary infection score 40
Clonidine 92
Cobb's angle 156
Codeine 70
    to morphine, conversion of 70f
Colchicine 111
    prevents myocardial injury 111

Colonoscopy 218
Common carotid artery 320f
Common neurosurgical entities 153
Community-acquired pneumonia 25
Complete blood count 158
Comprehensive geriatric assessment 277
Concomitant hydrocephalus 161
Congestive heart failure 38
Continuous positive airway pressure 19, 63, 226
Conventional lung ventilation 37
Conventional mechanical ventilation 34
Convolutional neural network 330f
Coronary artery disease 82, 105, 210
Cotton and Myers classification 189f
Cough 187
COVID-19 1, 13, 18, 28, 29
    pandemic 230, 336
Cranial nerve injury 121
Craniofacial anomalies 66
Craniovertebral junction anomalies 156
Cricothyroid membrane 318f
Cricotracheal resections 192
Critical care units 1
Critically ill 1
    patients 14
Cross-field ventilation 185, 194f
Cytomegalovirus 211

D

Death 356
    rattle 359
Decreased mixed venous O_2 content 11
Deep brain stimulation 140, 141, 144
    anesthetic considerations for 144
    implantation 145, 146
    procedures 146
Deep brain stimulators 141, 149
Deep cervical plexus block 118
Delirium 361
Desflurane 162, 259f
Dexamethasone 88, 95
Dexmedetomidine 69, 93, 176, 223
Diabetes mellitus 206, 207, 208t
    classification of 209
    type 1 10, 209
    type 2 209
    types of 209t
Diastematomyelia 155
Difficult airway 171
Difficult Airway Association 202
Difficult Airway Society 174, 202
Direct laryngoscopy 177

Dobutamine stress echocardiography 82
Drone-delivered automated external defibrillators 347
Drones and basic life support 343
Drug
    overdose 12
    residual effects of 37
Duke activity status index 279
    score 106
Dukes Activity Severity Index 79
    score 79
Dural arteriovenous fistulas 157
Dyspnea, exertional 186
Dysraphism 153
Dystonia 140-143

E

Earth atmosphere 258
Earth energy expenditure 259, 259f
Echocardiography 314
Edema 12
Ehlers-Danlos syndrome 157f
Electrocardiogram 104, 163, 241
Electroencephalography 120, 333
Electronic health record 298, 332
Embolization 131
Emergence and tracheal extubation 166
Emergency medical service 344
End-expiratory lung volume 41
Endobronchial intubation 11
End-of-life care 354-356, 357f, 359t, 360, 362
    components of 358
    comprehensive 354
    flow of steps to 359f
    management 357
Endoscopic retrograde cholangiopancreatography 219
Endoscopy 218
Endotracheal intubation 18, 19
Endotracheal tube 161, 177, 179f, 194f, 196f, 199, 201, 336f
    cuffed 188
Endovascular embolization, anesthesia for 128
End-tidal carbon dioxide 241
Energy adenosine triphosphate 2
Enhanced recovery after surgery 276, 296
Enhanced surgical recovery programs 274, 275
Environment 257
Environmental hazards exposure 266
Epidural analgesia 55
Epinephrine 91

Esophagogastroduodenoscopy 219
Essential tremor 140, 142, 143
Estimated blood volume 165
European Carotid Surgery Trial 115
Euthanasia 365
Evidence-based strategies 41
Excessive intravenous fluid administration 11
Excessive positive end-expiratory pressure 11
Exercise stress echocardiography 82
Expiratory esophageal pressure 42
Extracorporeal membrane oxygenation 50, 191
    intraoperative 54
    venoarterial 348
Extreme tracheal lesion 200, 201f
Extubation 202

F

Fentanyl 90, 223
Fiberoptic bronchoscopy 177, 195
Fiberoptic-guided intubation 178
Flail chest 12
Fluid electrolyte management 164
Fluid management 59, 282
Focused cardiovascular ultrasound 309
Focused ultrasound
    indications for 149
    thalamotomy 140
Foreign body airway 12
Free-standing bispectral index monitor 241f
Freitag classification 190f
Fresh frozen plasma 158
Friedberg's triad 239, 240, 240f, 249, 252
Functional capacity 79
    assessment of 78
Functional neurosurgery 140, 141
    anesthetic considerations for 140
Functional residual capacity 35

G

Gamma-aminobutyric acid 223
Gartner hype cycle 330, 330f
Gas flow rates 83
Gastric point-of-care ultrasound 316f
Gastric ultrasound 309
Gastroenterological interventions 218, 224
Gastroenterological procedures, organizational logistics of 222
Gastroesophageal reflux disease 38

Gastrointestinal system, ultrasound of 315
Gastrolaryngeal tube 224, 229, 229f
Gastrostomy tube 219
General anesthesia 35, 38, 45, 116, 117, 136, 137, 172, 187, 221, 221t, 242
Gestational diabetes mellitus 208
Glasgow Coma Scale 133
Global warming potential 257, 260, 265
Globus pallidus internus 141, 144
Glossopharyngeal nerve block 175
Good death, concept of 364t
Graft dysfunction, primary 50, 55, 57
Graft rejection 50
Greenhouse gas 257, 258
Guardian stitch 203f
Guillain-Barré syndrome 1, 12

H

Halogenated anesthetic agents 261
Handwashing 258
Head and neck surgery 66
Heart 189
    rate 81, 109
Hemispheric multielement 147
Hemodynamic
    management 58, 124
    optimization 282
    status, unstable 24
Hemoglobin saturation, low 11
Hemoptysis 187
Hemorrhage 12
    grading subarachnoid 133t
    intracranial 144
    massive 362
Hepatic system 160
Hepatitis
    B virus 210
    C virus 210
High positive end-expiratory pressure 53
High-flow nasal cannula 25
High-flow nasal oxygen 18, 19, 199, 231
    cannula 232f
High-frequency jet ventilation 191, 199
High-ventilator driving pressure 39
Holliday-Segar's formula 164
Human leukocyte antigen 52, 210
Hydrocephalus 134, 153
Hydrocodone 71
Hydroxyethyl starch 283
Hypercapnia 16, 188
Hypercapnic respiratory acidosis 20
Hypertension 120, 121
    deliberate 130
    intracranial 134

Hypotension 24, 120, 121
    deliberate 130
    intraoperative 108
    rapid ultrasound for 317
Hypothermia 284
    perioperative 111
Hypoventilation 11
Hypoxemia 12
Hypoxemic nonhypercapnic respiratory failure, acute 21
Hypoxemic respiratory failure, acute 19

I

Illness trajectory 357
Immunocompromised patient 22, 27
Immunosuppressants 56, 211
Inadvertent perioperative hypothermia 285
Incremental shuttle walk
    distance 82
    test 82
Individualized positive end-expiratory pressure 34, 41
Infection and sepsis management 59
Infectious exposure 266
Inhaled anesthetics 257
In-hospital cardiac arrest 344
Inspired oxygen concentration 43
Insulin autoantibodies 207
Intended oncologic treatment 286f
Intensive care unit 167, 190, 213, 230, 298
Internal jugular vein 200
Internal pulse generator 146
International pancreas transplant registry 207
International Society for Heart and Lung Transplantation 57
Interstitial fibrosis 11
Interventional neuroradiology 127
Intra-abdominal fluid extravasation 317
Intracranial aneurysm 132
    rupture, management of 137
Intracranial pressure 129, 157
Intraoperative complications 166
Intraoperative lung protective ventilation, benefits of 40
Intraoperative mechanical ventilation, inappropriate 39f
Intratracheal tumor 12
Intravenous regional anesthesia 96
Intubation refusal 24
Invasive blood pressure monitoring 213
Invasive cardiovascular monitoring 58

Index

Invasive mechanical ventilation 19
Invasive nerve blocks 175
Ionizing radiation 269
Ionotropic agent 59
Islet autotransplantation 206
Islet cell transplantation 206
Isoflurane 259f
Isolated carinal resections 200f

J

Jet ventilation 185, 191
Jugular venous bulb monitoring 119

K

Ketamine 69, 88, 94, 223, 239
    dosing 249, 250
Kidney 207
    injury, acute 102, 109
    pancreas after 207
    transplantation procedure 212f
Kyoto protocol 260
Kyphoscoliosis 161
    severe 157f

L

Langerhans cells 210
Laryngeal block, superior 175
Laryngeal mask airway 191, 245, 246, 265
Laryngospasm, ketamine-
        associated 249, 251
Left main bronchus 199
    tumor 200f
Left ventricular ejection fraction 210
Leg fatigue 81
Lifecycle assessment 257
Local anesthesia 122, 145
Local anesthetic 87
    systemic toxicity 91
Loop anesthesia delivery system 333f
Low carinal resection 195
Low tidal volume 41
Low-flow devices 224
Low-hemoglobin saturation, effect of 9
Lumbar lipomeningomyelocele 154f
Lung
    disease, end-stage 50
    function, improved 40
    injury 37
        ventilator-induced 19
        protective strategies 196
    sonography 311
    transplantation 50, 51, 60t
    ultrasound of 309, 311
Lung protective ventilation 34, 38, 43, 44
    intraoperative 38, 41
    physiology 39
Lung transplant 50, 60
    intensive care management for 50
Lymphocyte globulin 56

M

Machine learning 328
Magnesium 88, 94
Mask ventilation, difficult 202
Maturity-onset diabetes of young 208, 209
McCaffrey classification 189f
Mean arterial pressure 102, 283
Mechanical circulatory support 54
Mechanical ventilation 18, 34, 35
    intraoperative 34
    role of 37
    weaning of 58
Medical management, preoperative 108
Meninges 153
Meningismus 132
Meningoceles 154
Meningomyelocele 153
Mesenteric artery, superior 316f
Metabolic equivalents 78, 79
Metabolic rate, increased 11
Methane 259f
Microelectrode recordings 142
Midazolam 88, 93, 223
Middle-east respiratory syndrome 22
Mid-tracheal lesions 195, 196f
Mitigate hypoxemia 224
Montando tube 195
Morphine 70, 90
Motor evoked potentials 163
Mouth breathing 231
Mucus plug causing absorption
        atelectasis 7f
Multidisciplinary discussion 190
Multimodal pain management 284
Multimodal perineural adjuvant 96
Multiple sclerosis 12
Muscle relaxants 12
Muscular dystrophy 12
Myasthenia gravis 12
Myelocele 153
Myocardial depression 53
Myocardial infarction 79, 102-104
    classification of 104t
    perioperative 103

Myocardial injury 102, 104, 105, 107*t*, 111, 112
  after noncardiac surgery, risk of 106*b*
Myocarditis 103

N

Narcotics 12
Nasal
  airways 246*f*
  cannula 26
  mask 228*f*
Nasopharyngeal airway 224, 226, 226*f*, 227*f*
Nausea 361
Near infrared spectroscopy 119
Neck hematoma 121
Needle stick 267
Neostigmine 88
Nerve roots 153
Neural tube defect 151-153
Neuraxial anesthesia 319
Neurological assessment 116
Neurological mishaps, management of 131
Neurological monitoring 114, 119
Neurological stability 127
Neuromuscular blockade 334
Neuromuscular blocker agent, fast-acting 161
Neuromuscular blocking
  agents 191
  drugs 38
Neurophysiologic monitoring 135
  intraoperative 152, 163*f*
Neurosurgery 140
New neurological deficits 121
Nitrous oxide 259*f*, 261
N-methyl-D-aspartate 223
  antagonist drugs 88, 94
  receptor 242
Nociception level index 298
Noncardiac surgery 102, 104
  myocardial injury after 102, 103, 105*fc*, 111
  pilot study 111
Non-contrast computed tomography scans 132
Nonhypercapnic hypoxemic respiratory failure 27
Nonhypercapnic respiratory failure, acute 21
Noninvasive arterial blood pressure 248
Noninvasive blood pressure 163
Noninvasive positive pressure ventilation 18, 19, 20*f*, 21, 24

Noninvasive ventilation 18, 30
Nonionizing radiation 269
Nonsteroidal anti-inflammatory drugs 55, 69, 88, 96, 167, 284, 360
Nucleus, intermediate 144
Nutrition 280
Nutritional risk indicator 280

O

Obesity hypoventilation 29
Observational scales 360
Obstructive coronary artery disease 105
Obstructive sleep apnea 12, 29, 38, 62, 63*f*, 71, 106, 158
Occupational health hazards 257
Oncological therapies 285
One-lung ventilation 50, 53, 191
Operating room logistics 326
Operational terms, implications of 356
Operative room logistics 335
Opioid adjuvants 89
Opioid inclusive care 240
Opioid-free anesthesia 239, 240, 240*f*, 249
Optimizing oxygenation 28
Organ system 208
Organ transplantations 206
Original duodenal drainage 212*f*
Out-of-hospital cardiac arrest 343, 344, 346
Oxycodone 71
Oxygen
  blender 26
  delivery 224
  saturation 83, 241
  supplementation 224
Oxygenating mouthguard 225, 226*f*
Oxygenation 174
  catheter 195
  failure 10
Ozone layer, montreal protocol for 260

P

Packed red blood cells 158, 165
Pain 360
  management maintenance 285
  postoperative 334
  type of 360
Palliation 24
Palliative care, continuum of 357*f*
Palliative sedation 354, 366
Pancreas 212*f*
  allocation suitability score, pre-procurement 211

anatomy 209
anesthesia for 206
donor risk index 211
graft 212f
kidney transplant 206
physiology 209
surgical vascularization of 212f
transplant alone 206
transplantation 206, 215
Pancreatic tissue transplantation 206
Parkinson's disease 140, 142
Patient-centered medical home 296
Pediatric obstructive sleep apnea 62
Pediatric spinal neurosurgery 151
Percutaneous endoscopic gastrostomy 219
Perioperative surgical home 292, 296, 299, 300t
benefits of 302
elements of 298
team 296f
Perioperative surgical team concept 301f
Peripheral intravenous catheters, placement of 320
Personal protective equipment 258, 267
Platelets 158
Pneumocystis carinii 59
Pneumonia 11, 22, 312
ventilator-associated 19, 20
Pneumothorax 11
Point-of-care ultrasound 309-311, 317
Polymyositis 12
Polysomnography 62, 66
preoperative 66
Positive airway pressure therapy 66
Positive end-expiratory pressure 5, 19, 34, 39f, 43f
Positive pressure ventilation 5
Postanesthesia care 38
unit 38, 213
Postcardiac arrest 24
Postextubation respiratory failure 23, 203
Postextubation support 28
Postoperative care unit 309
Postoperative nausea and vomiting 162, 239, 281
prophylaxis 281
Postoperative pulmonary complications
pathophysiology of 35, 36fc
risk factors for 37
Postprocedure care 124
Preanesthetic evaluation 331
Pre-excision fiberoptic bronchoscopy 193
Pre-extubation assessment 202
Prehabilitation 278

Preoperative fasting 158
Pressure, combats increased closing 40
Pressure-controlled ventilation 43, 201
Primary graft dysfunction, grading of 57t
Prophylaxis 211
Propofol 176, 223
Protect airway, inability to 24
Pulmonary artery 213
Pulmonary capillary blood 3, 9
Pulmonary collapse 11
Pulmonary complications, postoperative 35, 36, 38t
Pulmonary congestion 12
Pulmonary edema 11, 312
diagnosis of 312
Pulmonary embolism 11
Pulmonary function
assessment of 14, 51
tests 187
Pulmonary hypertension 11
reduction of 53
Pulmonary infection, postoperative 34, 35
Pulmonary vascular resistance 54

Q

Quality of life 276
health-related 286

R

Radiation 269
Randomized controlled trials 247
Raniovertebral junction 156
Rapid sequence intubation 53
Receive donor pancreatic tissue 210t
Recognizing cardiac arrest, technologies for 345
Rectus sheath block 214
Regional and neuraxial anesthesia 87
Regional anesthesia 88, 116, 118
techniques 96
Remifentanil 223
Remote ischemic preconditioning 108
Renal allografts 212f
Renal anomalies 153
Renal system 160
Reperfusion pulmonary edema 59
Residual paralysis 12
Respiration, physiology of 1, 2
Respiratory failure 11, 16, 18
causes of type 2 12
classification of 10
diagnosis of 15

Index

postoperative 24, 28
   type 2 11
   type 3 12
Respiratory muscle 12
   disorders of 12
   weakness 29
Respiratory system 160
   overview of 2
Resuscitative endovascular balloon 348
Retrograde intubation 171, 178
   steps of 179f
Right ventricular dysfunction 50
Room preparation 129
Rotational thromboelastogram 166
Rupture, intraoperative 136

S

Saline solution, normal 250
Scoliosis 156
Sedation 176
   minimal 247
   pharmacological principles of 221
Segmental atelectasis, presence of 11
Seizures 132, 134
Severe acute respiratory syndrome 336
Severe prematurity, history of 66
Sevoflurane 162, 259f
Sharps safety 267
Shock, rapid ultrasound for 317
Shunt, intrapulmonary 11
Simple low-flow face mask 225f
Simultaneous pancreas 207
   kidney transplant 206
Single-heated circuit 26
Single-lumen tube 199f, 201f
   long 198
Six-minute walk test 81
Sleep
   disordered breathing 62
   endoscopy, drug-induced 62, 67, 68, 68b
Small airway obstruction 11
Smaller midline tumors 200f
Sodium bicarbonate 88, 95
Somatosensory evoked potentials 120, 163
Spina bifida 152
   occulta 154
Spinae muscles 320f
Spinal cord
   injuries 12, 152, 156, 161
   parenchyma 157
   tumors 152
      primary 155
   vascular malformations 157

Spinal deformity 156
Spinal lipomas 154
Spinal neural tube defects, closed 154
Spinal region 153
Spiritual distress 363
Split cord malformations 155
Spontaneous ventilation 199
Stair climbing test 81
Standard low-flow nasal cannula 225f
Standard precautions 258
Stenosis 185
Stress
   myocardial perfusion imaging 107
   testing 82
Stridor 186
Stroke 114
   volume 283
Subarachnoid hemorrhage 132, 133t
   complications after 134t
   scale 133t
Sublingual sufentanil lozenges 247
Suicide, physician-assisted 365
Supraglottic airway 190
   device 162, 172
Supralaryngeal airway devices 228
Supratentorial mass 12
Surgery, cancer patient before 280
Surgical apgar score 297
Surgical resection
   anesthetic considerations for 130
   complications after 132
Surgical site infections 298
Surgical smoke 269
Surgical steps 193
Surgical stress 102
Surgical technique, overview of 211
Syringomyelia, primary 155
Systemic anesthesia 160t
Systemic inflammatory response syndrome 158

T

Tachycardia 108, 120
Target-controlled infusion 223, 232
Temperature management 166
Terminal illness 356
Tethered cord syndrome 152, 155
Tetralogy of Fallot 153
Thalamic nucleus 141
Theater preparation 191
Therapeutic gastroenterological interventions 219
Thoracic epidural analgesia 55, 214

Thoracic surgery 111
Thromboelastogram 59
Tidal volume 25
Total intravenous anesthesia 162, 191, 263, 265
Total pancreatectomy 206, 211
Trachea 185, 186, 189
   and carina, lower 201*f*
   incision over 193
   lower 194*f*
Tracheal dilatation 189
Tracheal extubation 181
Tracheal intubation, ventilation during 28
Tracheal lesion, lower 195, 198, 199*f*
Tracheal reconstruction surgeries, anesthesia for 185
Tracheal resection
   anesthesia for 185
   surgery 195
      anesthesia for 191
Tracheal tumor, lower 201*f*
Traditional perioperative
   management 294
   period 294*fc*
Traditional surgical care 300*t*
Tramadol 71, 91
Transcarotid artery revascularization 122
Transcranial Doppler 119
Transesophageal echocardiography 52, 213
Transfusion requirements 165*t*
Transient ischemic attack 208
Transmission based precautions 267
Transthoracic echocardiogram 187
Transverse low-collar incision 193
Transversus abdominis plane 214
Trauma 24, 103
   patients, ultrasound for 316
   sonography for 316
Tubeless airway techniques 199
Tumescent analgesia 249, 250

U

Ultrasound 326
   guidance 335
   technology 310

Upper gastroenterological interventions 219, 231
Upper tracheal resections 192

V

Vascular access, ultrasound for 319
Vasoactive drugs 55, 91
Vasodilatation 53
Vasopressors agent 59
Vena cava, inferior 200
Venous air embolism 163, 166
Venous saturation, effect of decreased 4*f*
Ventilated alveoli 11
Ventilation 34, 53, 263, 265
   and perfusion
      mismatch 1
      mismatch, effect of 8*f*
      relationships of 7*f*
   and perfusion imbalance
      effect of 8
      evaluation of 9
   manual jet 199
   postoperative 40
   volume-controlled 43
Ventilatory failure 11
Ventilatory management 56
Video laryngoscopy 178
Visualizing lumbar vertebrae 320*f*
Vocal cord 201
   paralysis 121
Volatiles and environment, clinical chemistry of 259*f*
Vomiting 361

W

Wireless intelligent patient 326
Workplace stress 268

Z

Zero end-expiratory pressure 37